Digital Health, Welfare, and Care:

Technologies, Inequalities, and Social Inclusion

Gabriella Punziano
https://orcid.org/0000-0001-8783-2712
University of Naples Federico II, Italy

Domenico Trezza
https://orcid.org/0009-0003-0238-4458
University Pegaso, Italy

Giuseppe Luca De Luca Picione
University of Naples Federico II, Italy

IGI Global
Scientific Publishing
Publishing Tomorrow's Research Today

Vice President of Editorial	Melissa Wagner
Director of Acquisitions	Mikaela Felty
Director of Book Development	Jocelynn Hessler
Production Manager	Mike Brehm
Cover Design	Jose Rosado

Published in the United States of America by
IGI Global Scientific Publishing
701 East Chocolate Avenue
Hershey, PA, 17033, USA
Tel: 717-533-8845 | Fax: 717-533-7115
Website: https://www.igi-global.com E-mail: cust@igi-global.com

Library of Congress Cataloging-in-Publication Data

LCCN: 2026032032 (CIP Data Pending)
ISBN13: 979-8-2600-3043-1
Isbn13Softcover: 979-8-2600-3044-8
EISBN13: 979-8-2600-3045-5

British Cataloguing in Publication Data
A Cataloguing in Publication record for this book is available from the British Library.

Table of Contents

Detailed Table of Contents

The chapter presents the findings of a qualitative case study conducted within the project "Dalla digitalizzazione all'innovazione nei servizi alla persona erogati dagli enti del Terzo Settore. L'esperienza di Federsolidarietà Friuli Venezia Giulia" promoted by the Department of Humanistic Studies of the University of Trieste, funded by the Friuli Venezia Giulia Region under Regional Law 34/2015, and implemented in partnership with Confcooperative FVG-Federsolidarietà. The aim of the case study was to explore the approaches, expectations, concerns, and strategies through which these organizations are addressing digitalization. Drawing on a sociotechnical perspective on digital technologies and an institutionalist approach to organizational analysis, the study highlights the dynamics triggered by differences in power, technological knowledge, and capacities for the use of digital devices among the various actors involved

Digital welfare systems increasingly rely on data-driven infrastructures, yet these remain largely oriented toward clinical and pathological data. Information on healthy populations, early-stage risks, and preventive trajectories is often limited or fragmented. This imbalance—conceptualized as data asymmetry—constrains the development of preventive and inclusive welfare strategies. This chapter examines how advanced Artificial Intelligence methodologies—such as data augmentation, minority oversampling, transfer learning, and synthetic data generation—can partially address these structural gaps. The chapter conceptualizes these techniques as socio-technical and communicative processes that reshape how data are constructed, interpreted, and mobilized. The analysis shows how synthetic data and transfer learning enable future-oriented representations of risk and population health, while raising challenges to validity, representation, and governance. AI is thus understood

This chapter presents a systematic review of the scientific literature on digital health within welfare systems, analysing a corpus of 5,977 articles indexed in Web of Science between 2012 and 2025. Through Latent Dirichlet Allocation (LDA) topic modelling, eight thematic areas are identified, mapping the discursive configurations through which digital health is constructed as a sociotechnical object in contemporary academic production. The analysis reveals that the computationalisation of health constitutes a structural transformation of epistemologies, institutional rationalities, and power relations governing care - not a linear process of technical modernisation. The findings highlight an unresolved tension between emancipatory promises and dynamics of algorithmic stratification, exclusion, and control. The chapter concludes by identifying priorities for a sociological research agenda oriented towards equity.

Internet of Bodies (IoB) technologies are often presented as technical infrastructures for continuous sensing, data analytics, and early risk prediction. This chapter instead treats IoB as a communication system that shapes how health information flows between bodies, devices, clinicians, institutions, and publics. We explore how connected devices on, in, and around the human body transform occasional clinic-based encounters into continuous, everyday exchanges of data, alerts, and recommendations. Building on recent work on IoT, IoMT, and IoB in healthcare, we describe the main categories of IoB devices and the types of physiological, behavioural, and contextual data they generate, but focus especially on how these data are translated into risk messages, decision support, and public-facing narratives. Particular attention is given to public health policy issues, including regulatory communication on privacy and security, institutional accountability for algorithmic decisions, and the risk that IoB-driven monitoring could widen existing inequities.

The digitalisation of welfare systems is reshaping social protection in low- and middle-income countries, where digital platforms, biometric identification, social registries, and algorithmic tools are increasingly used to expand coverage and manage benefit delivery. This chapter argues that digital welfare is not simply a process of administrative modernisation, but a deeper transformation in how states identify vulnerability, classify populations, allocate entitlements, and mediate access to social rights. It introduces the concept of algorithmic inclusion as a framework for assessing whether data-driven welfare systems can recognise diverse forms of vulnerability, ensure transparency and contestability, and protect rights throughout the decision-making lifecycle. Drawing on cases from East Africa, India, and Latin America, the chapter shows that digital welfare can support inclusion, but may also reproduce exclusion through data gaps, biometric failures, weak grievance mechanisms, and limited institutional capacity.

This article examines how the digitalisation of welfare systems reshapes access to social rights, focusing on digital competences as a key condition of social citizenship. As public services are increasingly delivered through digital platforms, the ability to navigate online environments and interact with administrative procedures becomes crucial for accessing welfare. While digital welfare is often framed as a process of administrative modernisation that enhances efficiency and inclusion, it may also generate new forms of inequality. Focusing on the Italian case, the article highlights how digital welfare has developed within a fragmented institutional context characterised by territorial disparities and uneven levels of digital inclusion. Using secondary data on digital skills, the study identifies which social groups are more likely to access digitalised welfare services and which are more exposed to exclusion. The findings show that digital competences act as a stratifying resource, shaping unequal access to welfare and challenging the universalistic principles of social rights.

Preface

INTRODUCTION

The rapid integration of digital technologies into health, welfare, and care systems is profoundly reshaping how societies organize support, deliver services, and promote well-being. Across diverse contexts, digital platforms, artificial intelligence, data infrastructures, algorithmic systems, and connected devices are becoming integral components of healthcare provision, social protection, and public administration. While these developments offer unprecedented opportunities for improving efficiency, personalization, prevention, and access, they also raise critical questions about equity, participation, governance, and social justice. The digital transformation of welfare is therefore not merely a technological phenomenon but a deeply social process that influences the distribution of resources, opportunities, and rights.

As editors, we conceived this volume in response to the growing need for interdisciplinary scholarship capable of examining both the promises and the contradictions of digital transformation in health and welfare. The increasing reliance on data-driven decision-making, automated systems, and digital service delivery requires careful reflection on how technological infrastructures interact with existing social inequalities and institutional arrangements. Questions concerning digital citizenship, algorithmic governance, digital literacy, inclusion, privacy, representation, and accountability have become central to understanding the future of welfare and care systems. This volume seeks to contribute to these debates by bringing together perspectives from sociology, communication studies, public policy, information systems, health studies, and related disciplines.

The chapters collected in this book investigate digital health, welfare, and care through a critical lens that emphasizes the interconnectedness of technology and society. Rather than viewing digitalization as a neutral process of modernization, the contributors examine how digital infrastructures shape social relationships, institutional practices, and access to rights. Together, these chapters demonstrate that achieving socially inclusive digital welfare requires more than technological innovation; it demands attention to governance, participation, ethics, and the diverse experiences of citizens navigating increasingly digital environments.

CHAPTER OVERVIEW

Chapter 1, Information Asymmetries and Power Dynamics in the Digitalization of the Third Sector, by Anna Zenarolla, explores how social cooperatives engage with digitalization and examines the information asymmetries and power dynamics that emerge during technological transformation. Drawing on findings from an ongoing participatory research project, the chapter highlights the absence of strategic approaches to digitalization and discusses the potential role of public institutions in fostering collaborative and socially oriented digital innovation.

Chapter 2, Artificial Intelligence, Synthetic Data, and the Socio-Technical Reconfiguration of Data Infrastructures, by Monica Murero, investigates the problem of data asymmetries in healthcare systems. The chapter analyzes how artificial intelligence techniques, including synthetic data generation and transfer learning, can address gaps in health information while simultaneously raising important questions concerning representation, validity, and governance within digital welfare systems.

Chapter 3, Configurations of Digital Health Citizenship, by Ferdinando Iazzetta, examines how healthcare data infrastructures shape digital health citizenship across Europe. Through comparative analysis, the chapter reveals significant differences in data ecosystem development and access policies, demonstrating how digitalization generates new forms of infrastructural inequality within contemporary healthcare systems.

Chapter 4, Digital Well-Being in Healthcare Services, by Maria Frezza, proposes a welfare-oriented analytical framework for understanding digital transformation in healthcare. Focusing on electronic health records and broader processes of health datafication, the chapter explores the implications of digital technologies for healthcare organization, doctor–patient relationships, and equitable access to services.

Chapter 5, The Sociotechnical Reconfiguration of Care, by Noemi Crescentini and Giuseppe Padricelli, presents a systematic review and topic-modeling analysis of nearly 6,000 scholarly publications on digital health. The chapter identifies major thematic trends and critically examines how algorithmic governance and digital infrastructures reshape knowledge production, care practices, and social inequalities.

Chapter 6, Continuous Monitoring, Early Prediction, and Public Health Policy using IoB, by Kathirvel Ayyaswamy and Naren Kathirvel, focuses on the Internet of Bodies as an emerging communication and health-monitoring infrastructure. The authors discuss how continuous data collection transforms healthcare interactions while addressing concerns related to privacy, security, institutional accountability, and social inequality.

Chapter 7, Beyond Datafication: Algorithmic Inclusion and Welfare in Low- and Middle-Income Countries, by Dario Russo, Piero Falorsi, and Ahmad Hussein, examines the growing role of digital welfare systems in developing contexts. Through international case studies, the chapter introduces the concept of algorithmic inclusion and evaluates how digital technologies can simultaneously enhance and constrain access to social rights.

Chapter 8, Digital Welfare and Digital Competence, by Caterina Ambrosio, Ciro De Falco, and Giulia De Florio, analyzes the relationship between digital skills and welfare access in Italy. The chapter demonstrates how digital competences increasingly function as a stratifying resource that shapes citizens' ability to navigate digitalized welfare systems and exercise social rights.

Chapter 9, Rethinking the Family/Public Divide in Older Adults' Digital Facilitation, by Giulia Melis and Mino Novello, explores the social practices that support older adults' engagement with digital services. Using qualitative case studies, the authors examine the interplay between family-based assistance and institutional digital facilitation initiatives, revealing the social and relational dimensions of digital inclusion.

Chapter 10, The Challenges of Digital Transformation in Rethinking Welfare, by Daniele Battista, Emiliana Mangone, and Giuseppe Masullo, addresses innovative digital strategies for preventing and combating gender-based violence. The chapter emphasizes the need for integrated approaches that combine technological innovation, social justice, victim protection, and rights-based welfare policies.

Chapter 11, Welfare and AI: Female Representation and Social Inequalities, by Mirella Ferrari, concludes the volume by examining gender inequalities embedded within artificial intelligence systems. The chapter investigates issues of representation, bias, and exclusion while advocating for participatory and reflexive approaches that can support more equitable AI-driven welfare services.

CONCLUSION

The contributions assembled in this volume demonstrate that digital transformation is redefining the foundations of health, welfare, and care systems across the globe. From healthcare data infrastructures and artificial intelligence to digital welfare platforms and algorithmic governance, the technologies examined throughout this book are reshaping how needs are identified, services are delivered, and social rights are exercised. At the same time, the chapters reveal that technological innovation often reproduces existing inequalities while creating new forms of exclusion, dependency, and power asymmetry.

A recurring theme throughout the volume is the importance of viewing digital technologies as socio-technical systems rather than purely technical tools. The contributors consistently show that digital infrastructures are embedded within institutional arrangements, policy frameworks, cultural practices, and social relationships. Whether examining digital health citizenship, algorithmic inclusion, digital competences, gender inequalities, or support for older adults, the chapters underscore the necessity of inclusive governance, transparency, accountability, and citizen participation in shaping digital futures.

As editors, we hope this book encourages further dialogue among scholars, policymakers, practitioners, and civil society actors concerned with the future of digital welfare. The challenges explored here cannot be addressed through technological solutions alone. Building equitable and socially inclusive digital health and welfare systems requires sustained interdisciplinary collaboration, critical reflection, and a commitment to protecting human dignity, social justice, and democratic participation. We trust that this volume will contribute meaningfully to these ongoing conversations and inspire future research and action in this rapidly evolving field.

Gabriella Punziano
University of Naples Federico II, Italy

Domenico Trezza
University Pegaso, Italy

Giuseppe De Luca Picione
University of Naples Federico II, Italy

Chapter 1
Information Asymmetries and Power Dynamics in the Digitalization of the Third Sector:
Early Findings From a Qualitative Case study

Anna Zenarolla
http://orcid.org/0000-0001-5487-6313
University of Trieste, Italy

ABSTRACT

The chapter presents the findings of a qualitative case study conducted within the project "Dalla digitalizzazione all'innovazione nei servizi alla persona erogati dagli enti del Terzo Settore. L'esperienza di Federsolidarietà Friuli Venezia Giulia" promoted by the Department of Humanistic Studies of the University of Trieste, funded by the Friuli Venezia Giulia Region under Regional Law 34/2015, and implemented in partnership with Confcooperative FVG-Federsolidarietà. The aim of the case study was to explore the approaches, expectations, concerns, and strategies through which these organizations are addressing digitalization. Drawing on a sociotechnical perspective on digital technologies and an institutionalist approach to organizational analysis, the study highlights the dynamics triggered by differences in power, technological knowledge, and capacities for the use of digital devices among the various actors involved

DOI: 10.4018/979-8-2600-3043-1.ch001

INTRODUCTION

The Third Sector, a key partner of public authorities in the provision of services within the Italian welfare system, has also been affected by the digitalization process that has been reshaping the country, particularly following the COVID-19 pandemic and the implementation of the National Recovery and Resilience Plan.

Initially introduced gradually and largely through the autonomous initiatives of individual organizations, digitalization became a compulsory step during the pandemic, which forced many Third Sector organizations to transfer and/or adapt their services to digital formats in order to ensure continuity of provision and, ultimately, their own organizational survival (Trapani, 2022). This led to a "hasty and contingency-driven" digital transformation (Punziano et al., 2023), which was not accompanied by adequate awareness of the opportunities and constraints of digital technologies, nor of the skills required for their effective use. Since then, the situation appears to have changed only partially and remains largely unresolved.

The Third Sector, a key partner of public authorities in the provision of services within the Italian welfare system, has been significantly affected by the digitalization processes reshaping the country, particularly following the COVID-19 pandemic and the implementation of the National Recovery and Resilience Plan.

Initially introduced gradually and largely through the autonomous initiatives of individual organizations—also in compliance with the Third Sector Reform (D.lgs. 117/2017) and the Social Enterprise framework (D.lgs. 112/2017), which promote technological innovation to enhance labour inclusion and administrative management—digitalization became unavoidable during the pandemic. The latter compelled many Third Sector organizations to transfer and/or adapt their services to digital formats to ensure continuity and, ultimately, organizational survival (Trapani, 2022). This resulted in a "hasty and contingency-driven" digital transformation (Punziano et al., 2023), not accompanied by adequate awareness of the opportunities and constraints of digital technologies, nor by the development of the necessary skills. Since then, progress has been only partial and many issues remain unresolved.

Recent studies (LegaCoop, 2023; Italia Non Profit, 2021, 2024) show that, despite some improvements, most organizations are still not fully digitalized, and only a minority have effectively integrated digital technologies into their practices and organizational culture. This process is characterized by the absence of a strategic approach among leadership, limited financial resources, and insufficient competences, often coupled with low levels of basic digital confidence (Cavotta et al., 2022; D'Alessandro et al., 2022).

These challenges must be understood within the broader national context (Busacca, 2022), where the Italian productive system continues to lag behind more advanced European countries—as indicated by the Digital Economy and Society Index

(DESI, 2022)—due to gaps in skills, human capital, and the uneven distribution of digital infrastructures. Moreover, despite recent growth in employment and active organizations, the Italian Third Sector—like the for-profit sector—is dominated by micro-enterprises (Istat, 2022), for which investing in digital technologies remains particularly difficult.

This context underpins the rationale of the research presented in the following sections, which examines the perspectives of senior management within these organizations regarding digital technologies and their adoption in their digitalization processes.

THEORETICAL FRAMEWORK

The theoretical assumptions guiding this research draw on the Unified Theory of Acceptance and Use of Technology (Venkatesh et al., 2003) and on the sociotechnical approach (Orlikowski, 1992, 2000, 2007; Orlikowski & Scott, 2008). These perspectives do not conceptualize digital technologies as neutral tools, nor as mere products of technical rationality applied to practical problem-solving. Rather, they view technologies as socially situated, insofar as they are interpreted and used in relation to the aspirations, interests, power relations, values, beliefs, and subjectivities of the actors involved in their implementation.

In the context of social cooperatives, these actors include Information and Communication Technologies (ICT) producers, administrators, managers, and cooperative members, as well as service beneficiaries and stakeholders, particularly administrators, managers, and professionals in the public social, health, and educational sector with whom cooperatives collaborate. Each of these actors holds specific assumptions and beliefs about technology and about how cooperatives should use it. Such assumptions and beliefs, sometimes formalized in more or less binding guidelines and directives, contribute to shaping the ways in which technologies are introduced into organizations, as well as the purposes and modalities of their use at different organizational levels and across different sectors. Consequently, these practices emerge from the interplay between technical and material dimensions and human and social dimensions. The situated nature of technology and organizations highlighted by the aforementioned theories justifies the adoption of an additional theoretical framework for interpreting the digitalization processes of social cooperatives, namely the institutional theory developed by Powell and DiMaggio (1991). Indeed, these authors introduce the concept of the organizational field, defined as a set of organizations that, taken together, constitute a recognized area of institutional life—that is, a plurality of actors who, more or less directly and consciously, contribute to processes of change, whether political, cultural, economic, or technological.

This concept directs research on change beyond the analysis of decision-making processes within individual organizations, extending attention to the role played by all actors involved in a given process, ultimately encompassing the ways in which the organizational field—composed of diverse types of organizations—is structured. Moreover, it highlights how the distinction between organizations that are subject to pressures and those that exert them becomes blurred, insofar as all organizations within the field simultaneously act as both recipients and sources of the pressures that traverse it. Consequently, the key issue is not to determine who conforms to what, but rather to understand how pressures circulate, how they are received, and the pace at which change occurs.

According to these authors, organizations are shaped by the values, norms, and rules circulating within the institutional environment in which they operate. These elements exert pressures that lead organizations to conform through processes of coercive, mimetic, and normative isomorphism, ultimately making them increasingly similar to one another. From this perspective, the adoption of digital technologies can also be interpreted as an adaptive response to legislative and regulatory constraints, rather than as a deliberate and intentional choice for change.

According to the socio-technical approach (Orlikowski, 2000), technologies can therefore be understood as "embodied structures" that, through the interaction between technological tools and their users, are enacted within specific contexts of application, giving rise to "technologies-in-practice," that is, to the technologies as they are actually used in everyday activities.

From this perspective, on the one hand, human actors interact with technologies to the point of becoming inseparable from and dependent on them; on the other hand, technologies become increasingly invisible in daily practice while simultaneously exerting a growing influence on it, often without users' full awareness. Despite this invisibility, technologies possess specific capacities and properties that shape how users perceive and act upon their surrounding reality. The action potentials of technology are therefore subjectively perceived, vary across individuals, and manifest themselves in everyday work practices over time. Similarly, technologies should not be understood merely as instruments serving organizational strategies, but also as factors that actively influence them (Orlikowski & Scott, 2008).

Within this framework, as emphasized by Venkatesh and colleagues (2003), mere possession of or access to digital technologies does not in itself solve the problems for which they are adopted (technological solutionism), nor does it necessarily lead to the behavioral changes required to address those problems (technological determinism). Both outcomes depend on the level of involvement of all actors engaged in their use, not only those operating at the decision-making level but, above all, those at the operational level.

These interactions also reflect a specific form of inequality associated with digital technology, namely the digital divide. Following van Dijk (2020), this should be understood not merely as a lack of availability of and access to digital technologies, but as a multidimensional condition in which the skills required to search for information, evaluate it, and effectively use digital content are intertwined with broader social inequalities (in terms of income, age, educational level, and gender). Together, these dimensions generate a gap between those who are able to actively exercise their citizenship rights and those who remain excluded from them.

This form of inequality affects both organizational staff and the users/clients of the services and goods they provide, manifesting as a factor that may either facilitate or hinder organizations' capacity to implement and integrate digital technologies within their structures.

An additional perspective through which to analyze the organizational field emerging around digital technologies is that of the so-called *digitalized welfare* or *data welfare state*. Despite the specificities that characterize different national welfare systems, this perspective highlights a broader convergence toward neoliberal logics emphasizing efficiency and the marketization of service delivery, greater scope for competition, and the involvement of both nonprofit and for-profit providers, alongside the diffusion of techniques and instruments associated with New Public Management (Henriksen et al., 2012), as well as the increasing proliferation and pervasiveness of digital technologies and artificial intelligence (Alexopoulou, 2024).

While these technologies ostensibly offer significant advantages, they also entail substantial risks and trade-offs. On the one hand, digital technologies have the potential to enhance accessibility, efficiency, effectiveness, and inclusiveness in the delivery of social services. On the other hand, they raise critical concerns related to the digital divide (Alexopoulou et al., 2022), the amplification of inequalities between a "digital oligarchy" and a "digital underclass" (Ragnedda, 2020), and, more broadly, the marginalization of individuals with limited digital literacy, restricted access to necessary resources, or conditions of vulnerability (Eubanks, 2018).

Moreover, in digital welfare states, systems of social protection and assistance are increasingly driven by digital data and technologies employed for a wide range of functions, including automation, prediction, identification, surveillance, detection, targeting, and sanctioning. These developments risk undermining the legal and ethical foundations of the democratic welfare state, while enabling new and potentially coercive forms of power (Ottman & Noble, eds., 2026). This transformation has contributed to a shift toward forms of "digital governance," also supported by neoliberal processes of privatization and managerialism (Abramovitz and Zelnik, 2026), in which key decisions are increasingly shaped by technocratic actors, corporate entities, and multinational companies, thereby weakening both citizen agency and state authority.

Finally, the progressive retreat of the state from a leading role in innovation and technological transformation (Hanna, 2018), together with broader processes of retrenchment often grounded in neoliberal principles, threatens existing systems of social protection and regulatory frameworks (Collington, 2022).

Finally, the introduction of both digital and non-digital technologies within an organization does not constitute innovation per se. To be considered as such, it must take the form of a change that, regardless of its origin, is capable of triggering a transformation in the organizational culture of the actors involved (Schein, 1999). This implies that innovation cannot be limited to superficial changes at the level of artifacts, such as digital technologies, but must reach the deeper level of basic assumptions, that is, the meanings attributed to artifacts and to their modes of use. In this sense, innovation can be said to occur only when the introduction of technology initiates a learning process.

With specific reference to social cooperatives, however, it was also considered necessary to adopt the perspective of social innovation, understood as the creation of new processes, products, and services that use technologies to meet societal digital social innovation that, combining digital innovation and social innovation, may be defined as the creation of new processes, products and services that use technologies to meet societal challenges hence, its aim is to do good while exploring new markets and customers and/or exploiting existing markets and existing customers, thereby focusing on creating social and economic value (Bonina et al., 2021; Buck et al., 2023). By their very nature and mission, social cooperatives aim not only to address social needs through their activities, but also to carry them out in ways that are responsive to the needs of those who perform them, consistently valuing the relational dimension of their work. In this context, therefore, even when it involves the introduction of technological tools, innovation necessarily takes the form of social innovation, aimed at responding more effectively to social needs while simultaneously fostering social relationships and collaborations that generate social value (Bureau of European Policy Advisers, 2011; Mulgan et al., 2007; The Young Foundation, 2012).

RESEARCH OBJECTIVES AND METHODOLOGY

The present study was conducted within the framework of a project funded by the Regional Authority Friuli Venezia Giulia pursuant to Regional Law 34/2015 and implemented in partnership with Confcooperative FVG-Federsolidarietà. As such, it takes the form of a case study focusing on a specific third-sector organization operating in the Friuli Venezia Giulia region. Notably, this organization represents the second largest federation in the regional sector, encompassing 176 cooperatives (type A, type B, and mixed) and employing 9,728 workers. Given its focus on this specific organizational context, the findings are inherently limited and cannot be generalized to the sector as a whole. However, generalizability was not the primary aim of the research; rather, the study sought to identify and explore the key issues that digitalization is imposing on these organizations. The objective, therefore, was to provide a broad and detailed representation of the challenges at stake.

The research aimed to elicit participants' perspectives on digitalization, while at the same time valuing their knowledge and experiences and promoting mutual exchange, also with a view to fostering a community of practice (Wenger, 1998).

In line with the qualitative approach adopted, the focus group was used as the research tool, a method based on structured yet spontaneous group discussion, in which a small number of participants are invited by one or more moderators to exchange views on a given topic. Such an approach facilitates the emergence of shared meanings, situated professional languages, situated rationalities, and narrative accounts, thereby enabling a richer and more multidimensional understanding of the phenomenon (Corrao, 2002; Cataldi, 2009).

Specifically, the objectives of the focus groups were to: explore the approaches adopted by cooperatives in addressing digitalization; elicit the meanings attributed to it, as well as the expectations, concerns, and fears associated with it; and investigate the perceived consequences of its implementation on organizational structures, service provision, staff, and service users.

This phase consisted of three focus groups conducted between November and December 2025 with twelve cooperative managers. Participants were selected through purposive sampling based on criteria of substantive rather than statistical representativeness. In particular, cooperatives represented in the extended Board of Directors of Federsolidarietà were invited to participate. All accepted the invitation, and the actual participants included twelve cooperative presidents: two from mixed type A and B cooperatives, one from a type B cooperative, and the remainder from type A cooperatives. Two participants also served as presidents of consortia bringing together both type A and type B cooperatives. They were representative in terms of headquarters location and the provision of public services in urban, peripheral, and mountainous areas of the region.

A semi-structured discussion guide was developed to explore the following areas: expectations and concerns regarding the digitalization of the organization; level of digitalization achieved, types of digital technologies introduced, and services involved; staff digital competences; training and support initiatives for digitalization; the impact of digitalization on staff and service users; and future perspectives.

To facilitate participation, two focus groups were conducted online and one in presence. The research adhered to the regulations established by the University of Trieste concerning personal data protection, in compliance with Regulation (EU)

2016/679 and Legislative Decree No. 196/2003. Prior to the commencement of each focus group, participants were informed that the sessions would be audio-recorded. Informed consent for recording and for the subsequent anonymized processing of data for research and scientific dissemination purposes was obtained from all participants, both orally and in writing through a dedicated consent form prepared for the study. Audio files and signed consent forms are securely stored in a dedicated university repository established for the project.

The focus groups were audio-recorded, transcribed verbatim, and subjected to thematic analysis (Braun & Clarke, 2017) aimed at identifying recurring patterns, divergences, and overarching interpretative themes. This methodology proved particularly suitable for capturing not only empirical evidence but also the symbolic meanings and cultural frameworks within which the interventions are embedded.

To ensure the trustworthiness of the analysis—specifically with regard to the criteria of credibility, transferability, and confirmability as defined by Lincoln and Guba (1985)—the focus group transcripts were initially analyzed and coded independently by the two researchers involved in conducting the sessions. The researchers then compared their respective analyses and coding schemes in order to identify convergences and divergences. This process revealed a substantial level of agreement, leading to the identification of 28 codes grouped into the following four macro-areas: internal and external factors underpinning the digitalization process; the role played by public authorities within this process; the impact of digitalization on staff and organizational structures; and approaches to artificial intelligence. The identified codes and macro-areas were subsequently examined in light of the theoretical framework and the literature reviewed and presented in the introduction.

It should be noted that the study did not include the perspectives of cooperative workers or service users. This constitutes an additional limitation, as it prevented a comparative analysis of these viewpoints and the identification of potential convergences and divergences among them.

RESULTS

Between Internal Needs and External Demands: Drivers of Digitalization

A first thematic cluster emerging from the focus group analysis concerns the factors that initiated the digitalization process within the cooperatives involved. The findings indicate that this process was launched and continues to develop primarily in response to contingent needs and external demands, rather than as the result of rational, internally shared decisions articulated within a more or less formalized strategy designed to guide progress toward predefined improvement goals and within predetermined timelines.

All the digital steps we have taken were actually born out of a need, as often happens when technology responds to needs. But in reality, sometimes these are the needs of certain parts of the organization, which have to coincide with the operational side that does not always feel the same need. (C11)

No, there was no plan at all. Every time a need arose, we intervened immediately, clearly, we discarded any kind of paper-based solution and automatically moved towards digital tools, but without any specific program. (C8)

We slipped into digitalization without really thinking about digitalization. [...] We really slipped into it, because of needs related to time, shared communication, and basically archiving. [...] We were guided by need, often the need of only one part of the organization and not shared by everyone. (C3)

Moreover, in most cases, the need that triggered the digitalization process does not stem from an internally perceived and collectively developed demand to improve organizational structures and/or service provision, but rather originates from external sources, particularly from public authorities for which the cooperatives operate. In line with this externally driven dynamic, cooperatives appear to respond by adopting three main types of behavior: actively seeking such demands, passively undergoing them, or accepting them—sometimes with passive resignation and, in other cases, with active curiosity.

[...] there is a part of digitalization that is 'imposed,' so to speak, and a part that is natural. The imposed one concerns everything related to our relationship with the Region, in the sense that, since we work on funded projects, the Region places everything—from project design to management and soon even schedules—on regional platforms. So, whether we liked it or not, we had to adapt, because otherwise it was impossible. [...] And by providing training to others, these needs are also stimulated by our instructors who teach our students." (C1)

We have more and more requests and obligations, so to speak. Without digital technology, we would be in serious difficulty, because even the Region, regional funding, INPS, child benefits, and all these different measures require us to stay constantly updated. [...] I would even try to anticipate things: in my view, we are in a phase in which digital technology offers many advantages. [...] It is something we are riding. (C2)

These accounts highlight how digitalization is largely shaped by external institutional requirements and operational pressures, rather than by proactive strategic planning, and how cooperative leaders navigate this process through a combination of adaptation, compliance, and selective appropriation.

Between Uncertainty and Unpredictability: Public Authorities as Drivers of Digitalization

Among the external factors driving the digitalization process, public authorities occupy a central position, not only because services and projects carried out through agreements and/or partnerships with public bodies account for a substantial share of cooperatives' revenues, but above all because, in several cases, public authorities require the adoption of specific reporting and/or data collection procedures, which in turn make it necessary for cooperatives to equip themselves with dedicated software systems. In some instances, such demands have also produced a multiplier effect, as they have contributed to further stimulating internal digital development by triggering processes of appropriation and adaptation of the technologies required by public authorities to the specific needs of each organizational context, on the one hand, and by extending their application to other areas of the cooperative, on the other.

The app we use for scheduling home care was originally created in response to a request from the contracting authority. [...] It was really their tool, where we just entered data; it did not draw on company data. We rewrote it and then made it retrieve data from our internal software and send them where they needed to go. So, we integrated it. (C9)

In prevalence, however, the demands formulated by public authorities often appear confused and contradictory, driven more by the contingent and constantly changing supply offered by the market than by a coherent, clear, and shared strategy. As a result, cooperatives are continuously required to adopt new applications or adapt those already in use, with significant organizational and financial implications.

With this whole issue of innovation, public authorities impose all kinds of unreasonable data-retrieval requests on us. We are overwhelmed by requests to recover data, by software that does not work, or by having to enter the same data three times. So, there is this moment of total schizophrenia, because everyone pursues their own software. It takes years before these processes become effective. But the public sector just throws this at us and says, 'Use this software.' And you say, 'Fine.' Then after six months they say, 'Let's make these changes.' And you say, 'Fine.' Three months later: 'Let's introduce another variable.' In practice, we live in a situation of constant staff training and continuous uncertainty and unpredictability, because the final data are always different, always incomplete. This is really exhausting and draining, because it has an immediate impact when we issue invoices. There are moments when conflicts arise because the authority says, 'Is this the data you collected?' And you reply, 'No, it's something else.' It's almost a nightmare. (C6)

There is a kind of widespread lack of knowledge that affects both our sector and public authorities. There is no particularly strong digital culture, so there is still the idea that if you introduce software, everything will be fixed in ten days, without understanding that there is an integration process. Software needs to be fed; it does not work on its own, data does not process itself. Data collection and entry systems are not trivial and cannot be implemented in a month. Then there are integration and interaction with external software, such as that of INPS. There are many issues to resolve in the dialogue with public authorities, and these are not always easy to address in a short time. (C7)

The absence of a coherent digitalization strategy, both within public authorities and within individual cooperatives, contributes to making its diffusion in this sector uneven and fragmented. Digital development thus appears highly differentiated both across cooperatives and among different sectors within the same organization. Some cooperatives have reached relatively advanced levels of digitalization, or are at least aligned with ongoing technological developments, while others struggle to keep pace and exhibit varying degrees of delay.

Between Enthusiasts and Resisters: The Impact of Digitalization on Staff

The impact of digitalization on cooperative staff is also uneven. Its effects vary according to professional profile—distinguishing among administrative, educational, care-related, and technical personnel—length of service, type of activity performed, and the type of technology introduced and used. Staff responses to the introduction and use of digital technologies can be traced back to three main attitudes: resistance, proactivity, and compliance, the latter being sometimes accompanied by difficulties, sometimes by enthusiasm, and sometimes by fear.

[...] there are many people who struggle and who even refuse, saying: 'No, you print it for me, because I'm really not suited for this, I don't like it, I can't do it, I hate technology.' (C8)

[...] I think there is a technical issue, a matter of competence, but also a matter of mindset. [...] First, a digital mindset has to be developed. Because there is resistance, there is real fear that leads people to think: 'They will replace us all.' There is a lot of imagination surrounding digital technology. (C3)

[...] we have a big gap between those who know how to manage and handle tools quite well and those who do not know them at all. [...] This gap is difficult to manage, because if I think about the ten people who are able to manage data well and maybe even produce projections, they say, 'This app is great, let's use it because it's fast,' but then I have to pull along the other forty. I always have to reason in terms of timing and accessibility. [...] It seems that you can do everything, but in reality, you cannot. [...] This is not trivial; it requires internal reflection. (C6)

Among the various sectors of cooperative activity, the administrative area is generally the one in which digitalization has reached the most advanced level of diffusion. This is not only because it is the area most directly affected by public authorities' digital requirements, but also because the benefits of digital technologies have emerged more clearly and rapidly within it. These benefits are mainly identified in time and paper savings, increased accuracy and volume of collected data, faster and more widespread dissemination of information, improved internal and external communication, and greater clarity of processes and procedures. For many cooperatives, therefore, the introduction of digital technologies in this area has played a significant driving role in promoting their adoption in other organizational sectors.

However, even among administrative staff, reactions to digital technologies are differentiated. The general heterogeneity of personnel in terms of familiarity with digital tools, propensity to use them, and willingness to learn represents one of the main obstacles to their introduction and implementation. As noted above, digitalization processes are often slowed down in order to proceed uniformly, seeking to respect everyone's pace and to avoid leaving anyone behind. In some cases, they are even halted altogether, despite their potential advantages for the cooperative and its members, as illustrated by the following excerpt:

[...] we would like to introduce digital meal vouchers, which would allow us to increase employee benefits. [...] But we can't manage to do it because many employees would not know how to handle the new card and the app properly or would not feel comfortable with it. [...] We are always blocked by the desire to move forward while having a reality that struggles to keep up. (C8)

As a result, many cooperatives devote considerable attention and effort to identifying the most effective ways and tools to foster among staff an adequate understanding and awareness of the real and not perceived risks as well as of the potential and usefulness of digital technologies, including for their own work.

Many people are not aware of their learning needs. They say, 'I've always done it this way.' [...] Very often, I have had to demonstrate that if you take this step, you gain a benefit, so in a way the need has to be created. [...] You have to do a lot of convincing, because they always have this attitude of low trust. [...] You really have to take small steps, and the goal is always to explain why you are doing things, because if you do it only for your own advantage, they say, 'That's your problem.' Instead, you always have to try to find their need. That is fundamental. (C4)

Among the concerns expressed by some staff members is also the fear that the use of digital technologies may undermine the quality and authenticity of relationships with service users.

We are now at the point where we would like families to receive an email, log in, enter their data, and upload all the necessary documents. Out of nine facilities, six do not want to do it. [...] They are afraid that interacting through technology will take away the relationship with families. [...] Coordinators and educators who are perhaps a bit older and less digitally oriented are very afraid of this. They cannot understand it. [...] We have a small blockage. [...] There is some resistance. (C2)

These findings highlight how the impact of digitalization on staff is mediated by professional roles, generational factors, skills, and organizational cultures, and how it entails not only technical adaptation but also deep processes of negotiation, learning, and identity redefinition.

Rising Costs, Market Dependence, and Privacy Constraints: The Impact of Digitalization on Organizational Structures

Additional factors identified as obstacles to the digitalization of cooperatives concern the costs associated with this process, including both the purchase of technological equipment and the organizational adjustments and changes required for its effective use. These costs are perceived not only as high, but also as constantly and progressively increasing, due to the rapid obsolescence of digital technologies, which consequently require frequent updating or replacement.

Digitalization is also increasing costs. We are witnessing what I think is called servitization: you no longer buy something once and for all, but you buy a service, you buy time-limited licenses. This has shifted costs from high but one-off to lower but permanent. (C5)

At first, you think it will make work easier, but then there is a phase in which the workload actually increases, because you have to find time to learn and make the transition. [...] As with any change, there is also an investment of time. (C3)

Very often, starting to use a tool involves a high initial investment, and only in the long run do you see the benefits. (C4)

In addition to acquisition costs, digitalization also generates forms of dependence on technological systems and, in particular on software providers. Once a specific platform or solution is adopted, cooperatives often become tied to it, which significantly reduces their bargaining power and discretionary margins in relations with ICT suppliers. As several participants emphasized, this awareness leads organizations to evaluate very carefully which systems and providers to choose, knowing that such decisions imply long-term constraints. This, in turn, contributes to further slowing down digitalization processes.

Dependence on a system makes you fragile, in the sense that if that system changes the rules and you are used to using something that no longer exists, as happened recently, you get upset, but that's it. You cannot really engage in dialogue with the designers. (C5)

A further aspect identified by focus group participants as a particularly significant barrier to digitalization concerns privacy regulations. Due to their interpretative complexity, these regulations often exert an inhibiting effect on potential initiatives aimed at digital implementation and innovation, especially when they directly involve actual or potential beneficiaries of services.

[...] How do you use Facebook, how do you use Instagram, what approach do you take? [...] It's not trivial, and immediately the whole issue of privacy comes into play, which in this area is endless. [...] The time required for these processes increases, and so do the costs, both in terms of working hours and management, because you can't improvise anymore; you have to consult a lawyer. (C6)

When it comes to critical issues, the doubt is always about sensitive data: which data can I ask for and which should I avoid? From my point of view, this greatly limits usage. (C10)

Overall, these findings indicate that digitalization places a growing financial, organizational, and regulatory burden on cooperatives. Rising and ongoing costs, dependence on market providers, and the complexity of privacy compliance combine to constrain organizational autonomy and to discourage rapid or experimental forms of digital innovation.

Approaches to Artificial Intelligence

A final aspect explored by the focus groups concerned participants' approaches to artificial intelligence (AI). In this area, respondents expressed a shared awareness that AI represents an unavoidable phenomenon. This awareness is accompanied by a generally cautious attitude which, in the absence of in-depth knowledge, currently leads cooperatives to exclude its use in direct interactions with service users.

Beyond the general enthusiasm surrounding this topic, I share this cautious attitude, because we deal with health, vulnerability, and people with support needs. So, clearly, initial experimentation should take place internally, to see how we can best use it in our daily activities. As for adopting it for external-facing actions, this prudence still prevails for now. (C7)

With regard to internal organizational use, the analysis revealed two main orientations: rejection and acceptance. Rejection tends to result in prohibitive practices. In some contexts, AI use is strictly forbidden, particularly at the recommendation of IT managers, who often feel that they lack adequate expertise in this area. As frequently occurs, however, such bans prove ineffective as deterrents and, in the absence of adequate monitoring, fail to prevent informal and concealed individual use.

We have an IT manager who is very strict. So, he said: There is no way you are going to use ChatGPT or any other nonsense out there without my complete control.' What is happening as a result? In reality, everyone who has to write texts is using it freely on their own. At the moment, we do not have a cooperative policy. We know people use it because it is actually useful. […] So right now, we are in a rather unregulated and unstructured situation. (C9)

The acceptance-oriented stance, by contrast, appears to lead to two prevalent patterns of behavior: unregulated use and cooperative-governed use accompanied by training. In some cases, cooperatives have not yet taken a formal position on AI, as they do not feel sufficiently prepared. While awaiting further training and recognizing the limited effectiveness of prohibitions, they tolerate free use by those who wish to adopt it.

[…] if you ban it, they will use it anyway. If they use it, all the data-related problems emerge and need to be managed. You cannot avoid it. So, we have already planned training for almost everyone, because access is now extremely easy, and given the sensitive services and contacts we deal with, this needs to be governed. We are also trying to understand how to use it in processes. Moving from data-entry software to artificial intelligence is a big leap, but we have already seen that moving from paper to software saves us 50% of time. If we make this leap, how much will we save? Or rather, how much will our overall work-related well-being improve? We believe it will, but we are leaving it as an open question and trying to understand. Above all, we will seek external support. (C6)

[…] we have application systems that we purchased for image production for external communication. As for production, I have happened to use ChatGPT, even professionally, […] but it is left to individual discretion. (C4)

Other cooperatives, by contrast, have identified several opportunities associated with AI for organizational improvement, alongside significant risks. Consequently, they have begun to use AI tools while preceding and accompanying their implementation with specific training programs addressed to all potentially involved staff members.

AI has helped us, and continues to help us, also in the internal training pathway we are developing. It is certainly useful for recurring bureaucratic tasks, reports, quality documentation, […]. We also use it for generative purposes: when we have a project idea, we consult it to see what emerges. Another area where it helps us is communication. We use artificial intelligence in its various forms, from ChatGPT to dedicated applications for producing images and slides to support trainers. At the moment, we are investing heavily in internal training. […] We all access the cooperative's subscription-based version, which was made available after a training initiative. It has helped us greatly. […] Having specific training and consultancy on artificial intelligence has reassured us and has allowed us to work more confidently, if not necessarily more efficiently. (C1)

As with other digital technologies, AI is predominantly used to enhance the efficiency of internal organizational processes. In relation to service users, however, as noted above, a cautious stance prevails. Even among those who accept AI, few employ it explicitly in user-facing activities, and when they do, its use is mainly limited to improving communication and the dissemination of information about cooperative activities and services.

As far as services are concerned, no, because at the moment we have not found a clear need or application. In administration, yes: for reports, summaries, quick reading, or extracting figures from 200-page documents. In that sense, it has been a considerable help. And also, for checking regulations, providing additional confirmation that supports the interpretation you are already developing. (C8)

Overall, these findings suggest that AI is currently positioned within social cooperatives primarily as an internal support tool, whose adoption is shaped by uncertainty, ethical concerns, and organizational learning processes, rather than as a technology directly oriented toward service delivery.

DISCUSSION

The results presented in the previous section not only confirm some of the evidence and trends already identified by previous studies but also allow a more in-depth examination of specific aspects and dynamics that contribute to a better understanding of these phenomena.

Overall, the findings confirm both the general backwardness of the sector in terms of digitalization and the marked heterogeneity of its development. While a small number of cooperatives have reached a relatively advanced stage or are broadly aligned with ongoing changes, many others continue to lag behind (Rogers, 1983). Further confirmation concerns the deterrent effect exerted by both direct and indirect costs associated with digitalization, which place a scarcely sustainable burden on the limited turnover that characterizes most of these organizations (LegaCoop, 2023; Italia Non Profit, 2024), as well as by privacy regulations (Trapani, 2022). With regard to the latter, the analysis highlights not only the constraining effect of regulatory requirements, but also the interpretative difficulties they entail. These difficulties often force cooperatives to rely on external consultants, generating additional costs and contributing to delays in both implementation and the overall digitalization process.

The findings also confirm that digitalization is proceeding in the absence of an emerging internal strategy within individual cooperatives (Mintzberg, 1978). The reflections of focus group participants help to clarify some of the underlying causes of this lack. These include, in part, the limited awareness among organizational leaders of the opportunities offered by digital technologies, as well as their persistent mistrust toward them. Such factors reinforce interpretations that attribute the low level of digitalization in this sector to the predominantly humanistic, rather than scientific or technological, background of organizational leaders. These profiles significantly influence economic and organizational investments in digitalization and, consequently, its outcomes (Cavotta et al., 2022; D'Alessandro et al., 2022).

In the absence of internal digital strategies, focus group analysis highlights how digitalization in this sector is largely driven by external pressures, particularly from the digital technology market and public authorities. Although this dynamic is to some extent expected, the analysis makes it possible to identify the interactions among these actors within the broader organizational field (Powell & DiMaggio, 1991) shaped by digital technologies. These technologies constitute a common element linking cooperatives, public authorities, and software providers. Indeed, they enable these actors to address many of the needs associated with their shared objective of providing welfare services. However, this common objective conceals partially divergent interests and is pursued from positions characterized by unequal distributions of power, technological knowledge, and capacities for technology use. These asymmetries among these actors result in differentiated pressures and varying possibilities for mutual influence.

A first contextual element contributing to the configuration of the organizational field in which these actors operate is represented by European and national regulations on digitalization. Reference is made to the legislative and regulatory framework promoted by the European Union within the EU Digital Strategy, including the General Data Protection Regulation (EU Regulation 2016/679), implemented in Italy through Legislative Decree no. 101/2018, as well as Legislative Decree no. 112/2017, Legislative Decree no. 117/2017, and the National Recovery and Resilience Plan (PNRR). These measures impose a range of compliance requirements on public bodies as well as private and non-profit organizations. Although such requirements are intended to foster improvement, they tend—at least in the short term—to constitute a burden for public administrations and for private and third-sector organizations providing personal services, particularly in light of the costs associated with acquiring new equipment and reorganizing internal processes.

Conversely, for software companies, the advantages prevail in both the short and long term. As a result, these actors exert stronger pressure toward compliance with the aforementioned regulations compared to public bodies and, especially, private and non-profit organizations. For the latter, moreover, there is a risk that compliance is conceived and implemented in a merely formal rather than substantive manner. This is also due to the often limited timeframes for implementation, which do not allow sufficient opportunity to fully understand the underlying rationale of these regulations or to identify ways of transforming them into opportunities for organizational development.

As also emerging from the focus group analysis, the prevailing perception of these regulatory frameworks is therefore predominantly constraining and negative, while their potential positive implications tend to remain in the background.

Moreover, software companies, public authorities, cooperatives, and service users differ significantly in their understanding of digital technologies and in their ability to select and purchase appropriate solutions. Software companies hold a position of epistemic superiority, as they are often the only actors able to fully assess the potential of the technologies they introduce to the market. This allows them to influence the choices of other actors by determining which technologies are available, which types of data may be collected and the modalities through which such data are processed and made available.

In addition, the convergence and generativity of digital technologies (Yoo et al., 2012), which enable the continuous addition of new functionalities and the development of increasingly multifunctional tools, allow single providers to meet a wide range of client needs through integrated products. This tends to generate oligopolistic market structures and forms of technological dependency, control and surveillance (Abramovitz & Zelnik, 2026).

Public authorities occupy a position of relative dependence on software companies in terms of technological knowledge and a partial dependence on cooperatives regarding organizational and user needs. At the same time, they retain substantial economic and decision-making power over which needs are addressed and how. As Abramovitz and Zelnik (2026) highlight, this power is significantly shaped by neoliberal policy pressures, which promote the reduction of public expenditure in favor of increased private spending. This shift is pursued through the expansion of market-based mechanisms in service provision and the introduction of managerial techniques and tools aimed at enhancing efficiency and productivity.

Cooperatives, in turn, are largely dependent on software providers for technological expertise, while possessing greater knowledge of user needs than public authorities. Nevertheless, they often remain subordinated to public authority in decisions concerning service funding and technological adoption. Moreover, like the third sector more broadly, these organizations are typically characterized by small to medium size, the particular fragility and complexity of the target populations they serve, and the relatively low professional profile of much of their workforce. As a result, they display a more limited entrepreneurial capacity compared to the private sector and encounter greater difficulties in sustaining the technological and training investments required by digitalization (LegaCoop, 2023; Italia Non Profit, 2021, 2024).

Service users generally occupy a position of epistemic and structural dependency, particularly those facing multiple social and health-related vulnerabilities. As discussed above, these conditions are compounded by inequalities in access to and use of digital technologies, contributing to the complex and multi-layered configuration of the so-called digital divide (van Dijk, 2020). This, in turn, exacerbates the risks of exclusion and marginalization that already affect many of these individuals. However, this perspective should not be generalized or applied in a stereotypical and prejudicial manner to the entire service user population. While a substantial proportion of users are indeed in a disadvantaged position with regard to the use of digital technologies, a non-negligible share appears receptive to their adoption and would, in fact, benefit from their implementation rather than be further disadvantaged. From the perspective of service utilization, while disadvantaged users are often constrained to rely on publicly funded or freely available services of uncertain quality, more affluent users can access privately provided, higher-quality services.

The different positions occupied by the four actors in terms of technological knowledge, decision-making power, and purchasing capacity generate interaction patterns that, if left unregulated, may reinforce existing asymmetries and inequalities (Powell & DiMaggio, 1991).

The digitalization process promoted by public authorities appears to be shaped more by market offerings and technical decisions made by software providers than by coherent strategies grounded in systematic knowledge of technologies and user needs. This, in turn, influences cooperatives' digitalization trajectories, which largely depend on the often ambiguous and contradictory choices of public institutions. The presence of an innovative strategy, developed through the reinterpretation of external stimuli and validated internally and externally, is a crucial factor for organizational success (Mintzberg, 1978; Birkinshaw & Mol, 2006). Moreover, the digitalization promoted by public authorities is strongly influenced by the neo-managerialist approach that prioritizes efficiency and productivity, often at the expense of service quality and effectiveness (Abramovitz and Zelnick 2026). Digital technologies have been mainly adopted to meet administrative and reporting requirements imposed by public authorities, within a context shaped by managerialist orientations (Lorenz, 2025; Burton et al., 2008; Devlieghere et al., 2020).

This orientation is also evident in the third sector and is reflected in participants' accounts which highlight that digitalization has mainly affected administrative and managerial processes within cooperatives, with limited impact on service delivery and user relationships. Only one respondent referred to the use of digital technologies to enhance service delivery, mentioning the continued use of video calls introduced during the COVID-19 pandemic to maintain contact between elderly residents and their families. Moreover, references to users have emerged primarily in relation to privacy concerns, which not only slow down digitalization but also constrains its developmental potential.

Another dimension concerns participants' perceptions of service users. Contrary to earlier findings (Punziano et al., 2023), respondents generally assumed that most users possess adequate digital skills. As anticipated, it is important to acknowledge that, despite the pervasiveness of digital technologies, significant segments of the population, particularly welfare service users, remain affected by digital exclusion. The intersection of limited digital skills with disadvantages related to gender, age, migration background, and economic conditions has disabling and disempowering effects, restricting autonomous access to digital welfare services (Buchert et al., 2023). This is a finding that should be taken into careful consideration. At the same time, as noted above, it cannot be generalized; it is equally necessary to recognize the presence of a non-negligible proportion of service users who appear both capable of and interested in using digital technologies, and who could potentially benefit from them in terms of access to and utilization of currently available services, as well as those that may be developed in the future. Social cooperatives must therefore address this issue both by ensuring accessibility and by promoting initiatives aimed at reducing digital inequalities. One participant expressed concern that digital technologies might weaken relationships between professionals and users, particularly between early childhood educators and parents. Although not widely shared, this concern deserves attention, especially in contexts where digitalization implies a redefinition of professional roles. However, these considerations need to be further substantiated by incorporating the perspectives of service users themselves, which, as noted above, this study was not able to capture.

Similarly limited was participants' awareness of the potential of digital technologies to improve staff well-being and work quality. Only two respondents reported improvements in internal communication and conflict mitigation. No explicit reference was made to the risks of marginalization and exclusion from the labor market faced by workers with limited digital skills, despite their broader social relevance.

With regard to the use of artificial intelligence (AI), the focus group analysis reveals dynamics similar to those observed in earlier phases of digitalization. A cautious, wait-and-see attitude—often rooted in skepticism or resistance—leads to organizational inertia. In the majority of cooperatives, AI-related knowledge remains limited across the workforce, including among individuals in managerial and executive roles. Furthermore, only in a small number of cases has the adoption of AI been formally introduced following structured and targeted training initiatives. Despite this, the accessibility and user-friendliness that characterize AI technologies are contributing to the emergence of informal and often unregulated forms of use, primarily driven by self-directed learning practices. As a consequence, the already substantial risks associated with AI implementation are further amplified. Given the rapid and pervasive advancement of AI, such an approach risks leaving its development in the hands of actors with greater technological and economic power. This, in turn, may undermine the capacity of public and social organizations to safeguard the rights of those most affected by AI-driven transformations, especially those unable to protect themselves autonomously.

Bridging the digital divide among organizational leaders in public authorities and cooperatives would also help to harness the interest and openness toward digital technologies present among some staff members. The analysis shows that expressions of curiosity and motivation are often not translated into practice, not primarily due to financial constraints, but rather because of difficulties in achieving broad organizational engagement, particularly among staff with lower levels of competence, interest, or confidence. This situation dampens innovative impulses and increases the risk of widespread demotivation. The focus group analysis revealed that levels of digital competence and readiness to use digital technologies in the workplace are highly differentiated within social cooperatives, being generally low among the majority of staff involved in service provision and moderate among administrative personnel. This uneven distribution inevitably affects the potential for the development of digitalization within these organizations. Indeed, for the introduction of digital technologies to result in their effective use by staff, organizations need to implement training pathways differentiated by professional category, alongside ongoing and tailored support processes for specific groups of workers.

In this respect, the recommendations put forward by Goldkind and Fink (2025) are particularly relevant. Focusing specifically on nonprofit human services organizations, the authors emphasize the importance of making AI use within organizations more visible and formally acknowledged, promoting open and critical dialogue on both the potential benefits and harms of AI, encouraging experimentation in low-stakes applications, supporting staff in the development of more efficient workflows, and considering the formulation of an organizational policy governing the use of AI.

Focus group analysis indicates that awareness of these disparities and dynamics is limited and unevenly shared. This lack of awareness hinders digital technologies from fully their innovative potential and suggests a risk that digital technologies may be treated as ends in themselves rather than as tools serving the social mission of these organizations, marginalizing interpersonal relationships and individual centrality (Busacca, 2022). For the social cooperative sector, it is therefore crucial to promote forms of digitalization that can be framed as processes of digital social innovation (Bria, 2015), in which technologies support collaboration, co-creation, and social value, rather than replacing face-to-face relationships or serving merely as instruments of impression management (Tracey & Stott, 2017).

To prevent the initial digital divide affecting each actor from deepening and transforming power asymmetries into structural inequalities, it is essential to develop shared approaches aimed at reducing these gaps, fostering mutual understanding of needs, and establishing effective governance mechanisms. Such mechanisms are necessary to promote inclusive digitalization capable of responding to the needs of both actual and potential service users and of the wider population. From this perspective, the role of public authorities in fostering a digital ecosystem is crucial for promoting shared vision, agile strategies, sustained commitment, and instituzionalized collaboration (Hanna, 2018; Collington, 2022).

CONCLUSION

As anticipated, this study took the form of a case study focusing on a specific third sector organization operating in the Friuli Venezia Giulia region and was aimed to identify and explore the key issues that digitalization is imposing on these organizations.

This study presents some limitations, as it is based on a case study involving a single confederation of social cooperatives in one Italian region. Moreover, it places greater emphasis on Type A cooperatives than on Type B ones and captures only the perspectives of managerial figures within a sample of cooperatives, without also exploring those of staff members and service users. These limitations constrain the scope and generalizability of the findings, while at the same time opening up promising avenues for further investigation into future research.

Despite these limitations, the findings offer a meaningful and relevant contribution to knowledge, not only for the federation under study but also for the wider field.

The results presented above depict a third sector that is slowly yet inexorably being reconfigured through the introduction of digital technologies. This reconfiguration, however, appears to be driven more by pressures from the market and by neo-managerialist demands for debureaucratization, efficiency, and control advanced by public authorities than by the intentional pursuit of a rationally defined strategy aimed at clear and shared objectives. As argued, this pattern can be traced back to the specific interactions generated by differing levels of knowledge and awareness of digital technologies, varying degrees of decision-making power over their adoption, and unequal capacities to finance their acquisition among social cooperatives, software providers, public authorities responsible for and funding the welfare system, and actual and potential service users.

These dynamics, combined with the predominance of a technocratic and deterministic approach to digital technology, appear to reduce its innovative potential—particularly in social terms—and to conceal several risks. These include, on the one hand, the marginalization and exclusion from cooperative organizations and, more broadly, from the labor market of socially and digitally disadvantaged workers, and, on the other hand, the marginalization and exclusion of socially and digitally vulnerable citizens from access to digital welfare services. At the same time, the economic impact of digitalization increases the risk that, if left solely to market mechanisms, its diffusion will lead to the gradual exit from the service system of third-sector organizations unable to sustain its costs and pace.

To prevent this outcome and to enable social cooperatives to understand and fully exploit the potential of digital technologies in pursuing their social missions, it is necessary for them to achieve sufficient organizational and economic growth to gain relevance and, in many fields, to compete with for-profit enterprises (Pastorelli, 2022). Only through growth can they invest not only in digital infrastructures but also in the training required to use them effectively, enhancing their potential for social innovation within a rationally developed and consistently implemented internal strategy.

However, the economic and digital-cultural development of social cooperatives must be accompanied by a parallel growth in the digital culture of public administrators, managers, and civil servants (Hanna, 2018). As the analysis shows, these actors play a crucial role in shaping the configuration of the welfare system, including its digital dimension. Without adequate knowledge and awareness of both the opportunities and limitations offered by digitalization, as well as of its effects on service providers and users, public authorities cannot ensure that digital transformation evolves in a direction consistent with system goals and user needs.

It is therefore essential to invest in training pathways aimed at reducing the digital divide that remains widespread across organizational levels in both the public sector and the social economy. At the same time, such initiatives should contribute to building communities of practice (Wenger, 1998) capable of accompanying digitalization processes in ways that foster genuine opportunities for social innovation and promote shared knowledge and empowerment among public institutions, software providers, social cooperatives, professionals, and service users. This approach can help prevent digitalization from evolving into forms of competition that generate divisions between included and excluded groups, winners and losers.

The perspective to be pursued is thus that of co-constructing ecosystems of social digital innovation (Bria, 2015; Hanna, 2018), in which political and technical decision-makers from public institutions, for-profit and non-profit organizations, and representatives of citizens can work together to: develop a shared understanding of the potentials and limits of digital technologies and of the multiple ways in which they can foster socially oriented innovation; agree on regulatory frameworks and interpretations of sector-specific and privacy regulations that protect digital service users without unduly constraining organizational initiative; and identify and attract accessible funding opportunities, particularly for small and medium-sized social cooperatives.

REFERENCES

Abramovitz, M., & Zelnik, J. (2026). Managerialism on steroids. The rise of Artificial Intelligence. In Ottman, G., & Noble, C. (Eds.), *AI and the Disruption of Welfare* (pp. 11–28). Routledge., DOI: 10.4324/9781003673675-2

Alexopoulou, S. (2024). Paradigm shift: Exploring the impact of digital technologies on the welfare state through a systematic literature review. *Social Policy and Administration*, *59*(1), 135–157. DOI: 10.1111/spol.13054

Alexopoulou, S., Åström, J., & Karlsson, M. (2022). The grey digital divide and welfare state regimes: A comparative study of European countries. *Information Technology & People*, *35*(8), 273–291. DOI: 10.1108/ITP-11-2020-0803

Birkinshaw, J., & Mol, M. J. (2006). How Management Innovation Happens. *Sloan Management Review*, *47*(4), 81–88.

Bonina, C., López-Berzosa, D., & Scarlata, M. (2021). Social, commercial, or both? An exploratory study of the identity orientation of digital social innovations. *Information Systems Journal*, *31*(5), 695–716. DOI: 10.1111/isj.12290

Braun, V., & Clarke, V. (2017). Thematic analysis. *The Journal of Positive Psychology*, *12*(3), 297–298. DOI: 10.1080/17439760.2016.1262613

Bria, F. (2015). *Growing a digital social innovation ecosystem for Europe, Digital Social Innovation Final Report*

Buchert, U., Kemppainen, L., Olakivi, A., Wrede, S., & Kouvonen, A. (2023). Is digitalisation of public health and social welfare services reinforcing social exclusion? The case of Russian-speaking older migrants in Finland. *Critical Social Policy*, *43*(3), 375–400. DOI: 10.1177/02610183221105035

Buck, C., Krombacher, A., Röglinger, M., & Körner-Wyrtki, K. (2023). Doing good by going digital: A taxonomy of digital social innovation in the context of incumbents. *The Journal of Strategic Information Systems*, 32(4), 101806. https://doi.org/ s.2023.101806DOI: 10.1016/j.jsi

Bureau of European Policy Advisers. (2011). *Empowering people, driving change: Social innovation in the European Union*. Publications Office of the European Union.

Burton, J., & van den Broek, D. (2008). Accountable and Countable: Information Management Systems and the Bureaucratization of Social Work. *British Journal of Social Work*, *26*, 1–17. DOI: 10.1093/bjsw/bcn027

Busacca, M. (2022). Imprese sociali e transizione digitale [Social Enterprises and Digital Transition]. *Impresa sociale*, 4, 27-28

Cataldi, S. (2009). *Come si analizzano i focus group* [How to Analyze Focus Groups]. Franco Angeli.

Cavotta, V., Grassi, E., & Toschi, L. (2022). Uso delle tecnologie digitali da parte degli imprenditori e innovatori sociali: Potenzialità e limiti. *Impresa Sociale*, *4*, 29–35.

Collington, R. (2022). Disrupting the Welfare State? Digitalisation and the Retrenchment of Public Sector Capacity. *New Political Economy*, *27*(2), 312–328. DOI: 10.1080/13563467.2021.1952559

Corrao, S. (2002). *I focus group* [Focus Groups]. Franco Angeli.

D'Alessandro, F., Landoni, P., & Marocchi, G. (2022). Le imprese sociali di inserimento lavorativo: Che rapporto hanno con le tecnologie [Work Integration Social Enterprises: Their Relationship with Technologies]. *Impresa Sociale*, *4*, 36–44. DOI: 10.7425/IS.2022.04.06

Devlieghere, J., Roose, R., & Evans, T. (2020). Managing the electronic turn. *European Journal of Social Work*, *23*(5), 767–778. DOI: 10.1080/13691457.2019.1582009

Eubanks, V. (2018). *Automating Inequality: How High-Tech Tools Profile, Police, and Punish the Poor*. St. Martin's Press.

European Commission. *Digital Economy and Society Index (DESI) 2022, Thematic chapters,* https://digital-strategy.ec.europa.eu/en/policies/desi

Goldkind, L., Ming, J., & Fink, A. (2025). AI in the Nonprofit Human Services: Distinguishing Between Hype, Harm, and Hope. *Human Service Organizations, Management, Leadership & Governance*, *49*(3), 225–236. DOI: 10.1080/23303131.2024.2427459

Hanna, N. (2018). A role for the state in the digital age. *Journal of Innovation and Entrepreneurship*, *7*(1), 5. DOI: 10.1186/s13731-018-0086-3

Henriksen, L. S., Smith, S. R., & Zimmer, A. (2012). At the Eve of Convergence? Transformations of Social Service Provision in Denmark, Germany, and the United States. *Voluntas*, *23*(2), 458–501. DOI: 10.1007/s11266-011-9221-5

ISTAT. (2022). *Censimento permanente. Struttura e profili del terzo settore in Italia* [Permanent Census: Structure and Profiles of Italy's Third Sector], https://www.istat.it/files//2022/10/Report-Non-Profit-2022.pdf

Italia non profit. (2021). *L'impatto della Riforma sugli enti non profit* [The Impact of the Reform on Non-profit Organizations]. https://italianonprofit.it/riforma-in-movimento/risultati/#intro

Italia non profit. (2024). *Terzo Settore & Digitale, Verso un futuro digitale* [Third Secor and Digital, towards a Digital Future]. https://italianonprofit.it/riforma-in-movimento/risultati/#intro

LegaCoop. (2023). *Indagine sulla digitalizzazione nelle imprese cooperative* [Survey on the Social Enterprises Digitalization].

Lincoln, Y. C., & Guba, E. G. (1985). Naturalistic Inquiry. *Sage (Atlanta, Ga.).*

Lorenz, W. (2025). Re-positioning the social mandate of social work. *Nordic Social Work Research*, 1–13. DOI: 10.1080/2156857X.2025.2478838

Mintzberg, H. (1978). Patterns in Strategy Formation Author. *Management Science, 24*(9), 934–948. DOI: 10.1287/mnsc.24.9.934

Mulgan, G., Tucker, S., Ali, R., & Sanders, B. (2007). *Social Innovation. What it is, why it matters and how it can be accelerated*, The Young Foundation Working Paper, The Young Foundation

Orlikowski, W. (1992). Rethinking the concept of technology in organizations. *Organization Science*, *3*(3), 398–427. DOI: 10.1287/orsc.3.3.398

Orlikowski, W. J. (2000). Using technology and constituting structures: A practice lens for studying technology in organizations. *Organization Science*, *11*(4), 404–428. DOI: 10.1287/orsc.11.4.404.14600

Orlikowski, W. J. (2007). Sociomaterial Practices: Exploring Techology at Work. *Organization Studies*, *28*(09), 1435–1448. DOI: 10.1177/0170840607081138

Orlikowski, W. J., & Scott, S. V. (2008). Sociomateriality: Challenging the Separation of Technology, Work and Organization. *The Academy of Management Annals*, *2*(2), 433–474. DOI: 10.5465/19416520802211644

Ottman, G., & Noble, C. (Eds.). (2026). *AI and the Disruption of Welfare*. Routledge.

Pastorelli, G. (2022). L'economia Sociale Digitale e la sfida dell'interoperatiblità. Verso una prossima economia sociale [The Social Digital Economy and the Interoperability Challenge. Toward a Further Social Economi]. *Impresa Sociale*, *1*, 87–91. DOI: 10.7425/IS.2022.01.12

Powell, W. W., & DiMaggio, P. J. (Eds.). (1991). *The new instituzionalism in organizational analysis*. The University of Chicago Press. DOI: 10.7208/chicago/9780226185941.001.0001

Punziano, G., & Acampa, S. (2023). Reti, digitale e processi di innovazione tra profili di resilienza e mutamento: i pilastri del fronteggiamento alla doppia transizione. [Networks, Digital and Innovation Processes between Resilience and Change: the Pillars to Cope with the Double Transition] In Punziano, G., Cicellin, M., & Zito, E. (Eds.), *Nuove risposte organizzative, innovazioni e impatti sociali del Covid-19 sul Terzo Settore* [New Organizational Responses, Innovations, and Social Impact of Covid-19 on Third Sector Organizations]. (pp. 110–123). Franco Angeli.

Punziano, G., Cicellin, M., Zito, E., Acampa, S., & Sorrentino, R. (2023). Role of the Digital for the Third Sector in the Campania Region (Italy): From the Side of Research to the Side of the Objects in the Aftermath of the COVID-19 Pandemic. *Italian Sociological Review*, *13*(X), 279–296. DOI: 10.13136/isr.v13i2.638

Ragnedda, M. (2020). *Enhancing digital equity: Connecting the digital underclass*. PalgraveMacmillan., DOI: 10.1007/978-3-030-49079-9

Rogers, E. M. (1983). *Diffusion of Innovation*. The Free Press.

Schein, E. H. (1999). *The Corporate Culture Survival Guide*. Jossey-Bass and Wiley & Sons.

The Young Foundation. (2012). *Social Innovation overview: A deliverable of the project: "The theoretical, empirical and policy foundations for building social innovation in Europe" (TEPSIE)*. European Commission.

Tracey, P., & Stott, N. (2017). Social innovation: A window on alternative ways of organizing and innovating. *Innovation (North Sydney, N.S.W.)*, *19*(1), 51–60. DOI: 10.1080/14479338.2016.1268924

Trapani, M. (2022). *L'impatto della digitalizzazione negli enti del terzo settore* [The Impact of Digitalization on Third Sector Organizations]. I Quaderni, Cesvot Edizioni.

Venkatesh, V., Morris, M. G., Davis, G. B., & Davis, F. D. (2003). User Acceptance of Information Technology: Toward a Unified View. *Management Information Systems Quarterly*, *27*(3), 425–478. DOI: 10.2307/30036540

Wenger, E. (1998). *Communities of Practice, Learning, Meaning and Identity*. Cambridge University Press. DOI: 10.1017/CBO9780511803932

Yoo, Y., Boland, J. R.Jr, Lyytinen, K., & Majchrzak, A. (2012). Organizing for Innovation in the Digitized World. *Organization Science*, *23*(5), 1398–1408. DOI: 10.1287/orsc.1120.0771

APPPENDIX

Ethics Approval and Consent to Participate

The study did not involve procedures that required formal approval from an ethics committee. All interview participants were informed about the purpose of the study and gave their written consent to participate and use their anonymized data for research and scientific dissemination purposes, in accordance with the University of Trieste regulations concerning personal data protection.

Chapter 2
Artificial Intelligence, Synthetic Data, and the Socio-Technical Reconfiguration of Data Infrastructures:
Data Asymmetries in Healthcare

Monica Murero
http://orcid.org/0000-0001-6693-8075
Università Federico II, Italy

ABSTRACT

Digital welfare systems increasingly rely on data-driven infrastructures, yet these remain largely oriented toward clinical and pathological data. Information on healthy populations, early-stage risks, and preventive trajectories is often limited or fragmented. This imbalance—conceptualized as data asymmetry—constrains the development of preventive and inclusive welfare strategies. This chapter examines how advanced Artificial Intelligence methodologies—such as data augmentation, minority oversampling, transfer learning, and synthetic data generation—can partially address these structural gaps. The chapter conceptualizes these techniques as socio-technical and communicative processes that reshape how data are constructed, interpreted, and mobilized. The analysis shows how synthetic data and transfer learning enable future-oriented representations of risk and population health, while raising challenges to validity, representation, and governance. AI is thus understood as a process shaping how health and prevention are defined and acted upon within digital welfare systems.

DOI: 10.4018/979-8-2600-3043-1.ch002

1. UNDERSTANDING DATA ASYMMETRY IN DIGITAL WELFARE SYSTEMS

The digital transformation of welfare systems is profoundly reshaping how data are collected, managed, and mobilized, creating new opportunities for prevention, personalization of care, and long-term system sustainability (D'Ancona et al., 2023).

However, this transformation is not simply a matter of technological innovation. Rather, it entails a broader reconfiguration of the epistemic, organizational, communicative, and socio-technical foundations through which health needs are identified, represented, and governed. This chapter does not present new empirical findings. Instead, it offers a conceptually informed and interdisciplinary discussion of emerging AI methodologies designed to address structural data limitations within healthcare and welfare systems, examining their epistemic, socio-technical, communicative, and governance implications.

These developments have contributed to the emergence of what may be described as data-driven welfare systems, in which decision-making processes are increasingly mediated by digital technologies, algorithmic models, and predictive analytics. At the same time, critical scholarship has emphasized that the datafication of welfare is not a neutral process. Rather, it produces new configurations of visibility, exclusion, and power, raising important questions about how individuals and populations are represented within digital infrastructures (Campedelli & Vesan, 2023; Dencik, 2022).

Within healthcare, a fundamental structural limitation emerges from the very architecture of contemporary data infrastructures. Digital welfare systems remain predominantly built around clinical and pathological data generated within institutional settings such as hospitals, specialist clinics, and healthcare organizations. As shown by Si and colleagues (2021) in their systematic review of deep learning applications using electronic health records (EHRs), contemporary healthcare AI is largely developed around EHR-derived patient representations and disease prediction tasks. This reliance on clinically generated data contributes to a healthcare data ecosystem that is particularly effective at modelling disease progression, treatment pathways, and healthcare utilization. However, because EHRs are primarily designed to document clinical encounters rather than represent population health (Ehrenstein et al., 2019), they provide a partial, reactive, and institutionally bounded representation of health and illness. Clinical datasets frequently reflect patterns of healthcare access, utilization, and documentation practices, introducing important representational limitations and forms of selection bias (Norori et al., 2021; Chen et al., 2023). Consequently, existing data infrastructures are generally better equipped to model illness than health, treatment than prevention, and clinical events than the socio-temporal trajectories that precede disease onset. By contrast, data describing healthy populations, early-stage risk conditions, preventive pathways, and everyday health behaviours remain comparatively fragmented, difficult to access, or insufficiently integrated into many AI development pipelines (Fahim et al., 2025). This imbalance gives rise to a condition that this chapter conceptualizes as data asymmetry: a structural disparity between the abundance of data on disease and the relative scarcity of data on healthy populations, prevention, and early risk conditions. While related to concepts such as data bias, data gaps, and data inequality, data asymmetry refers to a different phenomenon. Data bias concerns distortions in the composition or representation of existing datasets; data gaps refer to missing or unavailable information; and data inequality highlights uneven access to data resources across actors or populations. By contrast, data asymmetry focuses on the structural imbalance between categories of health-related data that are systematically overproduced and those that remain underproduced within digital welfare infrastructures. In this chapter, the concept specifically captures the disproportionate availability of disease-oriented data relative to data concerning prevention, healthy populations, and early risk conditions. Importantly, data asymmetry is not merely a technical limitation. It is also a socio-technical, epistemic, and communicative condition. Research in critical data studies has long demonstrated that data do not simply represent reality but actively participate in shaping what becomes visible, measurable, and actionable within institutional systems (Kitchin, 2014; boyd & Crawford, 2012). From this perspective, healthcare data infrastructures are not neutral repositories of information but socio-technical arrangements that privilege certain forms of knowledge while marginalizing others. As Ruckenstein and Dow Schüll (2017) argue in their analysis of the datafication of health, digital data practices increasingly define which dimensions of health, risk, and prevention become knowable and governable. Consequently, populations and phenomena that are poorly captured by existing infrastructures—such as healthy individuals, preventive trajectories, and pre-clinical risk conditions—may become not only statistically underrepresented but also institutionally and communicatively marginalized. What remains absent from data risks becoming less visible within decision-making processes, policy priorities, and AI-driven governance systems. As Cruz (2022) demonstrates, healthcare data infrastructures simultaneously capture, obscure, and shape understandings of care, reinforcing the need to critically examine how data availability influences the construction of health-related knowledge. If data asymmetry represents a structural limitation of contemporary digital welfare systems, an important question becomes how AI-based methodologies attempt to operate under conditions of incomplete, fragmented, or unevenly distributed data. It is within this context that methodologies such as data augmentation, minority oversampling, transfer learning, and synthetic data generation emerge as potentially important responses. Synthetic data, in particular, refer to artificially generated datasets that reproduce selected statistical properties of real-world data without directly replicating identifiable individual records. These methodologies can be understood not only as technical solutions to data scarcity but also as interventions that reshape how data are constructed, expanded, and mobilized. In doing so, they influence the conditions under which health phenomena become visible and the ways in which prevention and risk are conceptualized and operationalized. Rather than viewing these techniques as neutral reproductions of reality, this chapter approaches them as socio-technical and communicative mechanisms that contribute to shaping how future health scenarios are imagined, interpreted, and acted upon within digital welfare systems.The contribution of the chapter is therefore twofold. First, it examines how emerging AI methodologies can be deployed in contexts characterized by limited, fragmented, or imbalanced data, thereby expanding the analytical capacity of digital welfare systems. Second, it critically explores the broader implications of these approaches for knowledge production, healthcare organization, welfare governance, and decision-making processes in increasingly data-driven environments. In doing so, the chapter explicitly distances itself from technosolutionist narratives that frame AI as an inherently self-sufficient response to systemic challenges in welfare provision. Following Morozov (2014), technosolutionism refers to the belief that complex social and institutional problems can be effectively solved through technological innovation alone. By contrast, this chapter argues that the effectiveness of AI remains deeply dependent upon the characteristics, omissions, and asymmetries embedded within the data environments from which these systems learn. The focus is therefore not only on the technical capabilities of AI but also on the socio-technical conditions that shape what becomes visible, measurable, and actionable within digital welfare systems.

The remainder of the chapter is structured as follows. Section 2 situates data asymmetry within broader discussions on the datafication of welfare and digital health infrastructures. Section 3 examines emerging AI methodologies designed to address structural data gaps, including data augmentation, minority oversampling, transfer learning, and synthetic data generation. Section 4 explores the implications of these approaches for preventive welfare and healthcare transformation. Finally, Section 5 discusses issues of accountability, transparency, and governance in increasingly data-driven welfare systems.

2. DATAFICATION AND DATA ASYMMETRY

The digital transformation of welfare systems is increasingly understood not simply as the adoption of new technologies, but as a profound reconfiguration of the socio-technical infrastructures through which social needs are identified. In this context, data have become a central organizing principle of welfare systems, shaping how risks are classified, and how interventions are designed and implemented.

The concept of datafication provides a crucial entry point for understanding these transformations. As van Dijck (2014) argues, datafication refers to the process through which aspects of social life are translated into quantifiable data formats, enabling new forms of knowledge production, monitoring, and control. Within welfare systems, datafication operates through the construction of complex data infrastructures that connect, for example, administrative records, clinical information, and *digital traces* into integrated systems of analysis and decision-making. As Dencik (2022) highlights, the emergence of the "datafied welfare state" reflects a shift toward governance models that rely increasingly on algorithmic processing, and also on predictive analytics, and automated classification. These systems do not simply support decision-making; they actively shape the categories through which individuals and populations are understood.

In healthcare systems, data generation is predominantly organized around clinical encounters, diagnostic procedures, and treatment pathways. This is why the vast majority of available datasets are pathology-oriented, capturing information about individuals once they enter institutional care settings such as hospitals, specialized clinics, or emergency services. These data are indispensable for clinical decision-making, but they offer a fundamentally reactive representation of health, centered on disease manifestation rather than on its anticipation or prevention.

Healthy populations, early-stage risk conditions, and pre-clinical trajectories remain largely underrepresented within existing data infrastructures. Specifically, preventive dimensions of health—such as lifestyle factors, environmental exposures, social determinants, and longitudinal well-being—are often fragmented across multiple systems, inconsistently recorded, or entirely absent. This is not only a major challenge for AI design, but also results in a structural imbalance between what is visible and measurable within digital systems and what remains invisible or weakly captured. This condition can be conceptualized as data asymmetry, defined here as the *systematic overrepresentation of pathological data and the corresponding underrepresentation of preventive, longitudinal, and population-level health information.* Importantly, this asymmetry is not merely a technical limitation, but the outcome of historically sedimented institutional, and organizational priorities within healthcare systems.

From an epistemological perspective, data asymmetry also reflects a biomedical cultural model that prioritizes acute conditions, measurable symptoms, and clinically validated indicators. As Hoeyer and Wadmann (2020) suggest, the datafication of healthcare tends to extract forms of knowledge that are standardized, quantifiable, and compatible with existing data infrastructures. Similarly, Lupton (2018) highlights how digital health systems selectively amplify certain types of data while marginalizing others, thereby shaping the boundaries of what can be known and acted upon. From a socio-technical perspective, data asymmetry is embedded within the design and operation of data infrastructures themselves. As Kitchin (2014) argues, data infrastructures are not neutral repositories but complex assemblages that encode decisions about what should be collected, how it should be categorized, and for what purposes it should be used. In this sense, the relative absence of data on healthy populations is not accidental within welfare systems, but reflects systemic choices about where to invest in data collection, which actors are responsible for generating data, and which outcomes are prioritized. Recent research on the digital welfare state has further emphasized the ambivalent nature of these transformations. On the one hand, digital infrastructures promise greater efficiency, personalization, and anticipatory capacity in the delivery of welfare services. On the other hand, the risk is that they may introduce new forms of inequality, opacity, and control, raising critical questions about inclusion, accountability, and democratic oversight (van Toorn et al., 2024; Zakharova et al., 2024). In the field of digital health, scholars have shown how the increasing reliance on data-driven systems is transforming the production of medical knowledge and the organization of care. Lupton (2018) highlights how digital health technologies generate new forms of patient data while simultaneously reconfiguring relationships between patients, professionals, and institutions. Similarly, Hoeyer and Wadmann (2020) argue that the datafication of healthcare reshapes what is considered meaningful clinical work, privileging standardized, measurable outputs over contextual and experiential forms of knowledge. In recent contributions, these dynamics are also closely connected to broader concerns about data justice, which emphasize the uneven distribution of benefits, risks, and harms associated with data-driven systems (Dencik et al., 2022). Moreover, issues of representation, access, and participation become particularly salient in welfare contexts, where data are used not only to describe populations but also to allocate resources and define people's eligibility for services. As a result, data infrastructures can reproduce or amplify existing social inequalities, especially when certain groups remain underrepresented or invisible within datasets.

Against this backdrop, the problem of data asymmetry emerges as a central analytical concern in AI-modeling for preventive care, since data on healthy populations, early-stage risk conditions, and preventive trajectories remain scarce, fragmented, or entirely absent. This is a crucial point in the data asymmetry discussion that strongly limits the design of AI-based solutions in preventive care.

2.1 Data Asymmetry in Digital Health

In the previous section we have seen that a central yet underexplored issue in the digital transformation of healthcare and welfare systems concerns the structural asymmetry in the production and use of data. While contemporary data infrastructures are often described as increasingly comprehensive and granular, they remain profoundly uneven in what they can capture, represent, and make actionable. Data asymmetry has direct consequences for social inclusion and inequality within digital welfare systems. For example, populations that are less frequently captured within clinical datasets—such as individuals with limited access to healthcare, marginalized communities, or those in early stages of risk—remain underrepresented in the data used to train AI systems. As a result, these groups may be less likely to benefit from preventive interventions, and more exposed to systemic neglect or delayed care.

Crucially, data asymmetry also affects how prevention itself is conceptualized and operationalized. In the absence of robust data on early risk factors, prevention risks being reduced to a secondary or residual function, rather than becoming a central organizing principle of welfare systems. Preventive strategies remain constrained by the limited visibility of the populations they are intended to serve, as well as by the lack of longitudinal data needed to model future trajectories.

Understanding digital welfare through the lens of datafication and data asymmetry requires a shift from viewing data as neutral inputs to recognizing them as constructed, situated, and power-laden elements. As a consequence, digital welfare systems that rely predominantly on risk, reinforce a model of intervention that is predominantly reactive, rather than preventive. This perspective opens up critical questions about how data infrastructures might be reconfigured to support more inclusive, anticipatory, and equitable forms of welfare. Data do not simply represent reality; they participate in its construction by defining which populations are visible or prioritized, which risks are measurable, and which needs are recognized as legitimate. This has important implications for healthcare systems, where data infrastructures play a central role in shaping both clinical knowledge and broader welfare strategies.

2.2 Emerging Approaches to Address Data Asymmetry

The structural condition of data asymmetry outlined in the previous section calls for methodological approaches capable of operating under conditions of data scarcity, imbalance, and fragmentation. The implications of data asymmetry are particularly significant in the context of AI-driven decision-making. Machine learning models rely on large-scale historical datasets to identify patterns, predict risks, and support interventions (Feickert et al., 2024). This limits the potential of AI's dependance on data to support preventive welfare strategies, reinforcing a reactive model of care that intervenes only once problems have become visible within the system.

Addressing data asymmetry therefore requires more than expanding data collection; it entails a broader rethinking of how data infrastructures are designed, governed, and integrated within welfare systems. This includes recognizing that what is not collected is as significant as what is collected, and that absences in data are themselves socially and politically meaningful.

It is within this context that advanced AI methodologies—such as data augmentation, minority oversampling, transfer learning, and synthetic data generation—begin to emerge as potential socio-technical responses to structural data gaps, addressing existing data asymmetries while also introducing new challenges and risks. They can be more productively understood as interventions within data infrastructures that have the potential to reshape patterns of visibility, representation, and decision-making.

The techniques that we will see do not eliminate data asymmetry, but they can partially compensate for its effects by expanding representational capacity, simulating missing data, and enabling knowledge transfer across contexts. It is on this basis that the following section examines more closely how specific AI methodologies operate in contexts characterized by data asymmetry in healthcare.

2.2.1 Data Augmentation and Minority Oversampling

Data augmentation refers to the process of expanding existing datasets by generating modified versions of available data points. In healthcare contexts, this may involve transformations of medical images, signals, or clinical records to increase the variability and robustness of training data. For example, in radiology, datasets of chest X-ray images can be expanded through controlled transformations (e.g., rotation or contrast adjustment), enabling the training of advanced machine learning and deep learning models that would otherwise not be feasible due to limited data availability. In this sense, data augmentation does not simply improve model performance; it makes possible the very construction of AI systems under conditions of data scarcity. While these techniques are often discussed within technical and computational literatures, their implications extend far beyond model performance, as they directly affect issues of representation, inclusion, and epistemic authority within data-driven systems.

Closely related, *minority oversampling* explicitly addresses imbalances in class distribution within datasets by increasing the representation of rare events, conditions, or populations. In digital welfare systems, this technique has particular relevance for improving the detection of low-prevalence diseases, rare conditions, or marginalized groups that are often underrepresented in standard datasets. For instance, in the case of rare pediatric conditions such as cystic fibrosis, oversampling techniques make it possible to construct machine learning models capable of identifying these diseases, which would otherwise remain difficult to detect due to the scarcity of available data. By altering the statistical composition of data, oversampling techniques challenge the implicit assumption that majority patterns should dominate predictive models. Without such interventions, the limited presence of these cases would prevent the effective training of predictive models, reinforcing their invisibility within data-driven systems.

2.2.2 Transfer Learning, Circulation of Knowledge and Synthetic Data

Transfer learning introduces a different dimension to the problem of data asymmetry by enabling the reuse of knowledge across contexts. For example, models trained on large international datasets of brain MRI can be adapted to developing countries settings with limited data, enabling the development of deep learning-based diagnostic tools that could not otherwise be independently trained. In this way, transfer learning allows for the construction of advanced AI systems even in contexts where data scarcity would otherwise prevent their development. Models trained on large, well-structured datasets can be adapted to settings where data are scarce or fragmented, thereby facilitating the diffusion of analytical capacity across institutional and geographical boundaries. In welfare systems characterized by uneven data infrastructures, transfer learning can function as a mechanism for redistributing analytical resources, potentially reducing disparities between well-resourced and under-resourced contexts.

A central dimension concerns the role of *synthetic data* in addressing structural data gaps, particularly the absence of information on healthy populations and preventive trajectories. In AI system design synthetic data are artificially generated datasets that reproduce the statistical properties of real-world data without directly corresponding to identifiable individuals. Their increasing adoption in clinical settings to support decision-making reflects both a technical and a socio-technical shift in how data scarcity, privacy constraints, and representational gaps are addressed (D'Ancona et al, 2023). Synthetic data generation enables the simulation of plausible health scenarios, risk distributions, and population-level patterns without exposing sensitive personal information (Gonzales et al., 2023; Pezoulas et al., 2024). A particularly relevant example can be observed in the early stages of a pandemic, when available clinical data are limited and fragmented. In such contexts, synthetic data can be used to simulate transmission dynamics, risk profiles, and possible clinical evolutions, enabling the development of machine learning models at a stage in which real-world data are still insufficient. Without such techniques, the construction of predictive models would be significantly constrained during the most critical early phases of a crisis.

From an AI-driven perspective, synthetic data offer a promising solution to several well-known limitations of healthcare datasets, including data scarcity, class imbalance, and restricted access due to privacy regulations. By generating additional data points that approximate underrepresented populations or rare conditions, synthetic data can support the training of more robust and generalizable AI models. This is particularly relevant in preventive contexts, where data on early-stage risk conditions or healthy populations are often limited or fragmented. Recent literature has begun to highlight the dual nature of synthetic data. On the one hand, they are seen as a key enabler for addressing structural data gaps and improving model performance. On the other hand, they challenge traditional assumptions about the relationship between data and reality, particularly in contexts where decisions are made on the basis of simulated or augmented datasets. Moreover, research on synthetic healthcare data highlights its potential to address structural data gaps in health systems while simultaneously raising questions about data validity, governance, and ethical oversight. In this context, synthetic data not only help bridge data scarcity but also enable privacy-preserving forms of data sharing and analysis, making them particularly relevant in highly regulated healthcare environments. It is also within this perspective that synthetic data can be conceptualized not simply as a technical solution, but as an epistemic and communicative intervention that expands what can be known, modeled, and governed within digital welfare systems.

This tension underscores the need to move beyond purely technical evaluations of AI-based solutions and to consider the broader socio-technical and cultural implications of interventions within data infrastructures.

2.3 Towards the Socio-Technical and Communicative Reconfiguration of Data Infrastructures

We noticed so far that data asymmetry does not simply represent a limitation in data availability, but points to a broader need to rethink how data infrastructures are designed, interpreted, and governed within digital welfare systems. Addressing data asymmetry in AI-based interventions therefore requires moving beyond a purely technical understanding of data gaps and engaging with the socio-technical, cultural, and communicative processes through which data are produced, circulated, and made meaningful. Techniques such as data augmentation, minorty oversampling, transfer learning, and synthetic data generation should not be understood solely as tools for improving model performance. Rather, they can be seen as interventions within communicative and socio-technical systems, capable of reconfiguring how populations are represented, how risks are anticipated, and how decisions are justified within welfare infrastructures.

In this perspective, data infrastructures can be understood as communicative environments in which health, risk, and prevention are not only measured, but also constructed, framed, and negotiated. The absence or underrepresentation of certain populations and conditions within datasets is not simply a matter of missing information, but reflects deeper processes through which some realities are made visible, while others remain marginal or excluded. As a result, data asymmetry operates not only at the level of data distribution, but also at the level of representation, meaning-making, and institutional recognition.

This shift in perspective has important implications for how AI methodologies are conceptualized, applied and deployed. From this standpoint, the role of AI becomes closely intertwined with broader processes of knowledge production and communication. AI systems do not simply process data; they contribute to shaping the narratives, classifications, and categories through which health phenomena are understood. In doing so, they influence not only what is known, but also what becomes legitimate, actionable, and governable within institutional contexts.

At the same time, this reconfiguration introduces new challenges. From a socio-technical perspective, also data augmentation and minority oversampling can be interpreted in light of a strategy for enhancing the visibility of underrepresented patterns, allowing models to recognize conditions that would otherwise remain statistically marginal. In this framework, also transfer learning can be understood as a mechanism through which knowledge is redistributed, rather than newly produced. At the same time, data enhancement and redistribution is not neutral, as it involves the circulation of specific data regimes, classificatory frameworks, and interpretive logics across contexts. In this sense, for example, transfer learning can also be seen as a communicative process, through which particular representations of health, risk, and normality are transferred, translated, and recontextualized within different institutional settings. This raises important questions about whose data are used as a reference, which populations are considered representative, and how such transfers may reproduce or challenge existing hierarchies within welfare systems. The movement of models across contexts therefore includes a process of communicative and cultural translation, in which meanings, assumptions, and norms embedded in data are re-articulated within new socio-institutional environments that AI developers and decision-makers should take into consideration.

Within this framework, the significance of synthetic data extends beyond their technical function. Their introduction into healthcare systems represents a broader transformation in how knowledge, uncertainty, and future risk are constructed and communicated. Unlike traditional datasets, which are retrospectively derived from observed clinical events, synthetic data are inherently prospective and generative: they model possible scenarios, simulate trajectories, and anticipate conditions that may not yet be fully observable within existing data infrastructures.

In this sense, synthetic data can be understood as communicative and cultural constructs that contribute to shaping how populations are imagined, represented, and governed. They do not simply fill gaps in existing datasets; they actively participate in defining what becomes visible, plausible, and actionable within data-driven systems. The generation of synthetic data involves choices about which variables to model, which relationships to preserve, and which populations to simulate, thereby embedding specific assumptions about health, risk, and normality.

From a socio-technical perspective, synthetic data fundamentally challenge the boundary between observed and constructed knowledge. This has significant implications for preventive welfare, as it enables the modeling of future-oriented scenarios that are not yet visible within existing datasets. Preventive knowledge thus becomes increasingly mediated by simulated and projected representations, rather than solely grounded in retrospective clinical evidence. This shift introduces new forms of temporal orientation, moving from reactive models based on past events toward anticipatory frameworks that also rely on the construction of possible futures.

In sum, the use of AI-based methodologies to address data offers unprecedented opportunities but also raises questions about the validity, interpretability, and accountability of data-driven models, particularly when decisions are based on data that are partially constructed rather than directly observed. These challenges are not only technical, but also cultural, potentially biased and communicative, as they concern how uncertainty is represented, how results are explained, and how trust is established between systems, institutions, and users.

Understanding AI methodologies in this way allows for a more nuanced interpretation of their role within digital welfare systems. Rather than framing them as pre-existing problems, they can be understood as active components in the ongoing reconfiguration of data infrastructures, strategically contributing to the transformation of preventive strategies and to the reshaping of the relationship between data, knowledge, and governance.

This has important implications for the development of preventive welfare strategies. By enabling the representation of populations that are otherwise underrepresented or absent in empirical data, synthetic data, minority oversampling, data augmentation and transfer learning AI-based methodologies can support a shift from reactive, disease-centered models toward more anticipatory and preventive approaches. At the same time, they introduce new layers of mediation between reality and representation, raising critical questions about validity, bias, and the governance of artificially generated knowledge.

3. AI AND THE RECONFIGURATION OF WELFARE SYSTEMS

In the previous sections, the integration of advanced AI methodologies into healthcare showed the potential and duality of a broader transformation of these systems into data-driven socio-technical environments, in which cultural and communicative processes play a central role in shaping how health, risk, and care are represented, interpreted, and deeply intertwined with algorithmic processes. Within this transformation, AI does not operate as a neutral tool but as an active agent in the reconfiguration of institutional logics. By shaping how data are collected, processed, and interpreted, AI systems influence the categories through which populations are classified, the thresholds through which risks are identified, and the criteria through which interventions are prioritized. In this sense, AI participation in the construction of social reality within welfare systems, could contribute to the emergence of new forms of visibility and invisibility.

A key dimension of this transformation concerns the shift from reactive to anticipatory models of welfare. Traditional welfare systems have largely been organized around the management of existing conditions, responding with different degrees of reaction to needs once they become visible within institutional frameworks.

However, the increasing use of predictive analytics and AI-driven modeling may enable a move toward anticipatory governance, where interventions are informed by probabilistic assessments of future risks. This shift is closely linked to the expansion of data infrastructures and the incorporation of methodologies—such as synthetic data generation—that allow for the modeling of populations and scenarios beyond those directly observable.

While this anticipatory turn offers significant potential for improving prevention and resource allocation, it also must raise important questions about how uncertainty is managed and how decisions are justified within the decision-making process. Predictive models, by their nature, operate on probabilities rather than certainties, yet they may be used to inform decisions with tangible consequences for individuals and communities. This creates a tension between the promise of more efficient and proactive welfare systems and the risk of over-reliance on algorithmic outputs that may not fully capture the complexity of social and health realities.

Another critical aspect of this reconfiguration relates to the changing role of professional expertise. As AI systems become more deeply embedded in clinical and administrative processes, they increasingly mediate the relationship between professionals and the data on which they rely. Decision-making processes may become partially delegated to algorithmic systems, raising questions about professional autonomy, accountability, and trust. The integration of AI does not eliminate human decision-making, but it reshapes it, introducing new forms of dependency on computational systems that are not always transparent or easily interpretable.

These dynamics also intersect with broader issues of inequality and inclusion. As discussed in previous sections, the data on which AI systems are trained are often unevenly distributed, reflecting existing social, economic, and institutional disparities. The use of advanced methodologies to address data asymmetry—such as augmentation or synthetic data—may mitigate some of these imbalances, but they may also introduce new forms of bias if not carefully designed and governed. In this sense, the reconfiguration of welfare systems through AI is not inherently progressive; its outcomes depend on how these systems are implemented, regulated, and critically examined.

From a socio-technical perspective, it is therefore essential to understand AI not only in terms of its technical capabilities but also in relation to the institutional, cultural, and political contexts in which it operates. Welfare systems are not simply technical infrastructures; they are embedded within broader social arrangements that shape how needs are defined, how resources are distributed, and how responsibilities are assigned. The introduction of AI into these systems thus entails a rearticulation of these arrangements, with potential implications for power relations, governance structures, and public accountability.

In particular, the increasing reliance on data-driven decision-making raises questions about transparency and legitimacy. Algorithmic systems often operate as "black boxes," making it difficult for both professionals and citizens to understand how decisions are reached. This opacity can indirectly undermine trust in welfare institutions and complicate efforts to ensure accountability. At the same time, the complexity of AI systems may create asymmetries of knowledge between those who design and manage these systems and those who are subject to their outcomes.

The reconfiguration of welfare systems through AI also involves a transformation in how populations are represented and analyzed As data become central to the identification of needs and the allocation of resources, individuals are increasingly understood through their data profiles, risk scores, and predictive classifications. This process of datafication can enable more targeted and efficient interventions, but it may also reduce complex social realities to simplified representations, potentially obscuring contextual factors that are difficult to capture within data models.

These developments point to the emergence of what can be described as data-mediated welfare, where the functioning of welfare systems is deeply intertwined with the production, circulation, and interpretation of data. In this context, questions of governance become central: who controls the data, who defines the models, and who is accountable for their outcomes.wether These questions deserve greater attention within both policy and academic debates.

At the same time, it is important to recognize that these transformations are not uniform. Different healthcare systems, institutional settings, and regulatory environments shape how AI is adopted and integrated into welfare infrastructures. This variability highlights the need for context-sensitive analyses that take into account the specific configurations of technology, institutions, and socio-cultural practices in different settings.

Ultimately, the integration of AI into welfare systems represents a broader transformation in how societies understand and address social and health needs. It opens up new possibilities for efficiency and innovation, while also introducing new challenges related to inequality, accountability, and governance. Understanding these dynamics requires a critical and interdisciplinary approach that situates AI within the complex socio-technical systems through which welfare is produced and experienced.

4. AI IN THE PREVENTIVE WELFARE

4.1 Constructed Data for the Digital Welfare

Building on the conceptualization of AI-created data infrastructures, this section develops a deeper analysis of its role within the transformation of digital welfare systems, with particular attention to its implications for preventive healthcare. The deployment of innovative AI methodologies to partially address data asymmetry introduces significant ethical, social, and governance challenges. Techniques such as data augmentation, minority oversampling transfer learning, and synthetic data generation may enhance predictive performance, but they also risk reducing transparency, and even obscuring accountability (World Health Organization, 2021). Since these interventions introduce new forms of constructed data into decision-making processes, understanding their role requires situating them within the broader dynamics of digital welfare systems.

In particular, the normalization of *synthetic* representations within decision-making processes raises concerns about the relationship between simulated data and lived realities. When synthetic outputs are treated as equivalent to empirical observations, important differences between constructed and experienced realities may become blurred. If insufficiently scrutinized, these dynamics may contribute to new forms of exclusion or misrepresentation within welfare systems, relevant to ethical considerations. As we previously observed, critical scholarship on digital welfare suggests, data-driven governance is never neutral but reflects normative assumptions about risk and responsibility (Dencik, 2022).

Moreover, the use of advanced AI methodologies to compensate for data asymmetries may inadvertently shift attention away from the structural causes of data gaps. Instead of addressing why certain populations remain poorly represented, these techniques risk offering technically sophisticated but socially partial solutions, leaving underlying inequalities largely intact. Rather than relying exclusively on empirical observations, when digital welfare systems begin to incorporate simulated representations of populations and risks, may expand the scope of what can be analyzed and anticipated. In this sense, we observed that "synthetic data" can also be understood as communicative artifacts: they do not merely represent reality, but actively participate in shaping how future risks are framed, interpreted, communicated and made actionable within data-driven welfare systems. Ultimately, the integration of synthetic data into digital welfare infrastructures represents a reconfiguration of how data are selected, and mobilized, with direct consequences for how prevention, risk, and population health are governed, and even *not governed.*

By conceptualizing AI as a socio-technical and communicative infrastructure, methodological innovation must be accompanied by *governance innovation.* AI systems not only process data, but also mediate how information is interpreted, communicated, and acted upon across institutional contexts. This includes the development of transparent and accountable frameworks, the clarification of responsibility across the AI lifecycle, and the critical examination of how algorithmic systems reshape relationships between citizens, professionals, and institutions and the impact of using AI-based knowledge in the decision-making process. Whether digital welfare systems are ready to implement these challenges is a critical question.

The integration of advanced AI methodologies into digital welfare systems requires not only technical refinement, but a fundamental reconfiguration of data practices and governance models. Within this perspective, the dual framework developed in this chapter provides a critical lens through which to interrogate how digital transformation may enable more equitable, resilient, and sustainable welfare systems.

While this chapter develops a conceptual and interdisciplinary framework for understanding these transformations, it does not aim to provide an empirical validation of synthetic data applications. Rather, it seeks to identify key dynamics that warrant further empirical investigation. By simulating plausible data distributions, the construction of alternative narratives of *preventive welfare* can be observed.

As previously discussed, in the context of digital welfare, synthetic data could reshape the epistemic foundations of healthcare systems, influencing not only how data are generated, but also how future health needs are anticipated and potentially governed. Synthetic data does not only expand the availability of data for modeling purposes; it also reshapes the cultural and interpretive frameworks through which health, health risk, and future scenarios are understood. In this sense, synthetic data extends the scope of analysis beyond what is empirically observable, enabling the articulation of future-oriented scenarios that are not yet present in existing datasets. These scenarios function as well as cultural and communicative constructions that influence how risks are anticipated and how preventive strategies are imagined, legitimized and potentially modeled in AI-based systems.

A key contribution of synthetic data we observed so far, lies in its capacity to address one of the central challenges identified: the structural absence of data on healthy populations and early-stage risk conditions. As noted in recent literature, synthetic data can help fill critical data gaps by generating plausible representations of under-observed or entirely unobserved populations, thereby expanding the analytical space within which AI models operate. This capacity is particularly relevant in the context of preventive welfare, where the objective is not merely to respond to existing conditions, but to anticipate future risks and intervene before they fully materialize. Traditional healthcare data infrastructures, largely centered on clinical and pathological data, offer limited support for such anticipatory approaches. Synthetic data, by contrast, enable the construction of forward-looking datasets that incorporate hypothetical trajectories, probabilistic risk scenarios, and early-stage indicators that are not yet visible within empirical data.

In this sense, synthetic data can be conceptualized as an epistemic expansion mechanism. Rather than simply reproducing existing patterns, they allow welfare systems to explore alternative scenarios and to model populations that are currently little or entirely absent from data infrastructures. This shift has profound implications for how prevention is understood and operationalized: prevention becomes not only a policy objective, but a data-driven and model-based process, grounded in the simulation of possible futures. But the use of synthetic data also raises important questions regarding the relationship between simulation and reality. While synthetic datasets can approximate real-world distributions, they are ultimately constructed artifacts, shaped by the assumptions, parameters, and training data used in their generation. This introduces a layer of epistemic mediation, in which what is considered "knowable" is increasingly influenced by model-based representations rather than direct observation.

This dynamic has both enabling and constraining effects. On the one hand, synthetic data can support more inclusive and comprehensive models by incorporating populations that are otherwise invisible. On the other hand, they may introduce new forms of bias or distortion, particularly if the underlying assumptions reflect existing inequalities or incomplete knowledge. The use of synthetic data in healthcare must therefore be accompanied by careful consideration of issues such as data validity, representational accuracy, and governance.

Another key dimension concerns the role of synthetic data in addressing privacy constraints. In healthcare contexts, access to high-quality data is often limited by regulatory and ethical restrictions designed to protect patient confidentiality. Synthetic data offer a potential solution by enabling the sharing and reuse of data without exposing identifiable personal information. This can facilitate collaboration across institutions and jurisdictions, contributing to the development of more robust and generalizable AI models.

However, the framing of synthetic data as a privacy-preserving solution should not obscure the broader socio-technical implications of their use. The generation of synthetic datasets involves choices about which variables to include, which distributions to reproduce, and which populations to simulate. These choices are inherently normative and may have significant consequences for how risks are defined, how resources are allocated, and which groups are prioritized within welfare systems.

From this perspective, synthetic data should be understood as part of a broader transformation in how knowledge, uncertainty, and future risk are governed in digital welfare systems. They contribute to a shift from retrospective analysis toward anticipatory governance, where decisions are increasingly informed by modeled scenarios rather than solely by observed data.

This transformation raises critical questions for the future of welfare systems. If decision-making becomes increasingly based on simulated representations, how can we ensure that these models remain transparent, accountable, and socially grounded? How can we prevent the normalization of synthetic representations from obscuring the lived realities of individuals and communities? And how can we ensure that the expansion of data through synthetic means does not reproduce or amplify existing inequalities?

In sum, addressing these questions requires moving beyond a purely technical understanding of synthetic data and situating them within a broader framework of socio-technical governance. This includes developing standards for validation and accountability, fostering interdisciplinary collaboration between technical and social sciences, and critically examining the assumptions embedded within synthetic data generation processes.

In this sense, AI-created synthetic data occupy a pivotal position within the evolution of digital welfare systems. They offer new possibilities for addressing data asymmetries and supporting preventive approaches, but they also introduce new forms of epistemic and governance complexity. Understanding this dual role is essential for ensuring that digital welfare systems evolve in ways that are not only technologically advanced, but also socially inclusive, culturally and ethically grounded, and responsive to the needs of diverse populations.

These dynamics require systematic empirical investigation in order to assess how synthetic data-driven models operate in practice, and how their adoption may reshape preventive strategies within different welfare contexts.

5. ACCOUNTABILITY IN DATA-DRIVEN WELFARE SYSTEMS

The transformations outlined in the previous sections highlight the need for a critical reflection on the governance implications, and communicative dimensions associated with the integration of AI into healthcare and welfare systems. Digital welfare infrastructures become increasingly reliant on data-driven and algorithmic processes. Questions of governance can no longer be treated as secondary considerations; they become central to how these systems operate, evolve, and are legitimized. At the core of this issue lies a fundamental shift in the nature of decision-making. Welfare systems have traditionally been governed through institutional frameworks that rely on professional expertise, regulatory standards, and forms of public accountability. However, the increasing incorporation of AI introduces new layers of mediation, where decisions are partially shaped by computational models that are not always transparent, interpretable, or easily contestable.

This shift raises critical questions about *who is responsible* for decisions made within AI-mediated systems. Responsibility becomes distributed across a complex network of actors, including data providers, model developers, healthcare professionals, institutions, and regulatory bodies. In such distributed systems, traditional notions of accountability—based on clearly identifiable decision-makers—are increasingly difficult to sustain.

One of the key challenges in this context is the issue of algorithmic opacity. Many AI systems, particularly those based on machine learning and deep learning, operate as "black boxes," making it difficult to fully understand how specific outputs are generated. This lack of transparency complicates efforts to ensure accountability, as it becomes challenging to trace the reasoning behind decisions that may have significant consequences for individuals' health and access to care.

At the same time, the use of advanced AI methodologies—such as synthetic data generation—introduces additional layers of complexity. As discussed in previous sections, synthetic data blur the boundary between observed and constructed knowledge, raising questions about the validity and reliability of the data on which decisions are based. Governance frameworks must therefore address not only how data are used, but also how they are generated, validated, and interpreted.

In this respect, these developments also resonate with emerging ethical reflections on AI, particularly those emphasizing accountability, transparency and explicability in data-driven systems. Ethical considerations are equally central to this discussion. The integration of AI into welfare systems has the potential to improve efficiency, enhance prevention, and expand access to care. However, it also carries risks related to bias, discrimination, and unequal representation. If the data used to train AI systems reflect existing social inequalities, these inequalities may be reproduced or even amplified within algorithmic decision-making processes. In this context, the work of Floridi and colleagues (2018) is particularly relevant. They propose a widely cited ethical framework for AI—AI4People—grounded in principles such as beneficence, non-maleficence, autonomy, justice, and explicability. These principles provide a normative foundation for evaluating AI systems, particularly in sensitive domains such as healthcare and welfare, where decisions have direct implications for human well-being and social equity. Therefore, the increasing reliance on algorithmic decision-making requires normative frameworks capable of ensuring that such systems remain intelligible and socially accountable.

The principle of explicability, in particular, is highly relevant to data-driven welfare systems. It highlights the need not only for transparency in technical terms, but also for intelligibility and accountability in social contexts, ensuring that decisions can be understood, challenged, and justified. This aligns closely with the concerns raised in this chapter regarding the opacity of AI systems and the need for more accountable forms of data governance.

Efforts to address these risks have also been reflected in international policy frameworks, such as those developed by the World Health Organization (WHO, 2021), which emphasize principles including fairness, transparency, accountability, and human oversight. These frameworks underscore the importance of aligning AI systems with broader societal values and public health objectives.

However, translating these principles into practice remains a significant challenge. Ethical guidelines often operate at a high level of abstraction, while the implementation of AI systems involves complex technical and organizational decisions. Bridging this gap requires the development of operational governance mechanisms that can be embedded within the design, deployment, and evaluation of AI systems.

In this regard, governance should be understood not as a static set of rules, but as an ongoing and adaptive process that involves multiple stakeholders. This includes not only technical experts and policymakers, but also healthcare professionals, patients, and citizens more broadly. Participatory approaches to governance can play a crucial role in ensuring that AI systems reflect diverse perspectives and respond to the needs of different populations.

Another important dimension concerns the regulation of data infrastructures. As data become a central resource in digital welfare systems, questions arise about data ownership, access, and control. Who has the right to collect, use, and share health data? Under what conditions can data be combined, transformed, or simulated? And how can individuals retain meaningful control over their data in increasingly complex data ecosystems?

These questions are particularly salient in the context of synthetic data. While synthetic datasets can mitigate privacy risks, they also introduce new governance challenges related to data provenance, traceability, and accountability. Ensuring that synthetic data are generated and used responsibly requires clear standards and oversight mechanisms that address both technical and ethical considerations.

From a broader perspective, the governance of AI in welfare systems must also address issues of power and inequality. Data-driven systems can reinforce existing asymmetries between institutions and individuals, as well as between different groups within society. For example, those who have greater access to data and technological resources may be better positioned to influence how AI systems are designed and deployed, while others may be disproportionately affected by their outcomes.

Addressing these asymmetries requires a critical approach to governance that goes beyond technical fixes and engages with the political dimensions of data and

AI. This includes examining how decisions are made, and how different forms of knowledge are valued within data-driven systems.

Ultimately, the governance of AI in digital welfare systems must balance multiple and sometimes competing objectives: innovation and regulation, efficiency and equity, data utility and privacy, automation and human oversight. Achieving this balance is not simply a technical challenge, but a fundamentally social and political one. The development of inclusive, transparent, and accountable governance frameworks becomes essential for ensuring that the transformation of welfare systems through AI contributes to broader social goals. Rather than treating governance as an external constraint on technological development, it should be understood as an integral component of how these systems are designed and implemented.

The future of digital welfare will depend not only on the capabilities of AI technologies, but also on the capacity of institutions and societies to govern them effectively. This requires ongoing critical reflection, interdisciplinary collaboration, and a commitment to aligning technological innovation with the principles of public accountability, explicability, and human well-being.

Understanding these dynamics is essential for developing digital welfare infrastructures that are not only technologically advanced, but also socially inclusive, epistemically robust, and communicatively transparent, interpretable, and open to social negotiation.

REFERENCES

boyd, d., & Crawford, K. (2012). Critical questions for big data: Provocations for a cultural, technological, and scholarly phenomenon. Information, Communication & Society, 15(5), 662–679. DOI: 10.1080/1369118X.2012.678878

Campedelli, M., & Vesan, P. (2023). Welfare digitalizzato, welfare digitale e i nuovi rischi sociali digitali: Un'introduzione. Politiche Sociali/Social Policies, 10(2), 169–192. DOI: 10.7389/108019

Chen, I. Y., Pierson, E., Rose, S., Joshi, S., Ferryman, K., & Ghassemi, M. (2023). Ethical machine learning in healthcare. *Annual Review of Biomedical Data Science*, *6*(1), 123–144. DOI: 10.1146/annurev-biodatasci-092820-114757 PMID: 34396058

Cruz, T. M. (2022). The social life of biomedical data: Capturing, obscuring, and envisioning care in the digital safety-net. *Social Science & Medicine*, *294*, 114670. Advance online publication. DOI: 10.1016/j.socscimed.2021.114670 PMID: 35114488

D'Ancona, G., Massussi, M., Savardi, M., Signoroni, A., Di Bacco, L., Farina, D., Metra, M., Maroldi, R., Muneretto, C., Ince, H., Costabile, D., Murero, M., Chizzola, G., Curello, S., & Benussi, S. (2023). Deep learning to detect significant coronary artery disease from plain chest radiographs (AI4CAD). *International Journal of Cardiology*, *370*, 435–441. DOI: 10.1016/j.ijcard.2022.10.154 PMID: 36343794

Dencik, L. (2022). The datafied welfare state: A perspective from the UK. In Hepp, A., Jarke, J., & Kramp, L. (Eds.), *New perspectives in critical data studies* (pp. 145–165). Palgrave Macmillan., DOI: 10.1007/978-3-030-96180-0_7

Ehrenstein, V., Kharrazi, H., Lehmann, H., & Taylor, R. J. (2019). Obtaining data from electronic health records. In Gliklich, R. E., Dreyer, N. A., & Leavy, M. B. (Eds.), *Registries for evaluating patient outcomes: A user's guide* (3rd ed.). Agency for Healthcare Research and Quality., https://www.ncbi.nlm.nih.gov/books/NBK551878/

Fahim, Y. A., Hasani, I. W., Kabba, S., & Ragab, W. M. (2025). Artificial intelligence in healthcare and medicine: Clinical applications, therapeutic advances, and future perspectives. *European Journal of Medical Research*, *30*(1), 848. Advance online publication. DOI: 10.1186/s40001-025-03196-w PMID: 40988064

Feickert, S., Ewertsen, C., Rother, W., Ince, H., & D'Ancona, G. (2024). Pulsed field ablation and ultra-high-density mapping for PVI: Use of machine learning and data augmentation to guide procedure and identify recurrent tachycardia mechanisms at one-year follow-up. European Heart Journal, 45(Suppl. 1), Article ehae666.577. DOI: 10.1093/eurheartj/ehae666.577

Floridi, L., Cowls, J., Beltrametti, M., Chatila, R., Chazerand, P., Dignum, V., Luetge, C., Madelin, R., Pagallo, U., Rossi, F., Schafer, B., Valcke, P., & Vayena, E. (2018). AI4People—An ethical framework for a good AI society: Opportunities, risks, principles, and recommendations. *Minds and Machines*, *28*(4), 689–707. DOI: 10.1007/s11023-018-9482-5 PMID: 30930541

Gonzales, A., Guruswamy, G., & Smith, S. R. (2023). Synthetic data in health care: A narrative review. *PLOS Digital Health*, *2*(1), e0000082. Advance online publication. DOI: 10.1371/journal.pdig.0000082 PMID: 36812604

Kitchin, R. (2014). *The data revolution: Big data, open data, data infrastructures and their consequences*. SAGE Publications., DOI: 10.4135/9781473909472

Lupton, D. (2018). *Digital health: Critical and cross-disciplinary perspectives*. Routledge., DOI: 10.4324/9781315648835

Morozov, E. (2014). *To save everything, click here: The folly of technological solutionism*. PublicAffairs.

Norori, N., Hu, Q., Aellen, F. M., Faraci, F. D., & Tzovara, A. (2021). Addressing bias in big data and AI for health care: A call for open science. *Patterns (New York, N.Y.)*, *2*(10), 100347. Advance online publication. DOI: 10.1016/j.patter.2021.100347 PMID: 34693373

Pezoulas, V. C., Zaridis, D. I., Mylona, E., Androutsos, C., Apostolidis, K., Tachos, N. S., & Fotiadis, D. I. (2024). Synthetic data generation methods in healthcare: A review on open-source tools and methods. *Computational and Structural Biotechnology Journal*, *23*, 2892–2910. DOI: 10.1016/j.csbj.2024.07.005 PMID: 39108677

Ruckenstein, M., & Schüll, N. D. (2017). The datafication of health. *Annual Review of Anthropology*, *46*(1), 261–278. DOI: 10.1146/annurev-anthro-102116-041244

Si, Y., Du, J., Li, Z., Jiang, X., Miller, T., Wang, F., Jim Zheng, W., & Roberts, K. (2021). Deep representation learning of patient data from electronic health records (EHR): A systematic review. *Journal of Biomedical Informatics*, *115*, 103671. Advance online publication. DOI: 10.1016/j.jbi.2020.103671 PMID: 33387683

van Dijck, J. (2014). Datafication, dataism and dataveillance: Big data between scientific paradigm and ideology. *Surveillance & Society*, *12*(2), 197–208. DOI: 10.24908/ss.v12i2.4776

van Toorn, G., Henman, P., & Soldatić, K. (2024). Introduction to the digital welfare state: Contestations, considerations and entanglements. *Journal of Sociology (Melbourne, Vic.)*, *60*(3), 507–522. DOI: 10.1177/14407833241260890

World Health Organization. (2021). Ethics and governance of artificial intelligence for health. World Health Organization. https://www.who.int/publications/i/item/9789240029200

Zakharova, I., Jarke, J., & Kaun, A. (2024). Tensions in digital welfare states: Three perspectives on care and control. *Journal of Sociology (Melbourne, Vic.)*, *60*(3), 540–559. DOI: 10.1177/14407833241238312

KEY TERMS AND DEFINITIONS

Algorithmic Governance: Forms of governance in which decisions, classifications, and interventions are increasingly mediated by algorithmic systems. Such systems may embed assumptions about risk, responsibility, eligibility, and deservingness, thereby influencing institutional decision-making and social outcomes (Dencik, 2022; WHO, 2021).

Communicative Data Infrastructures: Data infrastructures understood not only as technical systems for storing and processing information, but also as communicative environments that shape how phenomena are represented, interpreted, and rendered meaningful. They influence which populations, risks, and social issues become visible, legitimate, and actionable within governance processes.

Data Asymmetry: A structural imbalance in data availability characterized by the overrepresentation of clinical and pathological data and the relative underrepresentation of healthy populations, preventive trajectories, and early risk conditions. This asymmetry shapes what becomes visible, measurable, and actionable within digital welfare systems and influences the production of knowledge, policy priorities, and decision-making processes.

Data-Driven Welfare Systems: Welfare systems organized around data-intensive infrastructures, digital platforms, and algorithmic models, where policy decisions and service provision are increasingly informed by predictive analytics and computational forms of knowledge.

Datafication of Welfare: The process through which welfare systems increasingly rely on data collection, processing, and analytics to organize decision-making, resource allocation, and service delivery. Through datafication, social needs are translated into measurable and governable categories, reshaping institutional practices and forms of social intervention (van Dijck, 2014; Dencik, 2022).

Epistemic Reconfiguration: The transformation of the processes through which knowledge is produced, validated, and mobilized. In the context of AI and synthetic data, epistemic reconfiguration refers to the growing shift from observational and retrospective forms of knowledge toward predictive, simulated, and future-oriented modes of knowing.

Preventive Welfare: An approach to welfare governance that prioritizes anticipation, early intervention, and long-term population well-being rather than reactive responses to already manifested social or health conditions.

Socio-Technical Systems: Configurations in which technological infrastructures, institutional arrangements, regulatory frameworks, and social practices are mutually constituted and continuously shape one another. Within digital welfare systems, socio-technical configurations influence how data are produced, interpreted, governed, and used (Bijker et al., 1987; Kitchin, 2014).

Synthetic Data: Artificially generated data that reproduce selected statistical properties of real-world datasets without directly corresponding to identifiable individuals. Synthetic data are increasingly used to address data scarcity, support model development, and enable data sharing, while also raising questions regarding validity, bias, and representational adequacy.

Transfer Learning: A machine learning approach through which knowledge acquired in one dataset, domain, or context is transferred to another. In healthcare and welfare applications, transfer learning enables model development in settings characterized by limited data availability.

Chapter 3
Configurations of Digital Health Citizenship:
Data Infrastructures and Inequality in European Health Systems

Ferdinando Iazzetta
http://orcid.org/0000-0002-5641-8823
University of Naples Federico II, Italy

ABSTRACT

This chapter examines the transformation of European healthcare systems in the context of digitalization and datafication. Drawing on sociological theories of digital infrastructures, welfare transformation, and digital inequalities, the chapter analyzes how digital health systems reshape access to healthcare data and the conditions of digital health citizenship. Using data from the European Commission's Digital Decade eHealth Composite Indicator, the study develops a comparative analysis of healthcare data infrastructures across European countries. The findings show that European health systems differ significantly in the integration of healthcare data ecosystems and in the inclusiveness of data access policies. These differences generate distinct institutional configurations of digital health citizenship. The chapter argues that digitalization does not simply expand access to healthcare information but also produces new forms of infrastructural inequality in data-driven welfare systems.

DOI: 10.4018/979-8-2600-3043-1.ch003

1. INTRODUCTION

Over the past two decades, European healthcare systems have undergone extensive processes of digitalization and datafication that are reshaping healthcare delivery, the management of clinical information, and the relationship between citizens and public institutions. The growing use of digital technologies in healthcare has often been associated with administrative modernization, organizational efficiency, and greater patient autonomy. Within this context, digital health has become a central category in national and supranational policy agendas, referring to the use of information and communication technologies to improve healthcare services, access to care, and the management of health information (World Health Organization, 2021).

This transformation has led to the expansion of electronic health records (EHRs), telemedicine services, electronic prescription systems, and online platforms through which citizens can access personal medical information. Electronic health record systems are particularly important because they enable the collection, storage, and circulation of clinical information across healthcare institutions (Kruse *et al.*, 2019). In several European countries, reforms promoting online portals and mobile applications have also encouraged more participatory forms of healthcare management and patient engagement (Markert *et al.*, 2021). Digital health infrastructures can therefore be understood not only as technical instruments for managing information but also as institutional arrangements that reshape how healthcare rights and medical knowledge are accessed and exercised.

At the same time, critical scholarship questions the assumption that the digitalization of welfare systems necessarily produces greater inclusion and equality. Several studies show that digital infrastructures may instead reproduce—or intensify—existing inequalities by introducing new forms of exclusion linked to technological access, digital skills, and the ability to interact with increasingly digitalized administrative systems (Greenhalgh *et al.*, 2017; Morley & Floridi, 2020). From this perspective, healthcare digitalization should be interpreted not simply as technological innovation but as an institutional transformation that redefines access to public services and health information.

Recent crises have further highlighted the strategic role of digital infrastructures in maintaining healthcare provision under conditions of disruption. During the COVID-19 pandemic, many healthcare systems rapidly expanded telemedicine and remote digital services to guarantee continuity of care despite mobility restrictions and pressure on hospitals (Shigekawa *et al.*, 2018). Similarly, in Ukraine, digital health infrastructures and telemedicine services played a crucial role in preserving access to healthcare during periods of severe infrastructural disruption and armed conflict (Malakhov, 2023). Taken together, these developments indicate that digital healthcare represents not only technological innovation but also a structural transformation in the infrastructures through which healthcare systems are organized. Examining the institutional conditions governing access to health data therefore becomes essential for understanding the changing forms of health citizenship emerging within data-driven societies. Building on these considerations, this chapter examines the European context as a relevant case for investigating the digital transformation of healthcare systems and the new forms of inequality emerging within data-driven welfare regimes. The central argument is that inequalities associated with healthcare digitalization cannot be reduced to the traditional notion of the digital divide understood as unequal access to devices or internet connectivity. Rather, these inequalities increasingly emerge through the institutional organization of health data infrastructures and the conditions governing access to digital health information. Different healthcare systems therefore produce distinct configurations of digital health citizenship, shaping unequal opportunities to access, use, and manage health data within contemporary welfare systems. To investigate these dynamics, the chapter combines critical theoretical discussion with a comparative empirical analysis of digital health infrastructures across European countries. Using institutional data produced within the framework of the European Union's Digital Decade strategy, the analysis examines how healthcare systems organize digital health infrastructures and how these arrangements shape different regimes of access to health data. In doing so, the chapter contributes to current debates on digitalization, welfare transformation, and social inequality, showing how digital healthcare has become a key arena for understanding the reconfiguration of social citizenship in the era of datafication.

2. DIGITAL HEALTH AND WELFARE TRANSFORMATION

To interpret sociologically the transformations affecting contemporary healthcare systems, it is necessary to situate healthcare digitalization within a broader framework connecting welfare sociology, studies on datafication, and research on digital inequalities. In European welfare systems, access to healthcare has traditionally been conceived as a fundamental social right guaranteed by public institutions and grounded in principles of equality and solidarity (Von Kersbergen & Vis, 2014). However, the digitalization of healthcare systems is progressively reshaping the ways these rights are exercised in practice. As Dahlgren and Whitehead (2021) observe, attention increasingly shifts from formally guaranteed rights to the infrastructural conditions that make healthcare access effectively possible. Access to medical services and health information now depends increasingly on digital systems capable of collecting, organizing, and circulating health data within welfare institutions. These transformations are embedded within broader processes of digital change affecting contemporary societies. The spread of the internet, smartphones, and digital communication technologies has profoundly altered how information is produced, circulated, and used within social and economic systems (Castells, 2010). The welfare sector has gradually been incorporated into these developments, often with the aim of improving efficiency, reducing organizational costs, and responding to growing expectations for accessible digital services (Hardey, Loader, & Keeble, 2009; Brynjolfsson & McAfee, 2014). As Hardey, Loader, and Keeble (2009) emphasize, the diffusion of services available anytime and anywhere has progressively reshaped expectations toward public institutions, including healthcare systems. Within academic debates, these developments are often framed through the concept of digital transformation, understood as an institutional and organizational change driven by the integration of digital technologies into everyday activities and decision-making processes (Bloomberg, 2018; Cochoy *et al.*, 2017). From this perspective, digitalization implies not simply the introduction of new technological tools but a broader restructuring of institutions and public service delivery systems (Van Dijk, 2012). In healthcare, this transformation is commonly described through the concept of digital health, referring to the set of technologies and information systems supporting healthcare delivery, clinical data management, and access to medical information (World Health Organization, 2021). Electronic health records (EHRs), digital prescriptions, online booking systems, and patient portals represent key components of these emerging infrastructures (Aceto, Persico, & Pescapé, 2018). The expansion of these technologies is also linked to broader structural pressures affecting welfare systems. Population aging, the increasing prevalence of chronic diseases, and concerns regarding the financial sustainability of public healthcare have encouraged governments to explore new organizational models for healthcare provision (OECD, 2016). At the same time, digital technologies are reshaping the role of citizens within healthcare systems. Patients are increasingly encouraged to participate actively in managing their own health through online services and digital platforms enabling them to monitor health conditions, consult medical information, and access clinical records. This development has led some scholars to emphasize the growing importance of the "digital patient," understood as an individual increasingly involved in the production and management of health information (Lupton, 2013; Powell & Deetjen, 2019). Within the European context, these dynamics are reflected in the growing use of the internet to search for health-related information. As illustrated in Figure 1, the proportion of individuals using online sources for medical information has steadily increased across the European Union in recent years. From a sociological perspective, this trend reflects the progressive digitalization of health citizenship. Access to healthcare services, medical knowledge, and personal health data is increasingly mediated by digital infrastructures organizing the production and circulation of health information. In this sense, healthcare digitalization should be understood not simply as technological innovation but as an institutional transformation reshaping how citizens access services, manage their health, and interact with welfare institutions (Van Dijk, 2012; Schmidt & Cohen, 2013).

Figure 1. Trend in the share of individuals using the internet to seek health-related information in the European Union

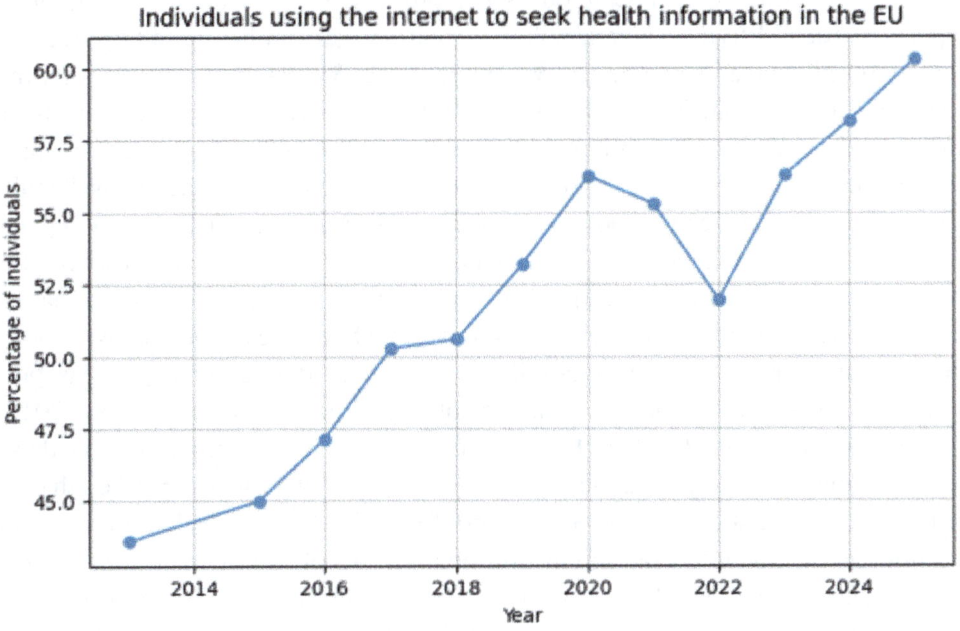

2.1 Datafication and Health Data Infrastructures

Sociological research on datafication and digital infrastructures has highlighted that data should not be understood simply as neutral representations of social reality but rather as active instruments of classification, selection, and governance (Bowker & Star, 1999; boyd & Crawford, 2012; Van Dijck, 2014). Digital infrastructures incorporate technical standards, classificatory categories, and operational protocols that define which information can be collected, recorded, and made visible within information systems (Bowker, 2014; Kitchin, 2014). From this perspective, data cannot be considered objective and pre-existing information but rather the result of processes of selection, modeling, and interpretation that reflect specific institutional, technological, and economic logics (Gitelman, 2013; Crawford *et al.*, 2014).Applied to the healthcare sector, this perspective highlights how access to healthcare services is increasingly mediated by data infrastructures that organize the collection, circulation, and use of clinical information. Healthcare delivery now depends to a growing extent on complex information systems that aggregate data from multiple sources, including electronic health records, administrative systems, digital platforms, and personal health monitoring devices (Hogle, 2016; Ruckenstein & Schüll, 2017). This transformation is often interpreted as part of a broader process of datafication, understood as the progressive translation of qualitative aspects of social life into quantifiable information that can be digitally processed and analyzed (Mayer-Schönberger & Cukier, 2013; Van Dijck, 2014). Within the healthcare domain, datafication operates at multiple institutional levels, ranging from biomedical research based on large datasets to public health infrastructures, clinical practices, and personal health monitoring technologies (Ruckenstein & Schüll, 2017). Consequently, contemporary healthcare systems are gradually evolving into complex informational ecosystems in which data represent a central resource for the organization, governance, and evaluation of health policies. Clinical databases, telemedicine platforms, and digital monitoring technologies generate continuous flows of information that make it possible to analyze epidemiological patterns, predict health risks, and support the management of healthcare resources (Topol, 2012; Hogle, 2016; Weber *et al.*, 2014). However, critical data studies emphasize that these systems cannot be interpreted merely as neutral technical tools. Rather, health data infrastructures constitute socio-technical configurations that embed specific power relations, economic interests, and institutional visions of health and illness (Iliadis & Russo, 2016; Kitchin, 2014). Within this context, new informational asymmetries emerge between actors with extensive capacities to collect and analyze data—such as public institutions, insurance companies, and digital platforms—and citizens who generate these data but have limited control over their use (Andrejevic, 2014; Beer, 2009). In the healthcare sector, these dynamics are particularly significant because data generated by patients through digital platforms, mobile applications, and self-monitoring devices can be collected, analyzed, and used by a wide range of institutional and economic actors, including technology companies, pharmaceutical industries, and insurance providers (Sharon, 2016; Van Dijck & Poell, 2016). The growing integration between healthcare systems and digital infrastructures therefore contributes to the emergence of new health data ecosystems in which information related to health acquires increasing informational, political, and economic value. At the same time, the growing availability of health data has fostered the development of algorithmic analytics and predictive models used to classify patients, estimate health risks, and support clinical or administrative decision-making processes (Gillespie, 2014; Mittelstadt *et al.*, 2016). Nevertheless, several studies have shown that these systems may incorporate biases deriving from the composition of the datasets used to train them, potentially affecting the distribution of healthcare resources and access to care (Beer, 2009; Cheney-Lippold, 2011). Taken together, these contributions suggest that the digitalization of healthcare cannot be understood solely as a process of technological innovation. Instead, it should be analyzed as a socio-technical transformation that reshapes the relationships between citizens, healthcare institutions, and data infrastructures. The datafication of health generates new forms of medical knowledge production, new configurations of informational power, and new institutional arrangements through which contemporary healthcare systems are organized.

2.2 Digital Health Divide and Inequality

The growing digitalization of healthcare systems has transformed the production, management, and use of health information. While digital technologies are often presented as tools capable of improving efficiency and expanding access to healthcare services, a growing body of critical literature highlights how these developments may also generate new forms of inequality. Within this debate, the concept of the digital health divide has gained increasing prominence, referring to inequalities in access to, use of, and benefits derived from digital health technologies (van Deursen & van Dijk, 2019; Robinson *et al.*, 2015). The digital health divide represents a specific dimension of the broader digital divide, originally developed to describe inequalities in access to information and communication technologies among social groups (van Dijk, 2005). In healthcare, however, these inequalities acquire relevance because they concern access to services and information directly affecting health conditions. Numerous studies show that access to digital technologies and online health services is unevenly distributed and tends to reproduce existing socioeconomic inequalities linked to income, education, age, gender, and ethnic background (Fiscella *et al.*, 2000; Agardh *et al.*, 2011). The introduction of digital technologies into healthcare systems has often been accompanied by narratives emphasizing democratization of medical knowledge and patient empowerment. Online health portals, telemedicine services, and mobile health applications are frequently presented as tools capable of strengthening patient autonomy and encouraging participation in healthcare decision-making (Dash *et al.*, 2019; Belle *et al.*, 2015). However, empirical research shows that these technologies tend to be used more intensively by individuals with higher levels of education, income, and digital skills, potentially widening pre-existing social inequalities (Robinson *et al.*, 2015).

A central factor underlying these inequalities concerns the unequal distribution of digital and health-related competencies. The effective use of digital health technologies requires a combination of cognitive, technical, and informational skills that are not equally distributed across the population. In this context, the concept of eHealth literacy represents a crucial analytical dimension for understanding processes of inclusion and exclusion within digital healthcare systems. Norman and Skinner (2006) define eHealth literacy as the ability to search for, understand, evaluate, and apply health information obtained from digital sources to make informed decisions about health. According to their model, eHealth literacy emerges from the interaction of multiple forms of literacy, including traditional literacy, information literacy, scientific literacy, media literacy, computer literacy, and health literacy. These competencies form the so-called "lily model" of eHealth literacy, illustrating how interaction with digital health technologies depends on a combination of cognitive, informational, and social resources (Norman & Skinner, 2006). The unequal distribution of these competencies contributes to new forms of stratification in access to digital health resources. Even in contexts characterized by widespread access to digital technologies, many individuals display limited levels of digital and health literacy, affecting their ability to use online medical information effectively (Institute of Medicine, 2004). Empirical studies also show that individuals with lower levels of health literacy tend to have less knowledge of disease prevention, make less frequent use of preventive healthcare services, and report poorer health outcomes (McCray, 2005). Inequalities in the use of digital health technologies are also connected to broader social determinants of health. Income, educational attainment, geographic location, and access to digital infrastructures significantly influence individuals' ability to use digital tools to obtain healthcare services (Saeed & Masters, 2021). In this sense, healthcare digitalization does not automatically eliminate existing inequalities but may reorganize them around individuals' capacity to interact with increasingly complex information systems. Another important area of reflection concerns the growing role of algorithms and data analytics systems in healthcare decision-making. With the diffusion of big data technologies and artificial intelligence, many clinical decision-support systems increasingly rely on predictive models developed from large health datasets (Dash *et al.*, 2019; Kruse *et al.*, 2016). Several studies have demonstrated that these systems may incorporate biases embedded in training datasets, potentially affecting the distribution of healthcare resources and access to treatment (Beer, 2009; Cheney-Lippold, 2011). For example, some algorithms used to estimate kidney function have been shown to overestimate the health status of African American patients, potentially delaying diagnosis and treatment (Diao *et al.*, 2021). Similarly, medical datasets characterized by gender imbalances may reduce the accuracy of diagnostic systems for underrepresented groups (Larrazabal *et al.*, 2020). These examples illustrate how health data analytics systems are not neutral but reflect broader social and institutional inequalities. Overall, the literature suggests that digital health technologies generate ambivalent effects on social inequality. On the one hand, telemedicine, remote monitoring systems, and digital health platforms may improve access to care and strengthen the efficiency of healthcare systems (Kruse *et al.*, 2016; Dash *et al.*, 2019). On the other hand, without appropriate inclusion policies and careful technological design, these innovations risk reinforcing existing inequalities by favoring groups already endowed with greater economic, cultural, and technological resources (Saeed & Masters, 2021). For these reasons, an expanding interdisciplinary literature emphasizes the need to interpret healthcare digitalization not only as a technological process but also as a broader social and institutional transformation involving issues of access, skills, and the distribution of informational resources. From this perspective, analyzing digital healthcare infrastructures also means examining the new forms of inequality emerging through the interaction between technologies, institutions, and social practices.

2.3 Digital Health Citizenship

Within the broader context of the digitalization of welfare systems, the relationship between citizens and healthcare institutions is increasingly mediated by digital infrastructures, information systems, and data management platforms. In this context, several studies have introduced the concept of digital citizenship to describe new forms of participation and interaction with public institutions in digital environments (Mossberger, Tolbert, & McNeal, 2008; Isin & Ruppert, 2015). Digital citizenship refers not only to access to digital technologies but also to the capacity of individuals to exercise rights, fulfill obligations, and participate in institutional processes through digital systems.

In healthcare, these transformations acquire particular significance. The expansion of electronic health records, online health services, and digital platforms for accessing clinical information has reshaped how citizens interact with healthcare systems and access medical information (Tapuria *et al.*, 2021). In many national contexts, access to personal health data is presented as a tool for strengthening patient autonomy, improving transparency, and promoting more participatory models of care (Goldzweig *et al.*, 2013; Kruse *et al.*, 2015; Risling *et al.*, 2017). However, critical scholarship emphasizes that these developments should not be interpreted merely as neutral technological innovations but as part of broader transformations in citizenship and governance within contemporary healthcare systems. In this chapter, digital health citizenship is defined as the set of institutional conditions through which citizens can access, understand, and use digital health data within increasingly datafied healthcare systems. From this perspective, digital health citizenship does not simply refer to the use of digital technologies in healthcare, nor does it fully coincide with broader notions of digital citizenship. Rather, it concerns the ways healthcare rights, access to medical information, and participation in healthcare systems are increasingly mediated by digital infrastructures and health data systems. Several studies show that welfare digitalization contributes to the emergence of new forms of citizenship based on interaction with digital platforms and public information systems (Dunleavy *et al.*, 2006; Schou & Hjelholt, 2017). Within these institutional arrangements, citizens are increasingly represented as active and responsible actors expected to manage access to public services autonomously through digital tools. According to Schou and Hjelholt (2017), policies promoting public-sector digitalization contribute to constructing a figure of the "digital citizen" characterized by expectations of autonomy, efficiency, and individual responsibility. These transformations should also be situated within broader changes in contemporary welfare systems, where neoliberal policy frameworks increasingly emphasize individual responsibility and the capacity to manage risks and opportunities autonomously (Brown, 2015; Dardot & Laval, 2013; Ong, 2006). In digital healthcare, these dynamics are particularly visible in the growing emphasis on individual access to health data and patient participation in managing care pathways. Access to electronic health records and patient portals is often framed as a strategy for promoting empowerment and participatory healthcare models (Winkelman *et al.*, 2005; Otte-Trojel *et al.*, 2014; Reed *et al.*, 2019). At the same time, several studies point out that these developments may also involve a transfer of responsibilities toward citizens, who are increasingly expected to manage complex health information and interact with digital systems to obtain healthcare services (Lupton, 2013; Davies, 2021). Research in infrastructure studies further emphasizes that these technologies are not simply technical tools but socio-technical systems incorporating specific logics of classification and representation (Bowker & Star, 1999). Health information systems define which data can be collected, how they are categorized, and which information becomes accessible to citizens and healthcare professionals. In this sense, digital infrastructures play a central role in structuring how health is represented, monitored, and governed within contemporary healthcare systems (Kitchin, 2014). These processes may also generate new inequalities in access to healthcare citizenship. Several studies show that digital health services tend to favor citizens with higher levels of digital literacy, health literacy, and socioeconomic resources, while more vulnerable groups often encounter greater difficulties in using these technologies (Sakaguchi-Tang *et al.*, 2017; Nahm *et al.*, 2020). Consequently, digital health citizenship may produce new forms of social stratification linked to individuals' ability to access and use the digital infrastructures of healthcare systems.

Building on these perspectives, digital health citizenship can be analytically understood through three interconnected dimensions. The first concerns legibility, referring to the extent to which individuals and their health conditions are represented within healthcare information systems. The second concerns autonomy, understood as the capacity of citizens to access, understand, and use digital health data in interactions with healthcare institutions. The third concerns responsibility, referring to the growing expectation that citizens actively manage health information and care pathways through digital platforms and online services. These dimensions provide an analytical framework for understanding how digital infrastructures reshape the institutional conditions of healthcare access and participation within contemporary welfare systems. From this perspective, digital healthcare emerges not only as a field of technological innovation but also as a space in which new forms of inclusion, exclusion, and data-mediated citizenship are institutionally configured.

3. THE EUROPEAN CASE: DIGITAL HEALTH INFRASTRUCTURES

The empirical analysis developed in this chapter is based on data from the Digital Decade eHealth Composite Indicator, a monitoring instrument developed by the European Commission within the framework of the Digital Decade strategy. The indicator is designed to assess the progress of European Union member states toward the strategic objective of ensuring that citizens have digital access to their Electronic Health Records (EHR).

The dataset represents one of the main institutional tools used at the European level to monitor the development of digital health infrastructures. It provides a comparative framework for examining the availability and diffusion of digital systems that enable citizens to access their health data across European healthcare systems. As such, the dataset offers a valuable empirical basis for analyzing cross-national differences in the development of digital health data infrastructures and in the institutional arrangements that regulate citizens' access to electronic health records.

3.1 The Digital Decade eHealth Composite Indicator

Data are collected through an annual institutional survey administered to the national authorities responsible for eHealth in the member states of the European Union, as well as in Iceland and Norway, using the European Commission's EU-Survey platform. The participating national authorities—identified through the eHealth Network and the Digital Decade Board—are responsible for completing the questionnaire and providing updated information on the state of implementation of digital health infrastructures within their respective countries.

The responses represent the development status of national systems as of December 31 of the reference year and are subsequently subject to a validation process conducted by the European Commission's research team.

From a methodological perspective, the dataset is not constructed based on behavioral data concerning the actual use of digital technologies by citizens. Instead, it relies on institutional self-reporting regarding the existence and implementation of digital health infrastructures. The indicators therefore describe the technical and organizational availability of systems that enable access to digital health data rather than the effective level of service utilization by the population.

Within this perspective, the dataset makes it possible to observe the infrastructural conditions that enable access to health data within European healthcare systems. This analytical approach is consistent with sociological research on digital infrastructures and datafication, which interprets information systems not merely as technical tools but as socio-technical configurations that structure access to information and contribute to defining the institutional conditions through which social rights are exercised (Bowker & Star, 1999; Kitchin, 2014; Van Dijck, 2014). Table 1 summarizes the structure of the indicator and the main analytical components on which it is based.

Table 1. Structure of the Digital Decade eHealth Composite Indicator

Thematic Dimension	Analytical Content	Sub-Indicators
Implementation of Data Access Services	Availability of digital services enabling citizens to access their electronic health data	Q1 – national or regional availability of the service
Types of Accessible Health Data	Categories of health data made available to citizens through digital systems	Q2 – patient summary data; Q3 – prescriptions and dispensations; Q4 – diagnostic results and clinical reports
Access Technologies and Coverage	Technical modes of access to digital systems and the degree of integration of healthcare providers	Q5 – authentication through digital identity; Q6 – access via portal or mobile application; Q7 – share of the population technically enabled to access the system; Q8 – connection of healthcare providers to national health data systems
Inclusion and Accessibility	Institutional mechanisms facilitating access to health data for specific population groups	Q9 – access for legal guardians; Q10 – access for authorized persons; Q11 – support services for disadvantaged groups; Q12 – compliance with web accessibility standards

3.2 Analytical Strategy

Building on this dataset, the analysis adopts a comparative approach to examine how European healthcare systems organize digital infrastructures for accessing health data. Rather than treating the composite indicator as a simple measure of technological maturity, the analysis reworks the original variables to identify key institutional dimensions and compare their configuration across countries.

The unit of analysis consists of the European countries included in the Digital Decade eHealth Composite Indicator dataset. The dataset includes twenty-nine national cases, corresponding to the member states of the European Union and several countries of the European Economic Area for which comparable information on the development of digital health systems is available.

The analytical strategy is descriptive and configurational rather than causal. The study relies on additive indices designed to capture the breadth of healthcare data ecosystems and the inclusiveness of access arrangements. Instead of employing inferential statistical techniques, the analysis compares recurring institutional configurations across European healthcare systems using theoretically informed composite measures. In a first stage of the analysis, the dataset underwent a data cleaning and restructuring procedure to ensure comparability across variables. The aggregated value representing the European Union average (EU27 Average) was removed because it does not constitute a national healthcare system comparable to the other cases included in the analysis. Subsequently, the variables were converted into numerical format and checked for consistency.

Some indicators in the original dataset take intermediate values between 0 and 1, reflecting partial territorial implementation in decentralized or regionalized healthcare systems. These values were retained because they capture meaningful variation in the institutional development of digital health infrastructures across national contexts. The analysis then examined the distribution of the main variables through descriptive statistics. This preliminary step allows the analysis to assess the diffusion of key infrastructural components across countries, including digital identity authentication systems, online access through portals or mobile applications, and the integration of healthcare providers into national health data systems.

Because many variables take values close to binary configurations indicating the presence or absence of specific services, the analysis does not employ complex inferential statistical techniques. Instead, it focuses on the comparison of institutional arrangements across healthcare systems.

The analysis is structured around three analytical dimensions. The first concerns the technical accessibility of digital health systems and provides contextual information on the infrastructural conditions enabling access to health data. The comparative analysis developed in the following sections focuses primarily on two synthetic dimensions: the breadth of the healthcare data ecosystem and the inclusiveness of access arrangements. These dimensions are theoretically connected to the broader concept of digital health citizenship introduced earlier in the chapter. Indicators related to accessibility and inclusion mechanisms capture institutional conditions associated with legibility and autonomy within digital health systems, while the breadth of healthcare data ecosystems reflects the extent to which citizens are incorporated into data-driven healthcare infrastructures. Table 2 summarizes the analytical dimensions, indicators, and their theoretical interpretation. The healthcare data ecosystem index is constructed from indicators measuring the connection of healthcare providers to national health data systems (Q8a–Q8k). These variables identify whether different categories of healthcare facilities—including general practitioners and primary care centers, public hospitals, rehabilitation centers, residential care facilities, mental health services, pharmacies, and their private-sector equivalents—contribute data to national electronic health record infrastructures. A provider category is considered integrated when at least 60% of facilities belonging to that category are connected to the national system. Based on these indicators, a synthetic index labeled Healthcare Data Supply Coverage was constructed by counting the number of provider categories connected to national health data systems. The index does not measure the quantity of data produced but rather the breadth of the informational ecosystem supporting national digital health infrastructures. Higher values therefore indicate a greater level of integration across the healthcare sector. The analysis also distinguishes between public and private healthcare providers to assess whether data integration relies primarily on public institutions or on more hybrid organizational arrangements involving private actors. This distinction helps clarify how different healthcare governance models shape the structure of digital health infrastructures. The second synthetic dimension, Digital Health Inclusion, is constructed from indicators related to inclusive access to health data (Q9–Q12). These indicators include access through legal guardians, access granted to authorized individuals such as family members or caregivers, the presence of support services for vulnerable groups or citizens with limited digital literacy, and compliance with European web accessibility standards (WCAG 2.1).

The Digital Health Inclusion index was constructed by summing these components. The index captures the extent to which healthcare systems incorporate mechanisms facilitating inclusive access to health information for different categories of users.

In the final stage of the analysis, the two synthetic dimensions were combined to construct a two-dimensional analytical space representing the distribution of European healthcare systems according to the breadth of their healthcare data ecosystems and the inclusiveness of their access arrangements.

This analytical space is represented through a scatterplot in which countries are positioned according to the values of the two indices. European mean values divide the space into four quadrants representing different configurations of digital health systems and making it possible to identify distinct infrastructural regimes emerging from the interaction between provider integration and inclusion mechanisms. This approach shifts the analytical focus away from the simple diffusion of digital technologies toward the institutional organization of health data infrastructures and the ways in which healthcare systems structure access to digital health information and emerging forms of digital health citizenship.

Table 2. Analytical Dimensions and Indicators of Digital Health Infrastructure

Analytical Dimension	Indicators	Interpretation
Technical Accessibility of Digital Infrastructures	Q5, Q6, Q7	Technological conditions that enable access to digital health data systems, including authentication through digital identity, access channels via web portals or mobile applications, and the share of the population technically enabled to use digital health services.
Healthcare Data Ecosystem (Healthcare Data Supply)	Q8a–Q8k	Breadth of the informational sources feeding digital health data systems, measured through the connection of different categories of public and private healthcare providers (general practitioners, hospitals, rehabilitation centers, residential care facilities, mental health services, and pharmacies). This dimension captures the degree of integration of the healthcare information ecosystem.
Digital Health Inclusion	Q9, Q10, Q11, Q12	Presence of institutional mechanisms that facilitate access to health data for different categories of the population, including legal guardians, authorized persons such as caregivers or family members, support services for vulnerable groups, and compliance with European digital accessibility standards.

3.3 Configurations of Digital Health Systems in Europe

Descriptive statistics show relatively high levels of diffusion of the main infrastructures enabling access to digital health data across European countries. Indicators such as authentication through digital identity (Q5), access through web portals or mobile applications (Q6), and the share of the population technically enabled to access digital health systems (Q7) display mean values above 0.85. This suggests that, in most European countries, the basic technological conditions required for accessing digital health data are already widely available.

The data therefore indicate a high level of diffusion of the core digital infrastructures that enable citizens to access health data within European healthcare systems. Authentication through digital identity (Q5) and access to health data through web portals or mobile applications (Q6) show mean values close to 0.9, indicating that these services are available in most of the countries analyzed. Similarly, the share of the population technically enabled to access digital health systems (Q7) also appears to be very high. In contrast, the connection of healthcare providers to national health data systems (Q8) shows greater variability across countries, suggesting significant differences in the degree of integration of national healthcare data ecosystems. While access infrastructures for citizens appear to be widely implemented, the extent to which healthcare providers contribute data to national digital health systems varies more substantially across national contexts. Table 3 presents the descriptive statistics summarizing the diffusion of the main digital infrastructures enabling access to health data in European healthcare systems.

Table 3. Diffusion of Digital Health Data Access Infrastructures in Europe

Indicator	Mean	Min	Max
Digital identity authentication (Q5)	0.89	0.00	1.00
Access through portal or mobile app (Q6)	0.88	0.12	1.00
Population technically enabled to access services (Q7)	0.93	0.08	1.00
Connection of healthcare providers to health data systems (Q8)	0.72	0.11	1.00

To analyze the degree of integration of the informational sources feeding digital health data systems, a synthetic index labeled Healthcare Data Supply Coverage was constructed. This indicator measures the breadth of the healthcare provider ecosystem contributing data to national electronic health record (EHR) systems. The index is derived from the survey items related to the connection of healthcare providers to national health data infrastructures (Q8a–Q8k). These variables capture whether different categories of healthcare facilities contribute to the production and sharing of digital health data. In particular, the dataset considers eleven categories of healthcare providers: public general practitioners and primary care centers, secondary and tertiary public hospitals, public rehabilitation centers, public residential care facilities for older adults, and public mental health services; the corresponding private-sector providers (private general practitioners and primary care clinics, private hospitals and clinics, private rehabilitation centers, private residential care facilities for older adults, and private mental health services); and pharmacies.

For each provider category, the variable takes a positive value when at least 60% of the facilities belonging to that category are connected to the national digital health data system. Based on these variables, a synthetic index was constructed by counting the number of provider categories connected to the national health data infrastructure. The index therefore ranges from 0 to 11, where higher values indicate healthcare systems characterized by a broader integration of providers in the production of digital health data. It should be noted that this indicator does not measure the amount of data actually produced nor the technical interoperability of health information systems. Rather, it captures the institutional breadth of the data sources contributing to digital health infrastructures. In this sense, the index can be interpreted as a measure of the extent of the healthcare information ecosystem supporting digital health data access systems across European countries. Table 4 presents the distribution of European countries according to the number of healthcare provider categories connected to national digital health data systems. The results reveal considerable variation across European healthcare systems in the degree of integration of the informational sources feeding digital health infrastructures. Some countries display relatively limited levels of integration of the healthcare data ecosystem. In Ireland and the Netherlands, for example, only one category of healthcare provider appears to be connected to national digital health data systems. Similarly, in several Western European countries—including Germany, Austria, and Italy—the number of provider categories integrated into health data systems remains relatively low. In these contexts, healthcare information infrastructures appear more fragmented from an institutional perspective. A second group of countries shows intermediate levels of integration. In healthcare systems such as Spain, Sweden, Norway, and Belgium, a larger number of provider categories contribute to the production of digital health data, suggesting more developed—although still incomplete—digital infrastructures. In these contexts, the integration of health data involves multiple components of the healthcare system but does not yet cover the entire ecosystem of healthcare services.

Finally, some countries exhibit very high levels of integration of health data sources. In Estonia, Denmark, Finland, and Lithuania, nearly all categories of healthcare providers are connected to national digital health data systems. These healthcare systems are characterized by highly integrated informational ecosystems in which a broad range of healthcare actors contributes to the production and sharing of digital clinical data.

Table 4. Healthcare Data Supply Coverage Across European Countries

supply_score	Countries
1	Ireland, Netherlands
3	Germany, Austria, Italy, Hungary, Romania
4	Luxembourg
6	Malta, Spain
7	Sweden, Norway, Croatia, Belgium
8	Iceland, Cyprus, Latvia
9	Slovenia, Portugal, Slovakia, Bulgaria
10	Poland
11	Denmark, Czechia, France, Finland, Greece, Estonia, Lithuania

To examine the degree of institutional inclusiveness in access to digital health data, a synthetic index labeled Digital Health Inclusion was constructed. The index is based on indicators Q9–Q12 from the Digital Decade eHealth Composite Indicator, which measure the presence of institutional mechanisms designed to facilitate access to digital health data for different categories of users.

Specifically, the indicators include the possibility of accessing health data through legal guardians (Q9), access granted to authorized individuals such as family members or caregivers (Q10), the availability of support services for vulnerable groups or individuals with limited digital skills (Q11), and the compliance of digital platforms with European web accessibility standards (Q12).

Based on these variables, a synthetic index was constructed by summing the components related to inclusive access to digital health data. The index ranges from 1 to 4, where higher values indicate healthcare systems characterized by greater institutional attention to inclusive access to digital health data. Table 5 presents the distribution of European countries according to the level of institutional inclusiveness in their digital health data access systems. The results show a distribution that is relatively concentrated toward the higher values of the index. Most of the countries included in the analysis display a value of 4, indicating the simultaneous presence of several institutional mechanisms aimed at facilitating access to digital health data for different categories of users.

Some countries, however, exhibit intermediate levels of inclusion. In contexts such as France, Greece, Croatia, and Slovakia, digital health data access systems incorporate only part of the measures considered in the index, suggesting the presence of access policies that are either less comprehensive or less uniformly implemented. In other cases, the level of inclusion appears more limited. Countries such as Cyprus and Sweden display values of 2, indicating that only some of the institutional mechanisms considered in the index are implemented. Finally, Ireland represents the case with the lowest level of inclusion, with a value of 1, suggesting a very limited presence of institutional instruments designed to facilitate access to digital health data for specific categories of the population.

Table 5. Digital Health Inclusion Across European Countries

inclusion_ score	Countries
1	Ireland
2	Cyprus, Sweden
3	France, Greece, Hungary, Latvia, Croatia, Slovakia, Romania
4	Czechia, Bulgaria, Estonia, Denmark, Belgium, Austria, Italy, Iceland, Finland, Germany, Netherlands, Lithuania, Luxembourg, Malta, Portugal, Poland, Norway, Slovenia, Spain

To jointly examine these two dimensions of digital health infrastructures, Figure 2 presents the distribution of European countries within a two-dimensional analytical space constructed from the indices Healthcare Data Supply Coverage and Digital Health Inclusion. The aim is to analyze how European healthcare systems combine the breadth of the healthcare information ecosystem with the degree of institutional inclusiveness in access to digital health data.

The horizontal axis represents the Healthcare Data Supply Coverage index, which measures the extent of the informational sources contributing to data production within national digital health data systems. As discussed in the previous section, this indicator is derived from survey items related to the connection of healthcare providers to national health data infrastructures (Q8a–Q8k) and captures the number of provider categories contributing data to electronic health record systems. Higher values of the index indicate healthcare systems characterized by broader information ecosystems and greater integration of different components of the healthcare sector in the production of digital health data.

The vertical axis, in contrast, represents the Digital Health Inclusion index, which measures the degree of institutional inclusiveness in access to digital health data. This indicator, derived from survey items Q9–Q12, reflects the presence of institutional mechanisms designed to facilitate access to health data for different categories of users, including legal guardians, authorized individuals such as family members or caregivers, support services for vulnerable groups, and the compliance of digital platforms with European web accessibility standards.

The horizontal and vertical dashed lines indicate the European mean values of the two dimensions and divide the analytical space into four quadrants. This representation makes it possible to observe how European countries differ in the combination of health data integration and inclusiveness of data access policies, allowing the identification of different institutional configurations of digital health systems. Countries located in the upper-right quadrant display high levels in both dimensions. In these contexts, digital health data systems are supported by a broad ecosystem of healthcare providers, and access to data is facilitated by institutional mechanisms that enable different population groups to use digital health services. These systems represent relatively advanced configurations of digital health infrastructures, where extensive informational ecosystems are combined with inclusive access policies. Countries such as Estonia, Denmark, Poland, and Lithuania fall into this category.

The lower-right quadrant includes countries where the coverage of health data sources is relatively extensive, while the inclusiveness of data access mechanisms is less developed. In these contexts, healthcare information infrastructures are supported by a wide range of providers, but institutional arrangements facilitating access for different social groups remain more limited. This configuration suggests cases in which the digitalization of healthcare infrastructures has progressed more rapidly than the development of digital inclusion policies. Greece and Slovakia represent examples of this pattern. The upper-left quadrant includes countries characterized by relatively high levels of inclusion in access to digital health data but more limited integration of the data sources feeding healthcare information infrastructures. In these systems, institutional policies supporting access to health data appear relatively well developed, but not all categories of healthcare providers contribute equally to the production and sharing of digital health data. This configuration reflects contexts in which the institutional dimension of data accessibility is more advanced than the integration of the healthcare system into digital data infrastructures. Germany, Austria, and Italy fall into this category.

Finally, the lower-left quadrant includes countries displaying relatively low values on both dimensions. In these contexts, both the coverage of health data sources and the institutional mechanisms facilitating access to data appear less developed, suggesting configurations in which both digital health infrastructures and data access policies remain relatively limited. Ireland represents the most prominent example of this configuration.

Figure 2. Configurations of Digital Health Welfare Systems in Europe

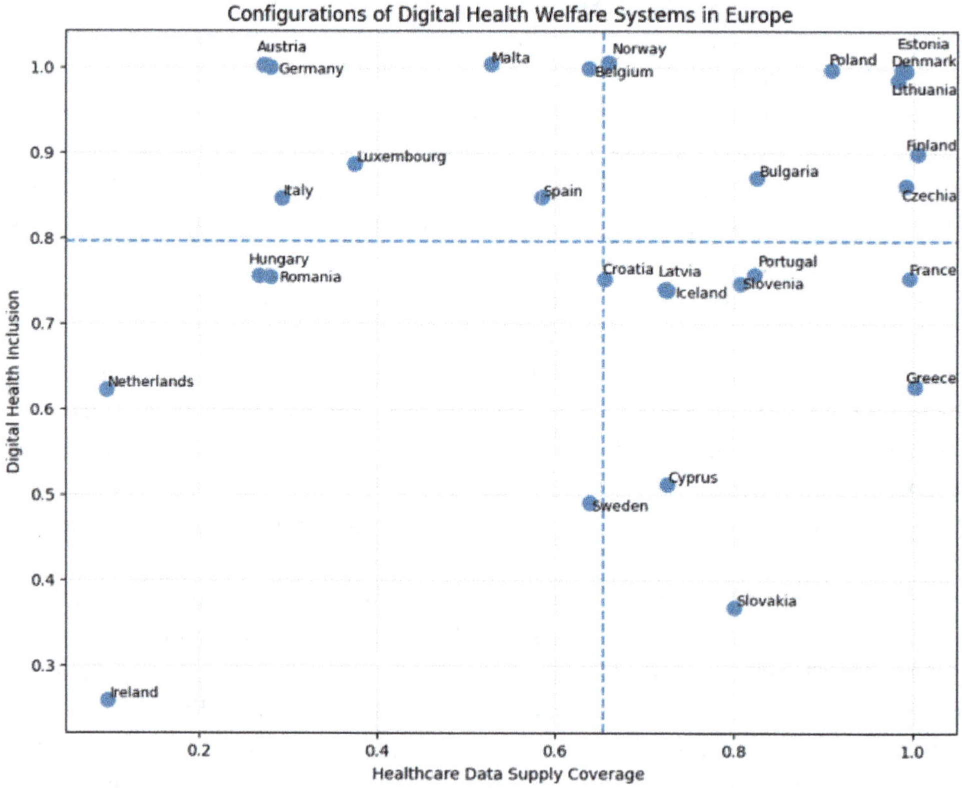

Overall, the distribution of countries within the analytical space shown in Figure 2 suggests the existence of differentiated trajectories in the development of digital health systems across Europe. These trajectories emerge from the interaction between the breadth of healthcare information ecosystems and the institutional policies designed to promote inclusive access to digital health data. Although a general trend toward the strengthening of digital health infrastructures can be observed, the results reveal significant heterogeneity in the ways national healthcare systems integrate different providers into health data production and define the institutional conditions governing access to such information. More specifically, the analysis indicates that the integration of health data sources and policies aimed at inclusive access to digital health data do not necessarily evolve in parallel across national contexts. Some healthcare systems exhibit highly integrated information ecosystems combined with relatively inclusive access policies. In other cases, however, the expansion of infrastructures supporting the production of digital health data is not accompanied by a comparable development of institutional mechanisms designed to facilitate citizens' access to these data. In yet other contexts, relatively inclusive access policies coexist with more limited integration of the informational sources feeding national digital health systems. These findings suggest that the digitalization of European healthcare systems cannot be interpreted as a linear or uniform process of technological diffusion. Rather, it appears as a field of differentiated institutional configurations reflecting both the organizational characteristics of national healthcare systems and the diverse strategies adopted to integrate health data and regulate access to such information. From this perspective, the analysis of digital health data access infrastructures makes it possible to observe how the data-driven transformation of European healthcare systems generates different configurations of digital health citizenship, in which citizens' ability to access their personal health data depends on how national healthcare systems organize the production, circulation, and accessibility of digital health information. Taken together, the results presented in Figure 2 show that European healthcare systems differ significantly in the ways they combine the integration of health data sources with institutional policies regulating access to digital data. The comparative analysis highlights that these two dimensions do not necessarily develop in parallel: healthcare systems characterized by broad informational ecosystems do not always exhibit high levels of inclusion in access to digital health data, while in other contexts relatively inclusive access policies coexist with more fragmented informational infrastructures. This variability suggests that the digitalization of European healthcare systems does not produce a single institutional model of digital health but rather a plurality of infrastructural configurations. From a sociological perspective, these differences can be interpreted by considering the two analytical dimensions examined in this study—the breadth of the healthcare data ecosystem (Healthcare Data Supply Coverage) and the degree of institutional inclusiveness in data access (Digital Health Inclusion)—as axes defining different configurations of digital health systems. By combining these two dimensions, four ideal configurations (Table 6) of digital health infrastructures emerge, reflecting different ways in which healthcare systems organize the production, integration, and accessibility of digital health data.

Table 6. Ideal Configurations of Digital Health Systems

Configuration	Characteristics
High Data Integration + High Inclusion	Relatively mature digital health systems characterized by broad healthcare information ecosystems and data access policies oriented toward citizen inclusion.
High Data Integration + Low Inclusion	Systems with well-developed health data infrastructures but more limited institutional mechanisms facilitating citizens' access to digital health data.
Low Data Integration + High Inclusion	Systems characterized by relatively inclusive data access policies but more fragmented or less integrated healthcare information ecosystems.
Low Data Integration + Low Inclusion	Systems characterized by more limited digital health infrastructures and less developed policies for access to digital health data.

4. DISCUSSION

The analysis developed in this chapter highlights how the digitalization of healthcare in Europe represents not simply a technological shift but a broader institutional transformation reshaping access to healthcare rights and health information within contemporary welfare systems. The findings show that European healthcare systems do not follow a uniform trajectory of digital development. Instead, they display different configurations in the organization of digital health infrastructures, particularly regarding the breadth of healthcare data ecosystems and the inclusiveness of access arrangements.

The combination of these dimensions reveals significant cross-national variation. Some countries combine highly integrated health data ecosystems with relatively inclusive access policies, while others display fragmented informational infrastructures or weaker inclusion mechanisms. These differences suggest that the development of digital infrastructures may evolve unevenly across healthcare systems, producing distinct institutional conditions for accessing and using health data.

The observed patterns appear broadly consistent with comparative research on welfare regimes and digital governance in Europe (Esping-Andersen, 1990; Dunleavy *et al.*, 2006). Nordic countries such as Denmark and Finland, for example, combine advanced digital infrastructures with inclusive access arrangements, reflecting long-standing traditions of universalistic welfare provision, strong administrative capacity, and high levels of institutional trust (Rothstein & Stolle, 2008; Schou & Hjelholt, 2017). By contrast, several continental and Southern European healthcare systems—including Germany, Austria, and Italy—display more fragmented patterns, where inclusion measures coexist with lower levels of provider integration, partly reflecting regional differentiation and more complex governance structures (Von Kersbergen & Vis, 2014). At the same time, some Eastern and Baltic countries, such as Estonia and Lithuania, appear to follow accelerated trajectories of digital state-building linked to broader modernization reforms (Margetts & Dunleavy, 2013).

These findings support broader sociological arguments emphasizing that digital infrastructures are not neutral technical systems but socio-technical arrangements shaping access to information, services, and social rights (Bowker & Star, 1999; Kitchin, 2014). As healthcare systems increasingly rely on digital platforms and health data ecosystems, access to health information becomes an increasingly important dimension of contemporary citizenship. The analysis also highlights the emergence of new forms of inequality linked to the organization of digital healthcare systems. While much of the literature on digital inequality has mainly focused on differences in digital skills or technological access at the individual level, the findings presented here suggest that inequalities may also emerge through institutional differences in the design and governance of digital infrastructures. Alongside the digital divide, it is therefore possible to observe the emergence of an infrastructural divide shaping unequal opportunities to access and use health data. Some limitations should nevertheless be acknowledged. The analysis relies on institutional data based on self-reporting by national authorities and therefore captures the formal availability of digital infrastructures rather than their actual use by citizens. In addition, the indicators examined here measure the existence and coverage of digital services rather than their practical effectiveness, quality, or interoperability. Finally, the analytical strategy is exploratory and comparative rather than causal.

Despite these limitations, the findings have important implications for the governance of digital health systems. If access to health data becomes increasingly central to healthcare provision, the design of digital infrastructures cannot be treated merely as a technical issue but must also be understood as a matter of institutional design with direct implications for social equity, transparency, and democratic governance.

5. CONCLUSION

This chapter has examined the transformation of European healthcare systems in the context of welfare digitalization and the growing datafication of health. Combining perspectives from welfare sociology, digital infrastructure studies, and research on digital inequalities with a comparative analysis of European health data infrastructures, the chapter has explored how digital systems reorganize access to health information and reshape the institutional conditions of healthcare citizenship.

The analysis demonstrates that European healthcare systems do not converge toward a single model of digital welfare. Instead, they display different infrastructural configurations shaped by varying levels of healthcare data integration and institutional inclusiveness. From this perspective, digital health systems should be understood not simply as technological upgrades but as institutional arrangements reflecting broader governance models and policy choices. The chapter also contributes to current debates on digital inequality by emphasizing the role of infrastructures in shaping unequal access to health information and services. Differences in provider integration, digital access mechanisms, and inclusion policies may generate unequal opportunities for citizens to interact with digital health systems and benefit from data-driven healthcare services. More broadly, the findings suggest that digital infrastructures are becoming a central component of contemporary welfare systems. As healthcare increasingly depends on digital platforms and health data ecosystems, the governance of these infrastructures will play an important role in shaping future forms of healthcare citizenship and the distribution of health-related opportunities in datafied societies. Future research should further investigate how citizens interact with digital health systems in everyday contexts and how factors such as digital literacy, trust, and socioeconomic inequalities influence the use of digital healthcare services.

REFERENCES

Aceto, G., Persico, V., & Pescapé, A. (2018). The role of information and communication technologies in healthcare: Taxonomies, perspectives, and challenges. *Journal of Network and Computer Applications, 107*, 125–154. DOI: 10.1016/j.jnca.2018.02.008

Agardh, E., Allebeck, P., Hallqvist, J., Moradi, T., & Sidorchuk, A. (2011). Type 2 diabetes incidence and socio-economic position: A systematic review and meta-analysis. *International Journal of Epidemiology, 40*(3), 804–818. DOI: 10.1093/ije/dyr029 PMID: 21335614

Andrejevic, M. (2014). The big data divide. *International Journal of Communication, 8*, 1673–1689.

Beer, D. (2009). Power through the algorithm? Participatory web cultures and the technological unconscious. *New Media & Society, 11*(6), 985–1002. DOI: 10.1177/1461444809336551

Belle, A., Thiagarajan, R., Soroushmehr, S. M. R., Navidi, F., Beard, D. A., & Najarian, K. (2015). Big data analytics in healthcare. *BioMed Research International, 2015*, 1–16. DOI: 10.1155/2015/370194 PMID: 26229957

Bowker, G. C. (2014). The theory/data thing. *International Journal of Communication, 8*, 1795–1799.

Bowker, G. C., & Star, S. L. (1999). *Sorting things out: Classification and its consequences*. MIT Press. boyd, d., & Crawford, K. (2012). Critical questions for big data. *Information Communication and Society, 15*(5), 662–679.

Brown, W. (2015). *Undoing the demos: Neoliberalism's stealth revolution*. Zone Books. DOI: 10.2307/j.ctt17kk9p8

Brynjolfsson, E., & McAfee, A. (2014). *The second machine age: Work, progress, and prosperity in a time of brilliant technologies*. W. W. Norton.

Castells, M. (2010). *The rise of the network society* (2nd ed.). Wiley-Blackwell.

Cheney-Lippold, J. (2011). A new algorithmic identity: Soft biopolitics and the modulation of control. *Theory, Culture & Society, 28*(6), 164–181. DOI: 10.1177/0263276411424420

Cochoy, F., Hagberg, J., McIntyre, M. P., & Sörum, N. (2017). Digitalizing consumption: Introduction. In *Digitalizing consumption*. Routledge. DOI: 10.4324/9781315647883-1

Crawford, K., Gray, M. L., & Miltner, K. (2014). Critiquing big data: Politics, ethics, epistemology. *International Journal of Communication, 8*, 1663–1672.

Dahlgren, G., & Whitehead, M. (2021). The Dahlgren–Whitehead model of health determinants: 30 years on. *Public Health, 199*, 20–24. DOI: 10.1016/j.puhe.2021.08.009 PMID: 34534885

Dash, S., Shakyawar, S. K., Sharma, M., & Kaushik, S. (2019). Big data in healthcare: Management, analysis and future prospects. *Journal of Big Data, 6*(1), 54. DOI: 10.1186/s40537-019-0217-0

Davies, B. (2021). Personal health surveillance: The use of mHealth in healthcare responsibilisation. *Public Health Ethics, 14*(3), 268–280. DOI: 10.1093/phe/phab013 PMID: 34899983

Diao, J. A., Wu, G. J., Taylor, H. A., Tucker, J. K., Powe, N. R., & Kohane, I. S. (2021). Clinical implications of removing race from estimates of kidney function. *Journal of the American Medical Association, 325*(2), 184–186. PMID: 33263721

Dunleavy, P., Margetts, H., Bastow, S., & Tinkler, J. (2006). *Digital era governance.* Oxford University Press. DOI: 10.1093/acprof:oso/9780199296194.001.0001

Esping-Andersen, G. (1990). The three worlds of welfare capitalism.

European Commission. Directorate-General for Communications Networks, Content and Technology & Capgemini Invent. (2025). *2025 digital decade ehealth indicator study: final report.* Publications Office of the European Union. https://data.europa.eu/doi/10.2759/2737039

Fiscella, K., Franks, P., Gold, M., & Clancy, C. (2000). Inequality in quality: Addressing socioeconomic disparities in health care. *Journal of the American Medical Association, 283*(19), 2579–2584. DOI: 10.1001/jama.283.19.2579 PMID: 10815125

Gillespie, T. (2014). The relevance of algorithms. In *Media technologies.* MIT Press. DOI: 10.7551/mitpress/9042.003.0013

Gitelman, L. (2013). *"Raw data" is an oxymoron.* MIT Press. DOI: 10.7551/mitpress/9302.001.0001

Goldzweig, C., Orshansky, G., Paige, N., Towfigh, A. A., Haggstrom, D. A., Miake-Lye, I., Beroes, J. M., & Shekelle, P. G. (2013). Electronic patient portals. *Annals of Internal Medicine, 159*(10), 677–687. DOI: 10.7326/0003-4819-159-10-201311190-00006 PMID: 24247673

Greenhalgh, T., Wherton, J., & Papoutsi, C.. (2017). Beyond adoption of health technologies. *Journal of Medical Internet Research, 19*(11), e367. DOI: 10.2196/jmir.8775 PMID: 29092808

Hardey, M., Loader, B. D., & Keeble, L. (2009). Introduction. In *Digital welfare for the third age*. Routledge.

Hogle, L. F. (2016). Data-intensive resourcing in healthcare. *Biosocieties, 11*(3), 372–393. DOI: 10.1057/s41292-016-0004-5

Iliadis, A., & Russo, F. (2016). Critical data studies: An introduction. *Big Data & Society, 3*(2), 2053951716674238. DOI: 10.1177/2053951716674238

Institute of Medicine. (2004). *Health literacy: A prescription to end confusion*. National Academies Press.

Isin, E. F., & Ruppert, E. (2015). *Being digital citizens*. Rowman & Littlefield.

Kitchin, R. (2014). The data revolution. *Sage (Atlanta, Ga.)*.

Kruse, C. S., Bolton, K., & Freriks, G. (2015). The effect of patient portals on quality outcomes. *Journal of Medical Internet Research, 17*(2), e44. DOI: 10.2196/jmir.3171 PMID: 25669240

Kruse, C. S., Goswamy, R., Raval, Y., & Marawi, S. (2016). Big data in health care. *JMIR Medical Informatics, 4*(4), e38. DOI: 10.2196/medinform.5359 PMID: 27872036

Kruse, C. S., Pesek, B., Anderson, M., Brennan, K., & Comfort, H. (2019). Telemonitoring for COPD. *JMIR Medical Informatics*.

Larrazabal, A. J., Nieto, N., Peterson, V., Milone, D., & Ferrante, E. (2020). Gender imbalance in medical imaging datasets. *Proceedings of the National Academy of Sciences of the United States of America, 117*(23), 12592–12594. DOI: 10.1073/pnas.1919012117 PMID: 32457147

Lupton, D. (2013). The digitally engaged patient. *Social Theory & Health, 11*(3), 256–270. DOI: 10.1057/sth.2013.10

Malakhov, K. (2023). Insight into the digital health system of Ukraine. *International Journal of Telerehabilitation, 15*(2). Advance online publication. DOI: 10.5195/ijt.2023.6599 PMID: 38162941

Margetts, H., & Dunleavy, P. (2013). The second wave of digital-era governance: a quasi-paradigm for government on the Web. *Philosophical transactions of the royal society A: mathematical, physical and engineering sciences, 371*(1987).

Markert, C., Sasangohar, F., Mortazavi, B., & Fields, S. (2021). Telehealth technology for older adults. *JMIR Human Factors*. Advance online publication. DOI: 10.2196/23796 PMID: 33512322

Mayer-Schönberger, V., & Cukier, K. (2013). *Big data*. Houghton Mifflin Harcourt.

McCray, A. T. (2005). Promoting health literacy. *Journal of the American Medical Informatics Association : JAMIA, 12*(2), 152–163. DOI: 10.1197/jamia.M1687 PMID: 15561782

Mittelstadt, B., Allo, P., Taddeo, M., Wachter, S., & Floridi, L. (2016). The ethics of algorithms. *Big Data & Society, 3*(2), 2053951716679679. DOI: 10.1177/2053951716679679

Morley, J., & Floridi, L. (2020). The limits of empowerment. *Science and Engineering Ethics, 26*(3), 1159–1183. DOI: 10.1007/s11948-019-00115-1 PMID: 31172424

Mossberger, K., Tolbert, C., & McNeal, R. (2008). *Digital citizenship*. MIT Press.

Norman, C. D., & Skinner, H. A. (2006). eHealth literacy. *Journal of Medical Internet Research, 8*(2), e9. DOI: 10.2196/jmir.8.2.e9 PMID: 16867972

OECD. (2016). *Digital government strategies for transforming public services in welfare areas*. OECD.

Ong, A. (2006). *Neoliberalism as exception*. Duke University Press.

Otte-Trojel, T., de Bont, A., Rundall, T., & van de Klundert, J. (2014). Developing patient portals. *Journal of the American Medical Informatics Association : JAMIA*. PMID: 26335985

Powell, J., & Deetjen, U. (2019). Characterizing the digital health citizen. *Journal of Medical Internet Research, 21*(3), e11279. DOI: 10.2196/11279 PMID: 30835238

Reed, M., Huang, J., & Brand, R.. (2019). Patient portal use and health outcomes. *Journal of Medical Internet Research, 21*(7). PMID: 31593546

Risling, T., Martinez, J., Young, J., & Thorp-Froslie, N. (2017). Evaluating patient empowerment in eHealth. *Journal of Medical Internet Research, 19*(9), e329. DOI: 10.2196/jmir.7809 PMID: 28963090

Robinson, L., Cotten, S., Ono, H., Quan-Haase, A., Mesch, G., Chen, W., Schulz, J., Hale, T. M., & Stern, M. J. (2015). Digital inequalities and why they matter. *Information Communication and Society, 18*(5), 569–582. DOI: 10.1080/1369118X.2015.1012532

Rothstein, B., & Stolle, D. (2008). The state and social capital: An institutional theory of generalized trust. *Comparative Politics, 40*(4), 441–459. DOI: 10.5129/001041508X12911362383354

Ruckenstein, M., & Schüll, N. (2017). The datafication of health. *Annual Review of Anthropology, 46*(1), 261–278. DOI: 10.1146/annurev-anthro-102116-041244

Saeed, S. A., & Masters, R. M. (2021). Disparities in health care and the digital divide. *Current Psychiatry Reports, 23*(9), 61. DOI: 10.1007/s11920-021-01274-4 PMID: 34297202

Schmidt, E., & Cohen, J. (2013). *The new digital age*. John Murray.

Schou, J., & Hjelholt, M. (2017). Digitalizing the welfare state. *Critical Policy Studies, 13*(1), 3–22. DOI: 10.1080/19460171.2017.1333441

Sharon, T. (2016). The Googlization of health research. *Personalized Medicine, 13*(6), 563–574. DOI: 10.2217/pme-2016-0057 PMID: 29754546

Shigekawa, E., Fix, M., Corbett, G., Roby, D., & Coffman, J. (2018). Telehealth evidence review. *Health Affairs*. Advance online publication. DOI: 10.1377/hlthaff.2018.05132 PMID: 30633674

Tapuria, A., Kalra, D., & Kobayashi, S.. (2021). Patients' access to electronic health records. *BMJ Open*.

Topol, E. (2012). *The creative destruction of medicine*. Basic Books.

van Deursen, A., & van Dijk, J. (2019). The first-level digital divide. *New Media & Society, 21*(2), 354–375. DOI: 10.1177/1461444818797082 PMID: 30886536

Van Dijck, J. (2014). Datafication, dataism and dataveillance. *Surveillance & Society, 12*(2), 197–208. DOI: 10.24908/ss.v12i2.4776

Van Dijck, J., & Poell, T. (2016). Understanding online health platforms. *Big Data & Society*. Advance online publication. DOI: 10.1177/2053951716654173

van Dijk, J. (2005). The deepening divide. *Sage (Atlanta, Ga.)*.

Van Dijk, J. (2012). *The network society* (3rd ed.). Sage.

Von Kersbergen, K., & Vis, B. (2014). *Comparative welfare state politics*. Cambridge University Press.

Weber, G. M., Mandl, K. D., & Kohane, I. S. (2014). Finding the missing link for big biomedical data. *Journal of the American Medical Association, 311*(24), 2479–2480. DOI: 10.1001/jama.2014.4228 PMID: 24854141

World Health Organization. (2021). *Global strategy on digital health 2020–2025*.

Chapter 4
Digital Well-Being in Healthcare Services:
A Welfare-Oriented Analytical Framework

Maria Frezza
http://orcid.org/0009-0008-1404-8503
University of Naples Federico II, Italy

ABSTRACT

This chapter, according to the authors, examines the transformations produced by digitalization processes in contemporary healthcare systems, focusing on the social, institutional, and relational implications of digital technologies in health management. It analyzes the role of the Electronic Health Record (EHR) as a socio-technical infrastructure capable of reshaping the organization of healthcare services, the circulation of clinical information, and citizen participation in care pathways. Adopting a qualitative approach based on a systematic review of sociological, institutional, and policy literature, the chapter explores three dimensions: the datafication of health, the transformation of the doctor–patient relationship, and digital inequalities in healthcare access. The analysis highlights the ambivalent nature of digitalization, which can enhance coordination, participation, and efficiency, but may also generate exclusion without adequate digital literacy and inclusive governance, supporting the need for policies promoting socially inclusive and equitable digital health models.

DOI: 10.4018/979-8-2600-3043-1.ch004

INTRODUCTION

The complex phenomenon of digitalization has implications and repercussions which, characterized above all by speed and pervasiveness, are at the center not only of the sphere of work, particularly of the healthcare system, but also of the most intimate and personal activities and relationships. «Digitalization, with its tools, platforms, algorithms, and artificial intelligence, is changing the structures of our society and of the economy, and indicates a new horizon, if not an already defined paradigm, also for the world of work» (Treu, 2021, p. 6).

Sociologists, psychologists, and anthropologists record and analyze a radical transformation of social interactions, which must therefore be reconsidered and redefined in light of the possibility of immediate, a-temporal, and non-localized connection, and of direct access to services, healthcare and beyond, taking into account the risks connected with this paradigm shift, which can be summarized in isolation and emotional and informational overload that individuals may encounter: «this new condition is explicitly represented by a sense of emptiness, disorientation, and lack of solutions» (Lo Schiavo & Giumelli, 2021, p. 14).

Such a scenario introduces the paradox of digital well-being, where informational overexposure may generate phenomena of "cyberchondria" (or digital hypochondria) in the patient and "technostress" in the operator, making the capacity for self-regulation an essential requirement for the balance of the system (White & Horvitz, 2009, p. 7; Gui et al., 2017, p. 160).

To navigate this paradox, it is necessary to establish a clear operational definition of digital well-being within this chapter. Digital well-being is defined here not merely as the absence of technology-induced stress, but as a multidimensional state of biopsychosocial equilibrium, mediated by digital technologies, where individuals possess the critical digital literacy and self-regulation capabilities required to inhabit digital environments autonomously and beneficially for their health journeys (Gui et al., 2017; Büchi, 2021).

Crucially, digital well-being must be distinguished from, yet added to, related but distinct notions. First, it differs from *digital health*, which primarily refers to the technological infrastructure, tools, and digitalized medical services themselves (Büchi, 2021). Second, it differs from mere *participation*, which denotes the formal access to and use of these platforms. Finally, it expands upon *patient empowerment*, which represents the motivational drive toward autonomy. Digital well-being encompasses all these dimensions, serving as the ultimate qualitative outcome: the subjective and collective capacity to exploit digital health resources without suffering from cognitive friction, alienation, or informational overload (Büchi, 2021).

Consequently, attention and continuous tension of contemporary society are directed toward the constant search for a balance between the benefits that technological momentum can offer and the well-being of individuals, which is recoded as digital well-being, that is, a condition of advantage conveyed by the web and by the infinite possibilities of connections. As Epifani argues, it is necessary to question and reflect on how relationships are increasingly dependent on and mediated by technology and "social media," and how it is gradually becoming more difficult to classify traditional moments of interaction from those carried out through the use of technological systems (Epifani, 2020, p. 43).

In the strictly healthcare field, these social, cultural, and economic implications and repercussions, with particular attention to the dimensions of personal well-being, must take into account certain dynamics concerning social inclusion, the redefinition of the delicate physician–patient relationship, the perception of security, and trust in the institutions of reference. In this sense, a transition can be observed from simple digitalization to the platformization of health, in which public administration opens itself to the digital process in an integrated manner: «the digitalization of public administration represents one of the main innovations that has affected both the organization of administrative activity and the regulation of individual procedures; moreover, it has entailed significant innovations in the relations with the users of administrative services» (Martines, 2019, p. 146).

The objective of the chapter is precisely to present the emerging new social paradigms and the practical implications analyzed in the proposed case study, with the intention of emphasizing the close correlation between the concept of digital well-being, mentioned above, and that of healthcare welfare, which finds implementation through the Electronic Health Record (FSE), which «has a temporal horizon that covers the entire life of the patient and is continuously fed by the subjects who take charge of the patient within the National Health Service» (Di Viggiano, 2014, p. 87).

Healthcare welfare is situated within a new digital ecosystem that cannot disregard the technological contribution and that, for this reason, must enhance the opportunities that arise in the dynamic between healthcare professionals at various levels—particularly with the reference physician—and patients, who increasingly acquire an active role that doubles the responsibility of choice but maximizes satisfaction (Barillà & Locatelli, 2013, p. 85–86).

It is essential to promote adequate levels of Digital Health Literacy (Azzopardi & Sorensen, 2019). Without real critical competence in inhabiting the digital environment, the risk is the creation of a second-level digital divide that would nullify the promises of inclusion of the new welfare system (Azzopardi & Sorensen, 2019).

BACKGROUND

It has thus been mentioned that there is an ongoing change not only in the organization of the healthcare system as a whole, in a perspective of integration with the most recent technologies, but also in the role of citizens within the welfare system itself. In this sense, it is interesting to recall the concept of the Capability Approach, that is, «the capability approach foresees the active and participatory role of individual subjects in promoting the achievement of their own goals, as members of society and responsible agents. This conception overturns the traditional view of the recipients of social policies as passive beneficiaries and provides the basis for a conception of an active welfare state» (Mocellin, 2023, p. 7).

Therefore, it is essential to understand the transition from resources made available to the opportunities that individuals encounter. Beginning in the 1980s, the Indian philosopher and economist Amartya Sen introduced the concept of the Capability Approach, according to which well-being cannot be reduced to the mere availability of resources or services, but must be understood as the real ability of individuals to transform these resources into concrete life opportunities: «defining equality in terms of equality of capabilities, or equality of real opportunities for effective social participation, means providing a concept of citizenship, or civic equality, consistent with the position of people with disabilities. This concept therefore promotes a more inclusive and just social and institutional arrangement compared to other perspectives» (Terzi, 2013, p. 43).

Applying this concept to the phenomenon of digital health emphasizes the difference between the possibility for certain individuals to access available technological tools, such as a digital platform, and the actual ability of citizens to use them consciously, autonomously, and advantageously for their own care pathway. When applied to the digital transition in healthcare, the Capability Approach directly underpins the concept of digital well-being. While patient empowerment emphasizes the theoretical agency of the individual in monitoring their health, digital well-being adds a crucial critical dimension, it represents the actual conversion of digital access into a well-balanced state of health, ensuring that the active role of the patient does not turn into an oppressive therapeutic burden or a source of digital anxiety.

Pasqualotto highlights how this concept is particularly linked to the dimension of disability, as originally conceived by Sen, but can be broadened to encompass a range of rights relevant to all individuals for a dignified and equal life that ensures physical health through legitimate and accessible healthcare treatments, as well as psychological well-being: «it is necessary to rethink, from this perspective, care and rehabilitation, school and work education, support after leaving the education system, targeted placements, and socio-assistance services for adult disability» (Pasqualotto, 2014, p. 284).

In addition, it is useful to introduce Deborah Lupton's critical reflection on digital health, which interprets healthcare technologies as sociocultural practices rather than neutral tools and choices. Today, alongside standard forms of healthcare provision, there is a strong push toward the use of telecommunications and virtual forms of consultation or data transmission, and all of this certainly has repercussions on the redefinition of social roles (Lupton, 2016). This involves considering the undeniable opportunities and advantages that telemedicine practices bring to the healthcare system, while also weighing the risks that users face in managing large amounts of data and technologies.

Lupton emphasizes that «these new techniques of telemedicine, monitoring, and self-management of personal data and tests represent a more subtle and insidious form of submission to biopolitical control by institutions, for economic and public order interests» (Lupton, 2016; Dadà, 2022, p. 38). Digitalization thus creates the figure of a new subject, which can be defined as the e-patient, increasingly involved in processes of self-monitoring, data collection and sharing, and self-management of health (Ferguson, 2007). One could argue that this consumer moves between two prospective horizons: on one hand, emancipation and autonomy; on the other, an ever-increasing demand for efficiency and functionality standards.

In this scenario, the biopolitical control mentioned by Lupton manifests today through the so-called datafication of health (Mayer-Schönberger & Cukier, 2013). The transformation of the patient's lived experience into continuous data flows—mediated by wearables or monitoring apps—introduces a third actor into the care relationship: the algorithm (Lupton, 2016; Pasquale, 2015). While automation promises efficiency, it also raises urgent questions about the transparency of decision-making processes. The risk is that the citizen's "active participation" may be reduced to a constant provision of data to opaque platforms, where the power to define health status shifts from human clinical judgment to computational logics oriented toward standardization, sometimes at the expense of the specificity of each individual case (Zuboff, 2019).

Consequently, digital well-being emerges as a counter-hegemonic capability: the capacity of the subject to resist algorithmic standardization and biopolitical control, safeguarding health as a dignified, non-alienated, and human-centered life project (Van Dijck et al., 2018). «As undeniable as the benefits brought by the advent of telemedicine are, in terms of greater patient independence, and as justified as the concerns of those who see a possible instrument of control over bodies may be, such considerations do not resolve our question; rather, they open a deeper reflection on the concept of autonomy» (Dadà, 2022, p. 40) and on the social well-being that is emerging and being investigated in this work.

Acting as a link between the reflections of Sen and Lupton, Nancy Krieger introduces her concept of ecosocial theory and embodiment (Krieger, 2011). According to

Krieger, the individual is not an abstract entity, but a body that biologically embodies the world in which it lives, including social and technological inequalities (Krieger, 2011). From this perspective, the digital divide is not merely a technical gap, but translates into an embodiment of disadvantages that directly impact physical health. If an individual does not possess the capabilities to navigate the digital ecosystem, their exclusion does not remain confined to the virtual sphere, but becomes a biological limitation, influencing clinical outcomes and the management of chronic conditions. Technology, therefore, is not an external addition, but a component of the ecosocial environment that actively shapes the body and the well-being of citizens (Krieger, 2011).

From a broader perspective, the phenomenon of healthcare digitalization can be situated within the multitude of structural transformation processes of contemporary society, which can be linked to the theory of the network society—a community that creates relationships through technological tools and networks. In today's society, strongly characterized by information conveyed through technological means, it is not sufficient merely to reorganize services; it is necessary, in order to present new paradigms, to examine the very concept of power, active participation in community life, and citizenship, and to acknowledge «the close, very close, correlation existing between communication (it should be clarified, understood as access, sharing, transparency, listening, service) and citizenship, between communication and democracy; but also between democracy and visibility/publicity of power» (Dominici, 2019, p. 98). «The relational dimension of information infrastructure is considered as the result, on the one hand, of existing interdependencies in the linkage between different technologies and applications, and on the other, of the adoption and use of these technologies and applications by organizational agents» (Cordella, 2005, p. 72). The healthcare domain is progressively assuming the pervasiveness of digital infrastructures, platforms for data sharing, and algorithmic logics that influence the modalities of access to social rights and the construction of trust toward public institutions.

Sociological and theoretical literature in recent years on these topics—the automation and increasingly extensive use of service platforms—highlights how these complex phenomena constitute two sides of the same, alongside greater efficiency, process standardization, and improved cost containment in diagnoses and therapies, there are forms of exclusion that force healthcare operators and more vulnerable citizens to navigate complex and opaque systems. The impact of new technologies thus appears ambivalent: inclusion, which is the goal to be pursued, does not always find full realization, and the individual does not always feel more actively engaged or collaborative. Literature evidence converges in considering that digital efficacy tends toward combating inequality, particularly economic inequality, promoting growth, but it also calls for reflection on training choices, often absent, which could compromise the effectiveness of digital innovation (Ciurleo et al., 2025, p. 17).

Social sciences must refocus attention on the individual because media and social networks have created a new ecosystem and a new anthropological vision, which also has direct implications for the healthcare system concerning two specific aspects, namely the digital divide and the new physician–patient relationship: «today the greatest possible innovation is ethics, that is, the possibility that through the digital economy a greater civic sense develops in the population» (Dècina, 2016, p. 10).

The first phenomenon represents a determining factor of the network society regarding inequalities in contemporary society: it does not concern only the worsening of inequalities in access to technologies, but as a multidimensional phenomenon that involves material and symbolic factors. Digitalization can have a strong and positive impact on patient care through telemedicine systems, electronic health records shared among multiple institutions, remote image-based diagnostics, and the increasing use of AI. However, if infrastructures are not adequate and cutting-edge, some populations may remain excluded, particularly, without doubt, the most vulnerable citizens, such as the elderly, chronically ill patients, people with disabilities, or residents in isolated or less accessible areas.

In addition, attention must also be given to the lack of training and digital skills, which limit access to the most advanced possibilities offered by digitalization: «the lack of digital tools, network access, and IT skills can be considered a particularly severe form of poverty. Those without access to the internet today are irreparably harmed in enjoying their fundamental rights. Being excluded from the internet—or not knowing how to use it—means being at the margins of society, with no hope of improving one's economic or existential condition» (Saraceni, 2019, p. 14).

Material access to the network is not sufficient; it is "eHealth Literacy" that determines whether technology will be a tool of emancipation or of decision-making confusion (Norman & Skinner, 2006, p. 2). Without adequate skills, the user slides toward passive provision of data to opaque platforms, transforming well-being into a process of algorithmic standardization (Pasquale, 2015). Therefore, in the absence of adequate digital skills, institutional support, and favorable social conditions, technology, which could serve as a driver of social opportunity, becomes an element of exclusion and limitation.

In light of the framework outlined so far, reference must also be made to the physician–patient relationship, a crucial element of relational well-being and the changes it is undergoing in the coming decades. Modes of remote assistance and patient monitoring are increasing, but it is necessary to maintain the unique relationship that allows the sick person not to live in isolation but to be part of a community that supports, understands, listens to them, and, through the physician, provides personalized and constant care, thanks to the new possibilities offered by technology: «innovative technologies will be able to perform all or almost all of the tasks of the physician. This is not just a way of speaking: some are equipped with functionalities that literally allow them to replace the physician in their professional activities» (Pravettoni & Triberti, 2019, p. 93).

The transition from the physical place of care, such as the hospital, to the virtual environment allows video calls or telemonitoring while preserving the human aspect of care (Fudim et al., 2025). Certainly, it is necessary to ensure that technology does not prevail and that machines replace human-to-human interaction, eliminating the relational dimension vital for proper patient management (Fudim et al., 2025). The remarkable opportunities offered by technology must not undermine the dimension of human care and attention exercised by physicians and nurses toward patients. Patients are no longer mere recipients of care but active participants in the healing process, endowed with a precise identity and inalienable rights (Fudim et al., 2025).

The challenge in the coming decades will therefore not be the replacement of humans with machines, but the transition toward a Human-Centered Digital Health model. In order for technology not to become an element of alienation, it must be designed based on the real needs and limitations of vulnerable individuals. Ethics, as cited by Dècina, must be translated into inclusive design, recognizing the physician as an interpreter of digital data and the patient as a co-author of their therapeutic path, preventing digitalization from becoming an additional burden of treatment on already vulnerable individuals (Dècina, 2016).

Table 1. Summary of theoretical frameworks applied to digital welfare

Theoretical Framework	Distinctive Analytical Focus	Specific Role in Welfare Transformation	Emerging Dimension of Digital Well-Being
Capability Approach*(Sen, Nussbaum)*	Conversion of technological resources into real opportunities for choice and action (*functionings*).	Overcoming passive welfare: the citizen becomes an active agent in their own care journey.	Critical self-management capacity to avoid digital anxiety or an oppressive therapeutic burden.
Critical Sociology of Digital Health*(Lupton)*	Medical technology as a socio-cultural practice and an apparatus of biopolitical control (*datafication*).	Risk of a welfare shift from universal/solidary to standardized and driven by metrics of profit/efficiency.	Counter-hegemonic capacity of the subject to resist algorithmic standardization.
Science and Technology Studies - STS *(Star, Bowker)*	Technological infrastructure (e.g., EHR) as a non-neutral socio-technical construct embedding power asymmetries.	Organizational reconfiguration of welfare: digital bureaucracy risks producing "infrastructural violence" by obscuring social factors.	Visibility of human needs beyond the rigid codification of software drop-down menus.

continued on following page

Table 1. Continued

Theoretical Framework	Distinctive Analytical Focus	Specific Role in Welfare Transformation	Emerging Dimension of Digital Well-Being
Eco-social Theory*(Krieger)*	The biological body as an entity that embodies the social and technological inequalities of the environment.	Redefinition of social determinants of health: the digital divide translates into biological limitation and exclusion from citizenship rights.	Distributive equity in access to digital resources and health protection for vulnerable groups.
Network Society Theory*(Castells, Dominici)*	Structuring of communities and power relations through networks and information flows.	Democratic transformation of welfare: transparency and access to services redefine institutional trust.	Web-mediated relational well-being and preservation of the human physician-patient bond.

METHODOLOGY

Starting from the theoretical frameworks and sociocultural reflections outlined in the previous section, it becomes necessary to examine how these concepts are addressed and operationalized in contemporary healthcare practices and digital infrastructures. In particular, the analysis of institutional documents, policy strategies, and scientific literature enables a broad understanding of how digital health technologies—such as the Electronic Health Record (EHR)—mediate access, participation, and well-being, as well as the conditions under which they promote inclusive forms of healthcare provision.

Consistent with these premises, this chapter adopts a qualitative and theoretical-interpretive approach to the literature and relevant documents, functioning as a conceptual analysis rather than a formal systematic review. This contribution is characterized as a qualitative analysis of theoretical and documentary sources. Accordingly, the approach does not rely on quantitative screening protocols typical of systematic reviews, but instead focuses on a critical and sociological reconstruction of the structural transformations of digital health.

Instead of offering an empirical or statistical assessment of EHR implementation at the national level, the objective is to develop a sociological reflection on the structural transformations that digital technologies are producing in access to care, in interpersonal and professional relationships among the various actors of the healthcare system, and in the concrete conditions through which citizens can effectively benefit from digital health services. From this perspective, the EHR is understood as a socio-technical device through which the broader digital transformation of healthcare welfare and its implications for digital well-being can be observed, with particular attention to the role of the «Electronic Health Record (EHR) as a central infrastructure of digital health» (Camera dei Deputati, 2024, p. 1).

In recent years, the digitalization of healthcare has assumed an increasingly central role in public policies and innovation strategies within contemporary welfare systems (Ministero della Salute, 2021). The growing diffusion of digital platforms, information infrastructures, and healthcare data management systems is radically reshaping the organization of healthcare services and traditional models of interaction between institutions, healthcare professionals, and citizens. In this context, the EHR represents one of the most relevant tools for the integration and sharing of clinical information, functioning as a complex information infrastructure designed to support continuity of care, the organizational efficiency of services, and greater active patient participation in care pathways (Camera dei Deputati, 2024). However, the spread of such technologies also raises important issues regarding universal accessibility, digital inequalities, the ethical governance of data, and citizens' actual capacity to use these technological resources to improve their overall well-being.

In light of these considerations, the research design is based on a targeted selection of secondary sources, identified according to their theoretical and institutional relevance to the themes of digital health, digital well-being, and the socio-technical transformations of welfare systems. The analysis critically integrates three different types of materials:

The first category of sources concerns institutional and regulatory documentation, including strategic plans, policy documents, guidelines, and reports produced by national and European institutions involved in the governance of digital healthcare. These documents make it possible to reconstruct the regulatory framework, strategic objectives, and policy trajectories guiding the development of digital infrastructures in healthcare systems.

The second category includes statistical data and monitoring reports from public observatories and national research institutions that analyze the diffusion of e-health technologies, telemedicine services, and digital platforms used within healthcare systems. These sources allow for an understanding of the level of implementation of digital infrastructures and the main trends characterizing healthcare digitalization processes.

The third category consists of national and international scientific literature, including peer-reviewed articles and academic contributions focused on digital health, the digitalization of healthcare systems, and socio-institutional transformations related to the management and circulation of health data.

The integration of these sources is not intended to achieve quantitative exhaustiveness but rather to develop a multi-level interpretive analysis. Guided by digital well-being as our central interpretive lens, the primary research question of this study is formulated as follows: To what extent can digital healthcare infrastructures foster inclusive forms of digital well-being within contemporary welfare and care systems? To answer this question, the analysis explores how the FSE impacts the qualitative equilibrium of care through three distinct dimensions: the datafication of the patient, the relational reconfiguration between doctors and patients, and the distributive implications of digital inclusion. This question successfully links the technological dimension of digital health to broader issues concerning access to services, citizen participation, and the quality of individual well-being in increasingly digitalized healthcare contexts.

Although the literature on digital health and healthcare digitalization is extensive, existing studies often remain fragmented across distinct disciplinary fields, including health sociology, science and technology studies, and welfare policy analysis. This chapter seeks to address this fragmentation by integrating these perspectives into a unified welfare-oriented analytical framework. In particular, the contribution of this chapter lies in explicitly connecting digital well-being to the governance transformations of contemporary welfare systems, highlighting how digital infrastructures simultaneously reshape access to care, institutional coordination, and the conditions of healthcare citizenship.

From a theoretical perspective, the interpretation of the materials is grounded in an integrated analytical framework combining three complementary perspectives. First, the Capability Approach provides the normative foundation of the analysis, enabling a distinction between the mere availability of digital infrastructures and individuals' actual capability to transform these resources into concrete opportunities for care and well-being (Sen, 1999; Nussbaum, 2011). Second, the perspective of the network society allows digital health to be interpreted as part of a relational informational system in which data, platforms, and technological infrastructures redefine relationships among healthcare institutions, professionals, and citizens (Castells, 2009). Finally, critical digital health sociology contributes to the analysis of health datafication processes, informational asymmetries, and emerging forms of individual responsibilization within healthcare systems based on the collection, processing, and circulation of clinical data (Lupton, 2018; Sharon, 2017).

Within this theoretical framework, the analysis develops along three main interpretive dimensions: patient datafication processes (Lupton, 2018); the reconfiguration of the physician–patient relationship (Lupton, 2018; Topol, 2019); and the institutional and distributive implications of digital health with respect to citizens' inclusion in digitalized care systems (van Dijk, 2005).

The methodological approach adopted is therefore exploratory and interpretive rather than quantitative or based on systematic protocols. The aim is not to measure the frequency of empirical findings but to critically analyze how digital health infrastructures are conceptualized in contemporary sociological and institutional debates.

ANALYSIS OF DIGITAL HEALTH TRANSFORMATION

Building on the theoretical and methodological framework outlined above, the following section presents an interpretative analysis of digital health transformation, focusing on how socio-technical infrastructures such as the Electronic Health Record (EHR) reshape healthcare practices, patient experiences, and institutional logics.

The digital transformation of health does not represent a mere administrative update or a simple evolution of the technological tools available to clinical practice, but rather constitutes a radical ontological and epistemological reconfiguration of contemporary medicine (Mori, 2019; Lupton, 2018). The transition from paper documentation to digital flows has triggered a profound metamorphosis in the way health and illness are conceptualized, measured, governed, and experienced (Mori, 2019). This transition dematerializes clinical information, detaching it from the physical constraints of the traditional hospital archive and transforming it into a continuous, ubiquitous, and computable flow. The patient's body is thus translated into strings of code, inaugurating a new era in which biomedical data becomes the primary lens through which the human condition is decoded (Mori, 2019; Lupton, 2016).

At the center of this informational architecture lies the Electronic Health Record (EHR). Although in public discourse the EHR is often reduced to a simple database, the sociology of innovation and Science and Technology Studies (STS) invite us to interpret it as a complex "socio-technical infrastructure" (Star & Ruhleder, 1996, p. 113). As theorized by Susan Leigh Star, infrastructures are never invisible and neutral "plumbing"; they actively incorporate cultural values, organizational logics, and power asymmetries (Star, 1999, p. 380). The EHR does not merely passively record clinical history but actively structures the field of action of healthcare professionals, defining which information is considered relevant and which, by contrast, becomes marginalized.

An emblematic example of this dynamic can be observed in the limits of standardized clinical coding. Many EHR systems are designed with rigid drop-down menus based on the ICD (International Classification of Diseases) classification (Pasceri, 2025, p. 45). This design forces the clinician into a binary or predefined choice that often excludes the complexity of lived experience. In this process, a form of invisibility of labor is produced: while quantifiable and codifiable medical acts are highlighted by the system, informal care work, empathy, and non-standardizable clinical nuances tend to disappear behind the digital interface (Pasceri, 2025). The EHR thus becomes a device that, in attempting to render everything readable and computable, risks expunging from official documentation the human and relational complexity of clinical practice (Pasceri, 2025, p. 47).

From a welfare governance perspective, the EHR should therefore be understood not merely as a technical repository of clinical information, but as a strategic infrastructure through which healthcare systems organize access to services, coordinate institutional responsibilities, and regulate interactions between citizens and public administration. By standardizing data circulation and integrating multiple healthcare actors within a unified informational ecosystem, the EHR contributes to the broader digital transformation of welfare governance, where rights, entitlements, and care pathways are increasingly mediated by digital infrastructures.

If the software decides that a social factor is not a medical datum because no field exists to enter it, that factor disappears from the official clinical history (Passeri, 2025, p. 51). During the opioid crisis or in the management of rare diseases, it emerged how the impossibility of recording determinants such as housing instability or social isolation rendered these factors clinically invisible. This generates what Geoffrey C. Bowker defines as "infrastructural violences" (Bowker & Star, 1999, p. 37): the patient is treated for the biological symptom, but the social cause remains invisible, fragmenting the subject's narrative in favor of a "virtual" patient composed of isolated parameters (Bowker & Star, 1999, p. 124).

In this context, the EHR acts as a boundary object: an entity that inhabits different communities of practice (physicians, programmers, administrators) and that is interpreted in different ways (Bottari, 2017). While for the programmer it is a data structure and for the administrator a cost report, for the physician it can become a constraint that fragments the unity of care (Bottari, 2017). Data integration is therefore not merely a technical challenge but an act of political coordination that imposes a rigid categorization of human suffering.

The infrastructural phenomenon is embedded within the broader macro-process of the datafication of health. Beyond the seminal definition proposed by Viktor Mayer-Schönberger and Kenneth Cukier, it is essential to introduce the concept of the "Googlization of health research" (GHR) proposed by Tamar Sharon (Sharon, 2016, p. 563). Sharon highlights how digital transformation is not merely a technical shift but is marked by the massive entry of Big Tech into the healthcare domain (Sharon, 2016, p. 566). This shift does not concern privacy alone, but the colonization of traditional medical values—such as solidarity and universality—by logics oriented toward profit, efficiency, and algorithmic prediction (Sharon, 2018).

The most striking example of this trend is the Project Nightingale case. In 2019 it emerged that Google, in collaboration with Ascension (one of the largest private healthcare systems in the United States), had collected identifiable health data from millions of patients without their explicit consent in order to train predictive algorithms. This case confirms Sharon's thesis: the shift of power is radical. The medical logic of care is replaced by the Big Tech logic of market prediction (Sharon, 2018). When a technology company analyzes clinical data, it does not do so with the objective of the universalistic solidarity of welfare but with that of algorithmic efficiency, transforming the public good of health into a private and computable asset.

Self-tracking technologies (wearables, monitoring apps) are not merely tools of empowerment but devices that establish what could be defined as the digital labor of care (Lupton, 2016). As the sociologist of time Judy Wajcman emphasizes, technology often does not save time but alters its perceptual quality. The patient becomes an incessant producer of biometric data, engaged in a form of self-surveillance that transforms life time into monitoring time (Wajcman, 2015). In this sense, health is no longer experienced as a silent state of well-being but as a project of constant optimization mediated by the numerical dashboards of the smartphone. The continuous production of data transforms everyday life into a diffuse clinical laboratory, where the boundary between healthy and ill becomes blurred by the need to constantly remain within the parameters of statistical normality imposed by platforms (Wajcman, 2015).

The convergence between the EHR infrastructure and the ecosystem of self-tracking produces a radical transformation of subjectivity: the patient is converted into a data subject (Pasceri, 2025). Their clinical identity and their rights of healthcare citizenship are mediated by the volume of information they are able to generate.

In this relationship, algorithms are not neutral tools but non-human actors endowed with their own agency (Pasceri, 2025). They determine who has access to certain treatments or who is considered high risk according to predictive logics that are often inscrutable. The study by Ziad Obermeyer provides definitive evidence (Obermeyer et al., 2019).

Technical analysis revealed that an algorithm widely used in the United States penalized Black patients because it used past healthcare expenditure as a proxy for future care needs (Obermeyer et al., 2019). This represents a socio-logical error: in contexts of profound inequality, poorer individuals spend less not because they are healthier but because they have less physical and economic access to services (Obermeyer et al., 2019). The algorithm, ignoring these barriers, mistook lack of spending for lack of illness.

As suggested by Cathy O'Neil, this produces a negative feedback loop: the vulnerable patient is labeled low risk, receives less care, their health worsens, but the system continues to see them as a low-priority subject (O'Neil, 2017). This is the "black box" described by Frank Pasquale: a decision-making process that has vital impacts yet remains inscrutable to both the citizen and the clinician (Pasquale, 2015, p. 18).

The transparency of algorithmic decision-making processes is therefore not a mere technical detail but a prerequisite of modern democracy (Pasquale, 2015). The patient thus becomes the victim of a form of "health surveillance" that does not protect them but categorizes them according to cost-efficiency logics, emptying the concept of healthcare citizenship of its ethical and solidaristic component (Pasquale, 2015, p. 26).

THE REDEFINITION OF THE DOCTOR–PATIENT RELATIONSHIP IN THE DIGITAL ERA

Having explored the socio-technical infrastructures and the processes of health datafication, the next section turns to their implications for human interaction in healthcare, examining how the doctor–patient relationship is being reshaped in the digital era.

In light of the infrastructural transformations and the processes of health datafication analyzed in the previous section, it becomes necessary to reflect on the implications that such dynamics produce in the relational dimension of care, particularly in the relationship between doctor and patient. The progressive digitalization of healthcare is in fact profoundly transforming this relationship, modifying not only its operational modalities but also its social and cultural meaning (Giarelli et al., 2023).

Historically, the therapeutic relationship developed within a strongly asymmetrical model in which the physician held the monopoly of scientific knowledge, while the patient occupied a predominantly passive position, limited to accepting diagnostic and therapeutic indications (Giarelli et al., 2023). This arrangement reflects what Talcott Parsons defined as the "sick role," a normative model in which illness is interpreted as a temporary deviation from the social order and in which the authority of the physician is socially legitimized by their scientific competence (Parsons, 1991, p. 193). Within this configuration, the patient is exempted from certain social responsibilities but has the duty to seek medical assistance and to cooperate with the healthcare professional in the process of treatment (Parsons, 1991).

This institutional balance between medical knowledge and the patient's position was later critically analyzed by Eliot Freidson, who described medicine as a profession characterized by "professional dominance," namely the «capacity to control the definition of illness, treatments, and the organization of care within the healthcare system» (Freidson, 1970, p. 233).

The patient no longer merely receives the diagnosis passively but increasingly tends to participate actively in the decision-making process, asking questions, comparing therapeutic options, and contributing their subjective experience to the definition of the care pathway. This transformation can also be interpreted in light of some classical contributions from medical sociology. Arthur Kleinman distinguished between *disease*, the biological and clinical dimension of pathology, and *illness*, the subjective experience of disease as lived by the patient in everyday life (Kleinman et al., 1978). In traditional practice, attention tended to focus primarily on disease, while the subjective experience of illness often remained marginal in the decision-making process (Kleinman et al., 1978). Today, the availability of digital tools and patient-generated data promotes the visibility of the patient's perspective, enabling individuals to share symptoms and narratives of their experience through digital platforms, monitoring devices, and online communities.

Similarly, Eliot Mishler described clinical communication as an interaction between two discursive registers: the "voice of medicine," based on technical and scientific language, and the "voice of the lifeworld," which reflects the patient's everyday experience and the social meaning of illness in their life (Mishler, 1984, p. 108–110). From the standpoint of digital well-being, the critical intersection of these two registers is heavily remediated by technology; the growing integration of data produced directly by patients contributes to making this experiential dimension more visible, transforming the doctor–patient relationship into a space of negotiation between biomedical knowledge and the situated knowledge of the patient, which requires new forms of communicative balance.

The emergence of digital technologies, telemedicine platforms, and the increasing availability of health information online has progressively eroded the traditional configuration, fostering the emergence of more articulated and participatory forms of interaction (Giarelli et al., 2023). At the same time, digital technologies are also transforming the temporal and spatial dimension of the therapeutic relationship. Tools such as remote consultations, health messaging systems, and remote monitoring platforms enable more continuous communication distributed over time, strengthening patient involvement in the management of their own health, particularly in the case of chronic diseases that require constant monitoring (Giarelli et al., 2023).

Within this scenario, the therapeutic pathway increasingly tends to take the form of «a process of co-production of health», in which the physician's clinical knowledge and the patient's subjective experience jointly contribute to the definition of therapeutic decisions and care practices (Batalden et al., 2016: 511). The therapeutic relationship thus becomes a space of collaboration among the different actors involved.

At the same time, the digital extension of the relationship introduces new organizational and relational pressures for healthcare professionals, who must manage a growing flow of digital communications and clinical data. From a sociological perspective, this dynamic can be interpreted as a process of technologically mediated relational intensification, in which opportunities for contact increase but are also accompanied by new forms of cognitive and emotional workload for both actors involved.

This relational and structural tension highlights why the conceptual framework of this chapter must constantly return to digital well-being as its central interpretive lens. Here, the lens of digital well-being clarifies that a successful digital transition does not equate to the maximization of virtual contacts (which is merely a metric of digital health utilization). Rather, digital well-being in the medical encounter is achieved only when the technology acts as a transparent mediator that reduces technostress for both parties, preserving empathy, mutual recognition, and systemic trust without substituting the fundamental logic of care (Mol, 2008). Consequently, digital well-being emerges as the indispensable equilibrium that prevents the active "voice of the lifeworld" from being crushed by digital alienation or transformed into an unsustainable cognitive burden of data management.

Another element of transformation concerns the symbolic dimension of trust that underpins the relationship of care. Traditionally, patient trust was primarily grounded in the professional competence of the physician and the institutional legitimacy of the healthcare system. Within the digital ecosystem, trust also extends to the technological infrastructures that manage health data (Giarelli et al., 2023). Citizens are called upon to trust not only the physician's expertise but also the security of digital platforms, the transparency of algorithms, and the reliability of the institutions that govern the use of clinical information (Giarelli et al., 2023).

This transformation can be interpreted in light of the theory of trust in complex systems proposed by Niklas Luhmann, according to which in modern societies trust is directed not only toward individuals but also toward the technical and institutional infrastructures that mediate social interaction (Giarelli et al., 2023).

The main challenge does not consist in replacing human interaction with technological systems, but rather in constructing models of digital healthcare capable of integrating technological innovation with attention to the relational dimension of care.

As emphasized by Annemarie Mol, contemporary medical practice can be interpreted as a *logic of care*, a continuous process of adaptation and negotiation among scientific knowledge, technologies, and relational practices (Mol, 2008). In this sense, the doctor–patient relationship remains the core of the therapeutic process even within a digitalized healthcare system, configuring itself as a space of negotiation among scientific knowledge, subjective experience, and technological mediation. The relational transformations described above cannot be fully understood without considering the structural inequalities that shape citizens' ability to access and navigate digital healthcare environments. For this reason, the following section shifts the analytical focus from interpersonal dynamics to the distributive and institutional dimensions of digital health transformation.

DIGITAL INEQUALITIES AND ACCESS TO DIGITAL HEALTHCARE

While the digitalization of the doctor–patient relationship reshapes communication and trust within care, these transformations are conditioned by broader structural factors. In particular, unequal access to digital infrastructures and disparities in digital literacy can significantly influence how patients experience and participate in digitally mediated healthcare.

The promise of a more participatory and data-driven healthcare system faces a critical challenge: unequal access to the infrastructures and digital skills necessary to effectively utilize such tools. While the digitalization of healthcare systems is often presented as a factor promoting the democratization of access to care, sociological literature demonstrates that these transformations can instead produce new forms of social stratification, reshaping the ways in which citizens access health rights and engage in care processes. In this regard, digital inequalities are not merely a technological issue but constitute a structural dimension of contemporary welfare systems, as information infrastructures increasingly serve as the primary channels through which public services are organized and well-being opportunities distributed.

Empirical studies confirm that the diffusion of digital health technologies proceeds at varying speeds across social groups and territories. According to the *Digital Decade 2025: eHealth Indicator Study* of the European Commission, by 2024 the average level of access to electronic health records (EHRs) in the European Union reached 83%, representing significant progress compared to previous years and approaching the policy objective of achieving digital access to health data for 100% of European citizens by 2030 (European Commission, 2025). However, this aggregated figure masks substantial territorial heterogeneity: while some countries, such as Belgium and Estonia, reach near-full digital maturity, others lag significantly behind, indicating that healthcare digitalization does not follow a uniform trajectory across Europe. Even in more advanced national contexts, formal access to infrastructure does not automatically translate into the actual capacity of citizens to use digital tools effectively (European Commission, 2025).

A critical factor concerns the social distribution of eHealth literacy—the ability to search, comprehend, and utilize health information through digital tools. Comparative analyses conducted across several European countries show generally modest levels, particularly among populations with lower educational attainment (Sørensen et al., 2012). In certain contexts, fewer than 10% of citizens are capable of effectively using digital tools for health management, revealing a significant gap between the availability of infrastructures and their actual appropriation (OECD, 2023). This suggests that the introduction of digital health services, if not accompanied by targeted digital literacy and inclusion policies, risks becoming an implicit mechanism of user selection.

Digital inequalities also manifest at the territorial level. Rural or peripheral areas often exhibit lower connectivity and limited access to digital services compared to major urban centers, creating a form of double marginalization for citizens already disadvantaged by the scarcity of traditional healthcare services (World Health Organization, 2021). In theory, telemedicine could reduce territorial disparities by overcoming geographic barriers to care. However, if digital infrastructures are underdeveloped or local populations lack the necessary skills, digitalization risks reinforcing existing inequalities rather than alleviating them (World Health Organization, 2021).

Empirical evidence highlights the role of digital skills as a primary source of inequality. OECD comparative data indicate that health-related digital literacy varies significantly with education level and age (OECD, 2023). In the European countries analyzed, the skill gap between individuals with high and low educational attainment often exceeds fifteen percentage points, confirming the decisive role of cultural capital in accessing digital healthcare (OECD, 2023). Similarly, approximately 40% of adults over the age of 65 report difficulties using digital health tools, compared to much lower percentages among younger generations (OECD, 2023). In the context of an aging population, this finding is strategically important, as the groups with the greatest healthcare needs are often the least equipped to use new digital infrastructures.

The sociology of digital inequalities emphasizes the multidimensional nature of the so-called digital divide, which goes beyond mere availability of connections or devices. As Jan van Dijk highlights, access to digital technologies develops through a cumulative sequence encompassing motivational access, material access, operational skills, and the ability to effectively use tools in everyday life (Van Dijk, 2020). From this perspective, digital inequalities tend to widen over time, reinforcing the advantages of already privileged social groups. The introduction of digital health services—from online appointment platforms to telemonitoring systems and electronic health records—can therefore create a paradox: tools designed to expand access to care may disproportionately benefit individuals with greater social, cultural, and technological resources. At this juncture, the distinction between participation and digital well-being becomes empirically urgent. Booking a medical appointment online or accessing a portal represents digital participation; however, digital well-being is only achieved when the citizen possesses the cumulative digital skills to navigate these interfaces critically, confidently, and without experiencing feelings of systemic exclusion, frustration, or cognitive disenfranchisement.

Empirical data confirm these dynamics. According to Eurostat, in 2023 approximately 42% of European citizens lacked basic digital skills, with higher percentages in several Southern European countries (Eurostat, 2023). In Italy, nearly half of the adult population demonstrates insufficient competencies to independently use complex online services, including health-related services. Increasing digitalization of public services requires not only the availability of internet connections but also the ability to navigate often complex and non-intuitive interfaces.

These inequalities are further compounded by territorial and socioeconomic factors: the distribution of digital infrastructures remains uneven between urban and rural areas and between economically developed regions and less technologically equipped territories. In many peripheral areas, limited connection quality or insufficient broadband coverage represents an obstacle to the use of digital health services, potentially exacerbating territorial disparities in access to care and penalizing the elderly and residents in isolated areas (Eurostat, 2023).

An additional transformation concerns the platformization of healthcare services. As noted by José van Dijck, Thomas Poell, and Martijn de Waal, digital platforms are becoming central infrastructures in social life, mediating interactions among citizens, institutions, and public services (van Dijck et al., 2018). In the healthcare sector, this dynamic manifests through digital ecosystems integrating appointment systems, clinical records, monitoring applications, and teleconsultation services. While these platforms may enhance efficiency and continuity of care, they also introduce new forms of technological dependency and informational asymmetry among users, institutions, and private actors (van Dijck et al., 2018).

The centrality of digital platforms transforms healthcare citizenship, increasingly mediated by technological competencies and the ability to navigate complex information systems. Access to healthcare services becomes a process of navigating institutional portals, mobile apps, and authentication systems, shaping the actual exercise of health rights. In this sense, digitalization redefines social citizenship, transforming access to public services into a practice increasingly mediated by technological competencies and information infrastructures.

The healthcare case is particularly significant because it anticipates broader transformations affecting contemporary welfare states. Similar dynamics of platformization, datafication, and algorithmic governance are increasingly visible in social assistance, education, employment services, and pension administration. Healthcare therefore functions as a paradigmatic domain through which to observe how digital infrastructures progressively redefine welfare governance, institutional trust, and citizens' access to social rights across multiple sectors of public service provision.

The consequences of these transformations became particularly evident during the COVID-19 pandemic, when the adoption of telemedicine and remote consultations accelerated. According to the World Health Organization, telemedicine use increased substantially, enabling millions of patients to maintain access to care despite restrictions (WHO, 2022). However, this also revealed profound inequalities: groups with fewer economic resources, lower educational levels, or limited familiarity with technology faced greater difficulties in access, demonstrating how digital healthcare may generate new forms of exclusion among vulnerable populations.

A critical aspect concerns the data underpinning innovations in digital medicine. The expansion of artificial intelligence and predictive systems relies on large clinical and behavioral datasets. However, the concept of data poverty highlights that certain social groups are systematically underrepresented in the datasets used to train algorithms (Birhane, 2021). This may produce biased outcomes, reinforcing inequalities in access to care or in diagnostic quality.

In light of this evidence, healthcare digitalization is not a technically neutral process but a socio-institutional transformation that reshapes how health systems produce knowledge, allocate resources, and build trust with citizens. Digital infrastructures embed conceptions of health, data governance models, and operational logics that profoundly influence access to care.

The principal challenge for digital health policies in the coming years will be to ensure that innovations are designed and implemented in a socially inclusive manner. This requires investments in technological infrastructure, digital literacy programs for the population, interface simplification, and the development of user-centered models that respond to real needs. Only by integrating technological, social, and institutional dimensions will it be possible to prevent digitalization from becoming a source of exclusion, transforming it instead into a tool that strengthens equity and quality in contemporary healthcare.

CONCLUSION

This chapter has examined the complex relationship between healthcare digitalization and digital well-being, highlighting the transformative role of technologies—particularly the Electronic Health Record (EHR)—within contemporary healthcare systems. From a sociological and interdisciplinary perspective, healthcare digitalization is not merely a technical innovation but a socio-technical transformation that reshapes care practices, redistributes responsibilities among institutional actors, and redefines citizens' roles in healthcare. Digital infrastructures function as both operational tools and knowledge mediators, influencing the organization, interpretation, and circulation of health information across professional and institutional networks.

Healthcare digital transformation must be understood within a broader societal context characterized by the proliferation of information infrastructures, digital platforms, and algorithmic decision-making systems. The EHR serves as a central infrastructure coordinating interactions among professionals, institutions, and patients, while structuring clinical practices and defining what counts as relevant medical information. Digital health systems carry epistemological implications, as the ways in which data are categorized and processed reflect institutional priorities and organizational logics. Technology shapes both the knowledge deemed legitimate and the organization of healthcare activities, highlighting its role beyond simple operational efficiency.

The increasing datafication of healthcare introduces new actors and dynamics, including algorithms, predictive analytics, and data-driven decision-making mechanisms. These technologies participate in identifying patient risk profiles, allocating resources, and shaping diagnostic pathways. Their growing influence raises critical questions about transparency, accountability, and equity. Research demonstrates that algorithmic systems may reproduce or exacerbate social inequalities when trained on incomplete or biased datasets. Consequently, integrating artificial intelligence and digital infrastructures into healthcare requires robust ethical governance frameworks capable of safeguarding fairness, universality, and equity, which are fundamental principles of public health.

A second critical dimension concerns the transformation of the physician–patient relationship. Historically hierarchical, with physicians holding epistemic authority and patients in largely passive roles, this relationship is evolving toward participatory and collaborative models. Digital health tools, patient-generated data, and online medical information empower individuals to participate actively in decision-making, fostering a more engaged form of healthcare citizenship. Patients increasingly manage their health conditions consciously, drawing on technological resources alongside professional guidance, thereby transforming the traditional power dynamics of medical encounters.

Nonetheless, this transition introduces new challenges. Expanded digital communication channels, telemedicine platforms, and remote monitoring technologies can increase the cognitive and relational workload of healthcare professionals, creating additional organizational pressures. Furthermore, access to abundant medical information does not always translate into clarity for patients; in some instances, it may result in information overload or phenomena such as cyberchondria. The design of digital healthcare solutions must therefore extend beyond expanding access to services, emphasizing technologies that strengthen the relational and interpretive dimensions of care. Healthcare professionals remain central as interpreters of clinical information and mediators who contextualize digital data within patients' lived experiences.

Digital inequality represents a third key issue. While digital technologies are often portrayed as democratizing instruments, empirical evidence demonstrates that their benefits are unevenly distributed across social groups and territories. Digital inclusion involves more than access to devices or internet connectivity; it encompasses factors such as digital skills, educational resources, socioeconomic status, and territorial infrastructures. Individuals with higher education and cultural capital are better equipped to navigate digital platforms, interpret online health information, and effectively utilize advanced digital services. The mere existence of digital infrastructures does not guarantee meaningful inclusion or equal opportunities for engagement.

The Capability Approach provides a conceptual framework for interpreting these dynamics. Well-being is not measured solely by the availability of resources or services but by individuals' real capabilities to convert these resources into meaningful opportunities for action. Applied to digital health, this perspective emphasizes that technological tools enhance well-being only when citizens possess the necessary skills, knowledge, and institutional support to use them effectively. Digital health literacy is therefore a crucial determinant of digital well-being. Without competencies to search for, interpret, and evaluate health information, citizens risk becoming passive users rather than empowered participants in their care pathways.

This challenge creates a "second-level digital divide," in which universal digital services disproportionately benefit already advantaged populations, while vulnerable groups—such as the elderly, less-educated individuals, or residents of peripheral areas—remain excluded from the potential benefits of digital healthcare. Addressing these inequalities requires not only technological investment but also institutional measures to promote digital literacy, simplify interfaces, ensure transparency, and guarantee equitable access to infrastructures across different social and territorial contexts. The inclusive potential of digital health infrastructures depends fundamentally on these social and organizational conditions.

The question of whether the EHR can expand citizens' capabilities cannot be answered purely technologically. Investments in digital systems must be accompanied by policies aimed at empowering users, strengthening support structures, and promoting fairness in access and use. In this framework, technology becomes a means of enhancing relational, organizational, and cognitive capacities rather than replacing human expertise. A Human-Centered Digital Health model envisions digital infrastructures as tools that support professional judgment, complement experiential knowledge, and foster meaningful patient engagement. By situating technology within the broader social and institutional ecosystem, healthcare systems can leverage digital innovation while preserving human-centered care.

Digitalization presents both extraordinary opportunities and significant challenges. If guided by ethical principles, social inclusion, and institutional accountability, digital technologies can improve quality, efficiency, and accessibility of healthcare services. Conversely, if implemented without attention to inequalities and relational dimensions, they may exacerbate exclusion, depersonalization, and inequity. The future of digital health hinges not only on technological innovation but also on the capacity of societies and institutions to integrate digital progress with democratic values, social justice, and a renewed commitment to the centrality of the human person in care.

Future research should empirically explore how diverse social groups interact with digital health infrastructures to understand the conditions under which technology contributes to more inclusive, equitable, and participatory healthcare systems. Examining variations in access, digital literacy, and engagement will provide insights into how healthcare systems can mitigate structural inequalities while harnessing the potential of digital innovation. Policies, educational initiatives, and institutional strategies that support digital literacy and equitable access will be essential to realize the full benefits of digital healthcare systems.

Ultimately, the development of digital healthcare should aim at a balanced integration of technological innovation and human-centered care. Digital infrastructures must be designed to support—not replace—professional judgment and patient knowledge, enhancing relational, organizational, and cognitive capacities. They should facilitate informed decision-making, empower patients to actively participate in care, and ensure that all citizens can convert available resources into meaningful opportunities for health management. In this vision, technology functions as an enabler of well-being rather than a substitute for human care.

By promoting digital literacy, ethical governance, and equitable access, healthcare systems can leverage digitalization to strengthen both individual and collective welfare. The inclusive potential of digital health is thus contingent on institutional foresight, social support, and ethical implementation. Digital technologies can serve as instruments of empowerment when embedded within human-centered, socially aware healthcare systems that prioritize accessibility, fairness, and relational integrity.

In conclusion, digitalization represents a dual opportunity and challenge for healthcare welfare. Properly governed, it enhances quality, efficiency, participation, and accessibility. Without careful attention to social inequalities, digital health risks generating new forms of exclusion and depersonalization. The future of healthcare will depend not solely on technological progress but on the ability of societies and institutions to integrate innovation with democratic values, social justice, and the centrality of the human person.

These findings carry important implications for public institutions and policymakers involved in the governance of digital welfare systems. First, digital infrastructures should not be evaluated exclusively according to criteria of efficiency and cost reduction, but also in relation to their capacity to promote inclusive forms of digital well-being and equitable access to healthcare services. Second, the development of digital welfare requires robust public governance capable of ensuring transparency, accountability, interoperability, and democratic oversight of healthcare data infrastructures. Third, policies aimed at strengthening digital literacy, supporting vulnerable populations, and simplifying access to digital services become essential conditions for preventing healthcare digitalization from reinforcing existing social inequalities. Finally, the healthcare sector demonstrates how digital transformation processes are likely to reshape the broader architecture of welfare states, making the governance of digital infrastructures a central issue for the future of social citizenship.

Through careful design, policy support, and educational initiatives, digital health can become a tool that strengthens relational practices, organizational coordination, and citizen empowerment. The success of digital healthcare relies on aligning technological capacities with social realities, ensuring that all citizens are equipped to benefit from advances in digital health infrastructures. Only by combining innovation with human-centered principles can digital health fulfill its potential to contribute meaningfully to inclusive and equitable healthcare systems.

REFERENCES

Azzopardi-Muscat, N., & Sorensen, K. (2019). Towards an equitable digital public health era: Promoting equity through a health literacy perspective. *European Journal of Public Health*, *29*(3, Supplement_3), 13–17. DOI: 10.1093/eurpub/ckz166

Barillà, L., & Locatelli, N. (2013). Welfare, tecnologie digitali e imprese sociali. *WelfareOggi*, *3*, 85–89.

Batalden, M., Batalden, P., Margolis, P., Seid, M., Armstrong, G., Opipari-Arrigan, L., & Hartung, H. (2016). Coproduction of healthcare service. *BMJ Quality & Safety*, *25*(7), 509–517. DOI: 10.1136/bmjqs-2015-004315

Birhane, A. (2021). Algorithmic injustice: Data poverty and social inequality in AI. *Patterns (New York, N.Y.)*, *2*(2), 1–9.

Bottari, C. (2017). L'inquadramento costituzionale del Fascicolo Sanitario Elettronico. *Salute e Società*, *2*(2), 65–70. DOI: 10.3280/SES2017-002005

Bowker, G. C., & Star, S. L. (1999). *Sorting things out: Classification and its consequences*. MIT Press. DOI: 10.7551/mitpress/6352.001.0001

Büchi, M. (2021). Digital well-being as a dynamic capability. *New Media & Society*, *23*(11), 3281–3301.

Camera dei Deputati. (2024). *Il nuovo Fascicolo Sanitario Elettronico*. https://temi.camera.it/leg19/post/il-nuovo-fascicolo-sanitario-elettronico.html

Castells, M. (2009). *Communication power*. Oxford University Press.

Ciurleo, E., Ceraso, D., Iaquinta, P., & Comite, U. (2025). Digitalizzazione e disuguaglianze: Un'analisi empirica sulle regioni italiane. *Regional Economy*, *9*, 15–31.

Cordella, A. (2005). Actor Network Theory per lo studio dei sistemi informativi. *Sinergie Rapporti di Ricerca*, *19*, 71–86.

Dadà, S. (2022). Autonomia in telemedicina. L'e-patient tra indipendenza e coinvolgimento. *Teoria*, *42*(2), 33–51.

Dècina, M. M. (2016). *Digital divide et impera: Il ritardo del digitale è un caso?* Editori Riuniti.

Di Viggiano, P. (2014). Sanità digitale e Welfare elettronico. *Rivista Elettronica di Diritto, Economia. Management*, *3*, 74–95.

Dominici, P. (2019). *Dentro la società interconnessa: La cultura della complessità per abitare i confini e le tensioni della civiltà ipertecnologica*. Franco Angeli.

Epifani, S. (2020). *Sostenibilità digitale: Perché la sostenibilità non può fare a meno della trasformazione digitale*. Digital Transformation Institute.

European Commission. (2025). *Digital decade 2025: eHealth indicator study*. Publications Office of the European Union. https://digital-strategy.ec.europa.eu/en/library/digital-decade-2025-ehealth-indicator-study

Eurostat. (2023). *Digitalisation in Europe – level of digital skills in 2023*. Eurostat News Release. https://ec.europa.eu/eurostat/web/interactive-publications/digitalisation-2024

Ferguson, C. J. (2007). The good, the bad and the ugly: A meta-analytic review of positive and negative effects of violent video games. *The Psychiatric Quarterly*, *78*(4), 309–316. DOI: 10.1007/s11126-007-9056-9

Freidson, E. (1970). *Professional dominance: The social structure of medical care*. Transaction Publishers.

Fudim, M., Feldman, D. I., & Sayed, A. (2025). Digital health: From remote monitoring to remote care. *Journal of Cardiac Failure*, *31*(2), 489–491. DOI: 10.1016/j.cardfail.2024.08.033

Giarelli, G., Genova, A., & Moretti, V. (Eds.). (2023). *Personalizzazione della cura e partecipazione dei cittadini nella società digitale sindemica*. Franco Angeli.

Gui, M., Fasoli, M., & Carradore, R. (2017). "Digital Well-Being": Developing a new theoretical tool for media literacy research. *Italian Journal of Sociology of Education*, *9*(1), 155–173.

Kleinman, A., Eisenberg, L., & Good, B. (1978). Culture, illness, and care: Clinical lessons from anthropologic and cross-cultural research. *Annals of Internal Medicine*, *88*(2), 251–258. DOI: 10.7326/0003-4819-88-2-251

Krieger, N. (2011). *Epidemiology and the people's health: Theory and context*. Oxford University Press. DOI: 10.1093/acprof:oso/9780195383874.001.0001

Lo Schiavo, L., & Giumelli, R. (2021). Dal sociale al social: Società in trasformazione. Una mappatura del campo analitico. *Sociologie*, *2*(1), 5–18.

Lupton, D. (2016). *The quantified self*. Polity Press.

Lupton, D. (2018). *Digital health: Critical and cross-disciplinary perspectives*. Routledge.

Martines, F. (2019). La digitalizzazione della pubblica amministrazione. *Medicine and Law*, *2*, 146–161.

Mayer-Schönberger, V., & Cukier, K. (2013). *Big data: A revolution that will transform how we live, work, and think*. Eamon Dolan/Houghton Mifflin Harcourt.

Ministero della Salute. (2021). *Fascicolo Sanitario Elettronico: stato di attuazione e prospettive*. https://www.salute.gov.it/portale/temi/p2_6.jsp?id=5323&area=fascicoloSanitarioElettronico&menu=vuoto

Mishler, E. G. (1984). *The discourse of medicine: Dialectics of medical interviews*. Bloomsbury Academic.

Mocellin, S. (2023). Il lavoro nel framework del capability approach: L'interpretazione di A. Sen. *Lavoro Diritti Europa*, *1*, 1–18.

Mol, A. (2008). *The logic of care: Health and the problem of patient choice*. Routledge. DOI: 10.4324/9780203927076

Mori, L. (2019). Il flebile bisbiglio degli organi. Datificazione della salute e processi di costruzione identitaria. *Rassegna Italiana di Sociologia*, *60*(3), 531–558.

Norman, C. D., & Skinner, H. A. (2006). eHEALS: The eHealth literacy scale. *Journal of Medical Internet Research*, *8*(4), 1–7. DOI: 10.2196/jmir.8.4.e27

Nussbaum, M. C. (2011). *Creating capabilities: The human development approach*. Harvard University Press. DOI: 10.4159/harvard.9780674061200

O'Neil, C. (2017). *Armi di distruzione matematica*. Bompiani.

Obermeyer, Z., Powers, B., Vogeli, C., & Mullainathan, S. (2019). Dissecting racial bias in an algorithm used to manage the health of populations. *Science*, *366*(6464), 447–453. DOI: 10.1126/science.aax2342

Organisation for Economic Co-operation and Development. (2023). *Health at a glance 2023: OECD indicators*. OECD Publishing. https://doi.org/.DOI: 10.1787/7a7afb35-en

Parsons, T. (1991). *The social system*. Routledge.

Pasceri, E. (2025). Knowledge Organization Systems come strumenti di sorveglianza sanitaria. L'applicazione della ICD in Italia. *AIDA Informazioni: Rivista di Scienze dell'informazione*, 43(1-2), 45–62.

Pasquale, F. (2015). *The black box society: The secret algorithms that control money and information*. Harvard University Press. DOI: 10.4159/harvard.9780674736061

Pasqualotto, L. (2014). Disabilità e inclusione secondo il capability approach. *L'integrazione Scolastica e Sociale, 13*(3), 278–284.

Pravettoni, G., & Triberti, S. (2019). *Il medico 4.0: Come cambia la relazione medico-paziente nell'era delle nuove tecnologie*. Edra.

Saraceni, G. (2019). Digital divide e povertà. *Dirittifondamentali.it*, 2, 1–19.

Sen, A. (1999). *Development as freedom*. Knopf.

Sharon, T. (2016). La Googleizzazione della ricerca sanitaria: Dall'innovazione dirompente all'etica dirompente. *Medicina Personalizzata, 13*(6), 563–574.

Sharon, T. (2017). Self-tracking for health and the quantified self: Re-articulating autonomy, solidarity, and authenticity in an age of personalized healthcare. *Ethics and Information Technology, 19*(2), 93–106.

Sharon, T. (2018). Quando la salute digitale incontra il capitalismo digitale, quanti beni comuni sono in gioco? *Big Data & Society, 5*(2).

Sørensen, K., Van den Broucke, S., Fullam, J., Doyle, G., Pelikan, J., Slonska, Z., & Brand, H. (2012). Health literacy and public health: A systematic review and integration of definitions and models. *BMC Public Health, 12*(1), 80. DOI: 10.1186/1471-2458-12-80

Star, S. L. (1999). The ethnography of infrastructure. *The American Behavioral Scientist, 43*(3), 377–391. DOI: 10.1177/00027649921955326

Star, S. L., & Ruhleder, K. (1996). Steps toward an ecology of infrastructure: Design and access for large information spaces. *Information Systems Research, 7*(1), 111–134. DOI: 10.1287/isre.7.1.111

Terzi, L. (2013). Disabilità e uguaglianza civica: La prospettiva del capability approach. *Italian Journal of Disability Studies, 1*(1), 41–58.

Topol, E. J. (2019). *Deep medicine: How artificial intelligence can make healthcare human again*. Basic Books.

Treu, T. (2021). *La digitalizzazione del lavoro: Proposte europee e piste di ricerca, conversazioni sul lavoro a distanza*. Cacucci Editore.

Van Dijck, J., Poell, T., & De Waal, M. (2018). *The platform society: Public values in a connective world*. Oxford University Press. DOI: 10.1093/oso/9780190889760.001.0001

Van Dijk, J. (2005). The deepening divide: Inequality in the information society. *Sage (Atlanta, Ga.)*. Advance online publication. DOI: 10.4135/9781452229812

Van Dijk, J. (2020). *The digital divide*. Polity Press.

Wajcman, J. (2015). *Pressed for time: The acceleration of life in digital capitalism*. University of Chicago Press.

White, R. W., & Horvitz, E. (2009). Cyberchondria: Studies of the escalation of medical concerns in web search. *ACM Transactions on Information Systems*, *27*(4), 1–37. DOI: 10.1145/1629096.1629101

World Health Organization. (2021). *Global strategy on digital health 2020–2025*. World Health Organization. https://www.who.int/publications/i/item/9789240020924

World Health Organization. Regional Office for Europe. (2022). *Equity within digital health technology within the WHO European Region: A scoping review*. World Health Organization. https://www.who.int/europe/publications/i/item/WHO-EURO-2022-6810-46576-67595

Zuboff, S. (2019). *The age of surveillance capitalism: The fight for a human future at the new frontier of power*. PublicAffairs.

Chapter 5

The Sociotechnical Reconfiguration of Care:

Digital Health, Algorithmic Governance, and Inequalities

Noemi Crescentini
http://orcid.org/0000-0002-4831-4987
University of Naples Federico II, Italy

Giuseppe Michele Padricelli
http://orcid.org/0000-0003-3096-1104
University of Naples Federico II, Italy

ABSTRACT

This chapter presents a systematic review of the scientific literature on digital health within welfare systems, analysing a corpus of 5,977 articles indexed in Web of Science between 2012 and 2025. Through Latent Dirichlet Allocation (LDA) topic modelling, eight thematic areas are identified, mapping the discursive configurations through which digital health is constructed as a sociotechnical object in contemporary academic production. The analysis reveals that the computationalisation of health constitutes a structural transformation of epistemologies, institutional rationalities, and power relations governing care - not a linear process of technical modernisation. The findings highlight an unresolved tension between emancipatory promises and dynamics of algorithmic stratification, exclusion, and control. The chapter concludes by identifying priorities for a sociological research agenda oriented towards equity.

DOI: 10.4018/979-8-2600-3043-1.ch005

INTRODUCTION

The digital transformation of welfare systems and public health represents one of the most significant challenges on the sociotechnical plane and, at the same time, one of the most contested of the contemporary era. Far from constituting a mere technical modernisation of bureaucratic infrastructures, it penetrates deeply into the normative, institutional and relational foundations of advanced democracies, redrawing the very categories of need, risk and vulnerability through which contemporary states organise access to care (Eubanks, 2018; Meijer & Bolivar, 2016).

Since the 1980s, four broad areas have progressively taken shape within the field of *digital health*: telemedicine, which made possible the remote delivery of care through information and communication technologies; *eHealth*, which transformed the ways in which health information is sought and exchanged; *mHealth*, which has mobilised portable digital devices for individual and public health purposes; and, more recently, *algorithmic medicine*, which incorporates advances in artificial intelligence into complex processes of diagnostic prediction and therapeutic personalisation (Marent & Henwood, 2021). In quantitative terms, the scale of this transformation is considerable: the global *digital health* market was estimated at approximately 176 billion dollars in 2023 and was projected to reach 449 billion by 2032 (SkyQuest, 2024); the OECD reported in 2023 that, following a pandemic-driven peak, the number of teleconsultations had stabilised at 1.0 per patient per year across member countries, signalling a structural - albeit uneven - integration of telemedicine within health systems (OECD, 2023).

Concurrently, according to an analysis conducted by the WHO European Region across 50 member states in 2024–2025, artificial intelligence is progressively being integrated into national health systems, albeit with profound disparities in governance frameworks, workforce preparedness, and data protection (WHO/Europe, 2025).

This historical stratification is not, however, simply technical: it reflects profound transformations in the power relations between patients, health professionals and institutions, in the epistemic structure of medical knowledge, and in the ways in which the body is surveilled, measured and governed (Lupton, 2017; Clarke et al., 2010). Digital health, far from constituting a neutral set of instrumental innovations, takes shape as a sociotechnical configuration that carries with it specific normative imaginaries, economic interests and governmental rationalities: a constellation that the sociology of health and Science and Technology Studies subject to critical disarticulation (Jasanoff, 2004; Winner, 2017).

It is precisely within this framework that one of the most consequential and still insufficiently examined transformations of our time takes hold: the progressive penetration of digital technologies into welfare systems, with profound effects on the modalities of access to social and health services, on eligibility criteria, and not least on the forms of institutional control.

This transformation rearticulates the principles of universality, de-commodification and stratification that Gøsta Esping-Andersen (1990) identified as the constitutive axes of twentieth-century welfare regimes, subjecting them to unprecedented pressures generated by the logic of *datafication.*

From a European standpoint, data from Eurofound (2025) document how at least ten EU member states now permit entirely digital applications for the vast majority of social services, at the risk of producing insurmountable barriers for digitally excluded segments of the population.

The scholar Virginia Eubanks (2018) has highlighted how automated systems for the management of health risk and poverty do not merely rationalise the delivery of services: they tend to transform welfare into a surveillance and control apparatus, concealing forms of structural discrimination behind a putative algorithmic objectivity. Against this backdrop, the technocentric optimism that pervades a large part of institutional discourse[1] risks obscuring the concrete dynamics through which digitalisation amplifies pre-existing inequalities, produces new exclusions and concentrates informational power in the hands of a small number of accountable actors.

Against this backdrop, the present contribution is guided by the following research question: *how is digital health as a sociotechnical field discursively constructed in international academic production, and what epistemic, institutional and governance tensions structure its operationalisation within contemporary welfare systems?* This question is addressed through a systematic review of the scientific literature combined with computational text analysis, with the dual aim of mapping the thematic configurations through which digital health is constructed as an object of academic inquiry, and of subjecting these configurations to a sociologically oriented interpretive reading capable of rendering visible the power dynamics, normative tensions and stratification processes that traverse the field. The choice of a corpus-based, empirically grounded approach responds to the need to move beyond both techno-optimistic narratives and aprioristic critiques, anchoring the analysis in the actual discursive landscape of international scholarly production on the nexus between digital health and welfare systems.

DIGITAL HEALTH AS A SOCIOTECHNICAL FIELD IN TRANSFORMATION

At the conceptual level, *digital health* does not take shape as an ordered and neutral set of technical innovations, but rather as a sociotechnical field traversed by profound epistemic, relational and power tensions, the understanding of which requires an analysis that goes well beyond the functionalist categories of efficiency and empowerment. The very notion, moreover, has proved historically unstable and semantically elusive: as the more critical literature has observed, it tends to operate as an empty signifier, mobilised strategically by institutional, industrial and political actors to attract investment and legitimise reforms, in the absence of adequate reflection on the social transformations it produces and reproduces (Marent & Henwood, 2023).

The historical depth of this field is sociologically significant: from the earliest experiments in the computerisation of medicine in the 1960s through the progressive development of electronic health record systems in the 1970s, it is with the diffusion of personal computers in the 1980s and the explosion of the Internet in the 1990s that digital health takes shape as a mass phenomenon. The notion of *eHealth* begins to circulate in institutional documents as the promise of a more accessible, efficient and patient-centred health system (Evans, 2016; Marent & Henwood, 2023).

It is within this historical arc that the most recent and structurally significant process for contemporary health sociology is inscribed: the entry of Big Tech into the health ecosystem, which expresses a new rationality of health governance founded upon the valorisation of health data as a strategic asset (Zuboff, 2019; Srnicek, 2017). Digital platforms institute new power asymmetries between those who produce data and those who control it, reconfiguring the patient as a data-producing user within commercial ecosystems whose valorisation logics are distinct from those of the public service (Sharon, 2018; Petersen, 2018). The fundamental paradox of this configuration lies in the fact that, whilst the dominant discourse celebrates the democratisation of access to health information, effective power structures consolidate around a restricted number of private actors who exercise asymmetric control over data flows and over the algorithmic architectures through which medical knowledge is produced - the problematic nexus around which the present contribution is articulated.

METHODOLOGY

The present contribution adopts the systematic literature review (SLR) as its research strategy, a choice motivated by the very nature of the object of inquiry and by the epistemological objectives that guide it. In a disciplinary field such as that of digital health applied to welfare systems that is characterised by a vast, multidisciplinary scientific output traversed by theoretical orientations frequently in tension with one another, the SLR proves to be the epistemically most appropriate instrument for constructing a critical, systematically grounded and intersubjectively controllable synthesis of the available evidence, overcoming the limitations of traditional narrative reviews which, whilst offering interpretative flexibility, are more exposed to the influence of the researcher's theoretical preconceptions in the process of selecting and organising the literature (Petticrew & Roberts, 2008).

The methodological architecture of this contribution integrates two complementary approaches. The SLR provides the procedural scaffolding through which evidence is selected and organised in an explicit, transparent and intersubjectively evaluable manner (Petticrew & Roberts, 2008). LDA topic modelling, by contrast, operates as an instrument of *discovery* rather than verification: it renders visible latent thematic structures that resist detection through manual reading of large-scale corpora (Boumans & Trilling, 2018). This dual movement - from the statistical identification of thematic configurations to their sociological reading through STS and critical health sociology frameworks - responds to the challenge of governing analytically a body of literature at once too vast for exhaustive qualitative reading and too discursively complex for purely quantitative reduction.

The process was conducted in adherence to the PRISMA 2020 guidelines (*Preferred Reporting Items for Systematic Reviews and Meta-Analyses*). The selection process for the analytical corpus followed the four sequential phases specified by the protocol: identification, screening, eligibility verification and definitive inclusion (as illustrated in the flow diagram presented in Figure 1). The graphical representation renders public and verifiable the chain of methodological decisions made at each stage, enabling the reader to evaluate the coherence between the criteria declared at the research design stage and the choices actually made during the selection of materials (Page et al., 2021).

The bibliographic search was conducted exclusively on Web of Science, chosen for its multidisciplinary coverage across the social sciences, health sciences and science and technology studies - the three areas most pertinent to the analytical framework adopted here - and for its indexing standards, which ensure a level of quality control consistent with the epistemological requirements of a systematic review (Petticrew & Roberts, 2008). The exclusive use of a single database constitutes a recognised limitation, as contributions indexed solely in Scopus or domain-specific databases such as PubMed may not be captured; however, this choice reflects a deliberate prioritisation of disciplinary breadth over exhaustive coverage, in keeping with the sociological rather than biomedical orientation of the inquiry. The adopted temporal horizon (2012–2025) responds to a precise historical-sociological rationale: it is from the early 2010s that the convergence between the computerisation of health systems, the diffusion of the Internet and the progressive digitalisation of social policies begins to take shape as an autonomous object of academic inquiry, producing a sufficiently extensive body of studies to render a systematic synthesis both necessary and scientifically justified (Marent & Henwood, 2023; Petticrew & Roberts, 2008).The inclusion of studies published up to 2025 also allows the most recent trajectories of international research to be captured, in particular those connected to the introduction of artificial intelligence into social and health service delivery systems, to the diffusion of major technological platforms in the field of care, and to the emergence of a critical debate on the algorithmic governance of welfare.

Figure 1. The process of data collection (own elaboration)

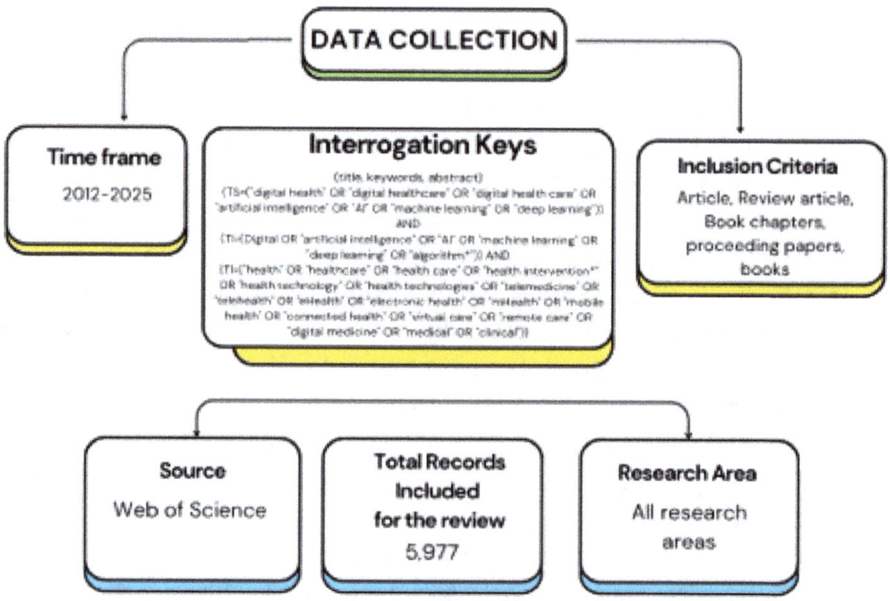

THE DATA COLLECTION PROCESS AND THE EMPIRICAL BASE

The construction of the search string required preliminary reflection of a conceptual rather than merely technical order. The field of *digital health* is characterised, as illustrated in the preceding paragraphs, by a pronounced semantic instability and by a lexical plurality that reflects the interdisciplinary and historically stratified nature of the field itself: the same practices and technologies are denoted by different terminologies depending on the disciplinary background of the authors, the historical phase of the studies' production and the institutional context of reference (Marent & Henwood, 2023). The search string was constructed through the combined use of the Boolean operators OR and AND, according to a two-level logic: within each conceptual cluster, the OR operator functioned expansively, saturating the semantic field through the aggregation of all synonymic or semantically contiguous descriptors; between the different conceptual clusters, the AND operator instead functioned restrictively, ensuring that the retrieved results satisfied simultaneously all of the predefined thematic conditions (Bramer et al., 2018).

At the operational level, the search string was structured around three distinct conceptual clusters, interconnected through the Boolean operator AND internally articulated by means of the OR operator. The first cluster delimited the perimeter of *digital health* in its broadest sense, aggregating the most widely used denominations in the international literature - *digital health, digital healthcare, digital health care* - with the principal technological descriptors that constitute its most recent applicative infrastructures, including *artificial intelligence, AI, machine learning* and *deep learning*. The second cluster, operating on the title field of publications, extended the technological coverage by including the term *algorithm*, particularly relevant in the sociological and STS literature that thematises the social implications of automated decision-making systems. The third cluster finally anchored the search to the health domain of reference, through an extended constellation of descriptors - from *health* and *healthcare* to *telemedicine, telehealth, eHealth, mHealth, connected health, virtual care, remote care* and *digital medicine* - covering the principal semantic configurations through which the international literature articulates the relationship between digital technologies and care systems, whilst acknowledging that the lexical boundaries of an emergent and rapidly evolving field such as digital health cannot be exhaustively delimited by any single search string

The temporal distribution of publications (Figure 2) reveals a pattern of progressive growth: up to 2018 scientific output remained at fewer than 100 articles per year, before accelerating sharply to approximately 500 in 2021, surpassing 800 in 2023, approaching 1,200 in 2024 and settling at over 2,000 in 2025. The inflection point of 2020–2021 coincides with the acceleration of health digitalisation induced by the Covid-19 pandemic, which acted as a catalyst for research processes already under way.

Figure 2. Distribution of publications 2012–2025 (own elaboration)

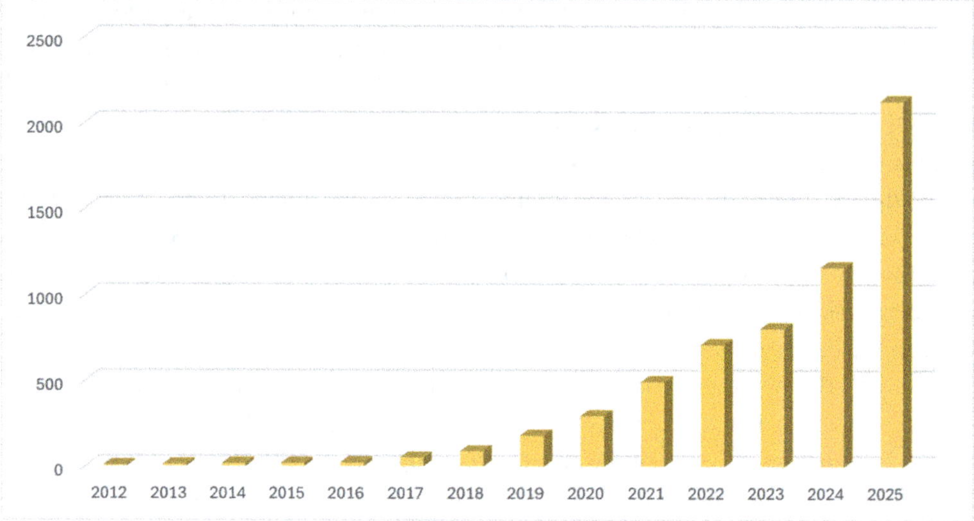

In greater detail, as evident from the summary presented in Figure 3, the field is dominated primarily by scientific production in the research areas of *Occupational health* (1161 articles) and *Science and technology studies (STS) (1,097 articles).* A significant contribution - the output of which has grown particularly in the last two years - is provided by the areas of *Healthcare sciences (740 articles), Social sciences (713 articles) and Education (530 articles),* in addition to the area of *Computer science (921 articles)* whose output is instead in decline in the 2024–2025 window. The residual portion of the dataset is composed of contributions from the areas of *Business and Economics (322 articles), Environmental science (233 articles), Government and Law (126 articles), Humanities (124 articles) and Public administration*[2] *(10 articles).*

Following the process of deduplication and cleaning of the bibliographic matrix - operations indispensable for eliminating duplicate records generated by the search and for ensuring the integrity of the selected corpus - the final corpus comprises 5,977 articles.

Figure 3. Publication trends by Research Area 2012–2025 (own elaboration)

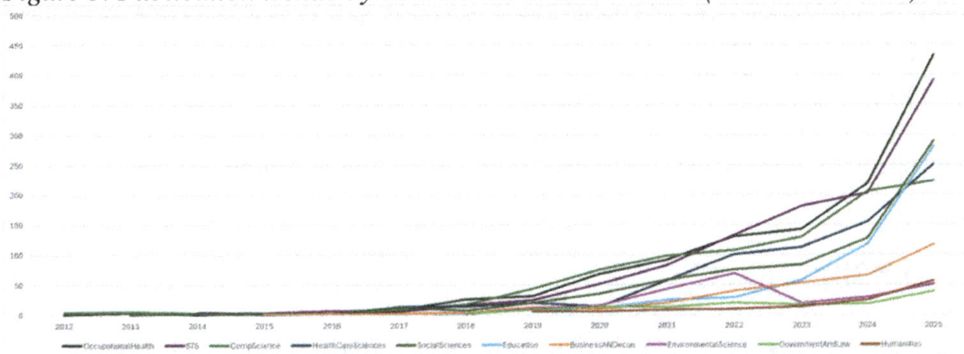

The analysis of the textual corpus was conducted through an integrated procedure combining content analysis techniques and computational text modelling, in line with the progressive affirmation of digital methods in the social sciences as instruments for the systematic exploration of large documentary corpora (Salganik, 2019; Boumans & Trilling, 2018). The theoretical-methodological point of departure resides in the recognition that scientific documents are not neutral objects but socially situated products oriented by specific institutional, disciplinary and discursive rationalities: an assumption consolidated in the tradition of social research that demands analytical instruments capable of rendering explicit this dimension of the social construction of knowledge (Prior, 2020; Amaturo & Punziano, 2013). In this perspective, content analysis is not reducible to a simple procedure of textual classification but takes shape as an analytical apparatus capable of mediating between the semantic dimension of texts and the social structures that orient their production (Krippendorff, 2018).

At the operational level, a systematic and categorical content analysis model was adopted, one that interrogates the corpus through a system of predefined analytical categories, organised into three distinct conceptual domains and constructed so as to translate the principal theoretical questions of the research into empirically observable and comparable indicators (Corbetta, 2003). The first domain pertains to general metadata and includes descriptive variables such as the language of publication, the diachronic distribution of articles and the institutional affiliation of authors, enabling reconstruction of the academic geography and temporal trajectory of scientific production in the field. The second domain pertains to the configuration of production and concerns the documentary typology, the disciplinary fields of belonging and the editorial venues, providing indicators useful for mapping the dynamics of scientific legitimation and the disciplinary boundaries of the field. The third domain pertains to semantic-content dimensions and concentrates the analysis on titles, abstracts and keywords - that is, the textual elements most dense with meaning and most directly representative of the authors' conceptual choices (Hsieh & Shannon, 2005).

Once the structuring of the corpus was complete, the *stop-words* were removed. Computational processing was conducted using T-Lab software, an analytical environment specialised in the exploration of complex discursive structures (Lancia, 2004).

ANALYSIS AND RESULTS

To identify the latent thematic structure within the corpus, *Latent Dirichlet Allocation* (LDA) was implemented, a generative probabilistic model now established as one of the most effective instruments for *topic modelling* on large-scale corpora (Blei et al., 2003). The underlying logic of the model assumes that each document is representable as a mixture of latent themes - the *topics* - and that each theme is defined by a probability distribution over the terms of the corpus vocabulary. From the application of this procedure, eight thematic areas emerged, whose labelling required an interpretive process grounded in the convergence between statistical parameters such as the relative frequency of terms and the distribution of shared lemmas across *topic*, as well as semantic criteria of internal coherence, in line with the methodological guidelines for the qualitative validation of *topic modelling* models (Chang et al., 2009; Roberts et al., 2014).

The first topic, relabelled "Normative and Governance Challenges"[3], takes shape as an analytical apparatus focused on the regulatory, ethical and institutional conditions that structure the processes of artificial intelligence adoption in the field of digital health. Observing the elementary contexts and high-frequency lexical co-occurrences -*AI*, *healthcare*, *intelligence*, *technology*, *challenge*, *innovation*, *framework*, *application*, *data*, *bias*, *governance*, *ethical/ethic* - it is possible to identify a normative problematisation of technological innovation that runs transversally through the corpus. In this sense, the semantic centrality of *AI* and *healthcare* does not simply refer to an applicative domain but contributes to discursively constructing a sociotechnical space in which the introduction of artificial intelligence is inseparable from apparatuses of regulation, standardisation and control, according to a logic consistent with what the STS literature has defined as the co-production of technical and social order (Jasanoff, 2004).

In a passage from Kumar et al. (2025) it is stated: «*Countries like Saudi Arabia are facing unique adoption challenges in their public healthcare, these challenges are specific to AI literacy, understanding and effective usage of AI technologies*» which signals that the challenges are not reducible solely to the technical dimension but are deeply rooted in differentiated institutional and cognitive conditions. In parallel, the passage from Nilsen et al. (2022) «*there are many knowledge gaps regarding how to implement and best use AI to add value to mental healthcare services, providers, and consumers*» highlights how knowledge gaps constitute a normative criticality in the broad sense: insofar as they obstruct the definition of shared standards and the elaboration of effective regulatory practices, they take shape as structural obstacles to the translation of innovation into institutionally recognised practice, in line with what is discussed in the literature on *implementation science* (Nilsen, 2022).

The properly normative dimension emerges with greater evidence in the recurrence of terms such as *data*, *bias*, *ethical/ethic* and *governance*, which contribute to discursively constructing artificial intelligence as an object of moral and juridical evaluation, as well as technical. The passage «*the use of AI in healthcare has potential risks that need to be mitigated*» (Kharisma et al., 2026, p. 226)), read in connection with references to «*algorithmic bias, accessibility of AI technologies, ethical and privacy concerns, unrepresentative training datasets, lack of transparency and interpretability*» (Ghanem, 2025), delineates a discursive repertoire articulated around risk management and the social production of trust. In this perspective, *data and bias* are not exhausted by their technical valence but become symbolic operators through which questions of distributive equity, institutional responsibility and the legitimacy of algorithmic action are articulated and negotiated, in line with the AI governance principles elaborated at the international level (WHO, 2021; Siala & Wang, 2022) and with the critical reflections on algorithmic justice developed within *critical data studies* (D'Ignazio & Klein, 2020).

Finally, the co-occurrence of *innovation*, *future* e *potential* with *challenge* and *issue* yields a structurally ambivalent representation of artificial intelligence in digital health: on the one hand, an enabling technology and transformative promise; on the other, an object of continual normative problematisation and a field of tension between expectations and constraints. Such ambivalence reflects dynamics widely documented in models of technological adoption, in which the diffusion of innovation is conditioned by multilevel determinants including regulatory, institutional and organisational constraints (Damschroder et al., 2009), and which refer more generally to the intrinsically conflictual nature of processes of sociotechnical stabilisation (Bodewitz et al., 1987).

Overall, the topic "Normative and Governance Challenges" portrays the adoption of artificial intelligence in digital health as a regulated and situated sociotechnical process, in which effective usage depends on the capacity of actors - institutional, professional and political - to construct, negotiate and legitimise governance frameworks that render innovation not only technically implementable, but also ethically sustainable and socially acceptable.

The topic designated "Attitudes of Future Doctors"[4] was understood as a discursive field in which the dispositions of medical students towards artificial intelligence emerge from the intersection between processes of professional socialisation, educational practices and institutional configurations of medical training. The lexical frequencies - in particular *student, education, medical, AI, curriculum, teaching, ChatGPT, educational, attitude, skill, perception, knowledge, training* - allow the identification of a semantics strongly anchored to the formative dimension as a space for the production and negotiation of meanings related to digital health.

The textual extracts contribute to delineating this configuration. The passage from Neittaanmäki (2025) «This survey study aimed to assess medical students' attitudes toward AI in medicine in general... and students' use of generative AI in medical studies» (Tung, 2023) highlights how students are not mere recipients of innovation but active subjects in the incorporation of generative AI tools into everyday learning practices, redefining the boundaries between the acquisition of *knowledge* and cognitive delegation to technologies. In parallel, the passage from Duan et al. (2025) «To analyse medical students' perceptions, trust, and attitudes toward artificial intelligence (AI) in medical education, and explore their willingness to integrate AI in learning and teaching practices» highlights the relevance of categories such as perception, attitude and trust as interpretive apparatuses through which actors attribute meaning and legitimacy to the use of AI, in a context structured by teaching practices.

The recurrence of *curriculum, course, training* and *university* furthermore indicates that such dispositions do not emerge spontaneously but are institutionally produced and regulated.

A further analytical element is constituted by the notion of *readiness*, made explicit in Arab-Borzu (2025) «it is essential to examine the perceptions and readiness of medical students... their ability to utilize this emerging technology effectively is crucial» and «evaluate their readiness to work with medical AI technology» (Tung et al, 2025). Such a concept does not refer to a simple individual predisposition but to a relational configuration that emerges from the interaction between formative resources, technological exposure and institutional expectations. The topic highlights a multilevel articulation in which cognitive dimensions (*attitude, perception*), practical dimensions (*training*, use of *ChatGPT*) and structural dimensions (*education, curriculum, university*) co-produce the conditions of possibility for the future adoption of AI. Such a configuration is consistent with sociotechnical models of innovation, which emphasise that adoption is the outcome of alignment processes between actors, technologies and institutional contexts, as well as with technology acceptance models that highlight the role of subjective representations and facilitating conditions (Venkatesh et al., 2003).

Overall, the topic "Attitudes of Future Doctors" may be interpreted as a discursive repertoire of professional prefiguration, in which digital health is anticipated and normatively oriented within educational contexts. The adoption of artificial intelligence in health systems thus appears rooted in processes of social construction that precede entry into the professional field, rendering medical training a crucial apparatus to produce competences, expectations and forms of legitimacy linked to the use of digital technologies.

The topic "Digital Health Literacy Inequalities and Behaviour"[5] may, by contrast, be considered as a discursive field focused on the social distribution of digital health literacy and its implications for health behaviours mediated by digital technologies. The predominance of terms such as *digital*, *health*, *literacy*, alongside *information*, *technology*, *access*, *user*, *online*, *service* and *public*, indicates that digital literacy in the health domain is discursively constructed as a practice situated at the intersection between technological infrastructures, access to informational resources and the capacity for use by social actors. In parallel, the presence of *social*, *community*, *factor* and *influence* signals a pronounced relational and structural dimension, in which competences are not uniformly distributed but rather are rooted in differentiated and historically determined social contexts (Zarcadoolas, Pleasant & Greer, 2006).

The elementary contexts confirm and articulate this configuration. Ji et al. (2024) argue that «*the limited proficiency in digital health behaviours among rural residents has emerged as a significant factor intensifying health disparities between urban and rural areas*» highlighting how digital health literacy is directly connected to structural factors and conditions of differentiated access, functioning as a mechanism for the production and reproduction of inequalities between groups and territories.

The cognitive and operative dimension of literacy is made explicit in the passage from König et al. (2024), «*Digital health literacy... describes the ability to seek, find, understand, and use health information from the internet to address health problems*» which directly evokes the co-occurrences *information*, *online* and *technology* and inscribes itself within the tradition of functional definitions of literacy as a multidimensional competence (Norman & Skinner, 2006).

The nexus between literacy and behaviour emerges with particular clarity in the passage from Ning et al. (2024), «*Investigating the digital health literacy of university students can facilitate their effective acquisition of health information and adoption of appropriate protective behaviours*» in which the capacity for accessing and utilising information translates into socially oriented health conduct. This relationship is further articulated in the passage from Georgantopoulos & Lamnisos (2025): «*health literacy and digital health literacy... have been associated with self-efficacy and improved health outcomes*» suggesting that literacy acts as a mediating variable between cognitive competences and incorporated practices, influencing both the intention to use and the capacity to perceive and manage health risk, according to a logic akin to socio-cognitive models of behaviour (Bandura, 2004).

The structurally unequal dimension of the phenomenon is further reinforced by the textual reference in Chung et al. (2024), «*disparities in digital health technology literacy exist among different generations, potentially exacerbating health inequities*», which brings to light how socio-demographic variables - including generation, geographical residence and social position - operate as differentiating factors in the opportunities for access to and use of digital health resources.

. They operate as differentiating factors in the opportunities for access to and use of digital health resources. In this framework, the co-occurrences of *pandemic* and *COVID-19* signal how such stratification dynamics were not only confirmed but amplified in contexts of systemic crisis, in which access to *online* services and digital health infrastructures became a necessary condition for participation in the management of public health, accentuating pre-existing inequalities (Beaunoyer, Dupéré & Guitton, 2020).

At the interpretive level, the topic delineates a configuration in which digital health literacy emerges as a form of sociotechnical capital distributed in an unequal manner that differentially structures the possibilities of access, use and interpretation of digital health information. The dimensions *social* and *community* indicate that such competences are produced and reproduced within specific relational and institutional contexts, whilst *technology* and *online* define the socio-material infrastructure through which such processes are articulated, configuring what Lupton (2014) has described as the intertwining of digital practices and health subjectivity.

Overall, the integration of co-occurrences and textual extracts allows the topic "Digital Health Literacy Inequalities and Behaviour" to be interpreted as a discursive repertoire of digital stratification in health, in which differences in competences between social groups translate into differences in behaviours, intentions to use and health outcomes.

The fourth topic, relabelled "Advanced Models for Health Data Analysis"[6] takes shape as a discursive field centred on the advanced computational modelling of clinical data, in which digital health is articulated through practices of *data analysis* based on *deep learning* architectures and complex algorithmic systems. The distribution of words as *deep*, *learning*, *model*, *data*, *algorithm*, *network*, *neural*, *dataset*, *classification*, *detection*, *segmentation*, *accuracy*, *system*, *monitor*, *image*, *medical*, *IoT*, *smart*, evidences a semantics strongly oriented towards the construction of analytical and predictive infrastructures, in which clinical data becomes the object of algorithmic transformation.

The textual extracts confirm this configuration. The passage from Sun et al. (2019) «medical health data has also increased dramatically… however… mixed medical big data format, many incomplete records, and a lot of noise… it is still difficult to analyse medical big data» highlights how *data* health data is characterised by structural heterogeneity (complex datasets), incompleteness and *noise*, rendering necessary the adoption of advanced *analysis* techniques. In this context, the centrality of *model* and *algorithm* emerges as a response to such criticalities, whilst the contrast "traditional machine learning methods can't effectively mine the rich information… while deep learning builds a hierarchical model» signals a transition towards approaches based on *deep learning* and *neural network.*

The systemic and infrastructural dimension of the topic emerges from the co-occurrence of *system*, *monitor*, *IoT* and *smart*, which indicate an extension of analytical techniques beyond the individual clinical case towards integrated digital ecosystems. This is consistent with the work of Huang et al. (2021), «a deep learning-based medical material inventory management model is constructed… effectively utilizes the data… establishes a corresponding inventory management model» which shows how models are not limited to diagnosis but are also employed in the management and *monitoring* of health processes.

A further element concerns the quality and availability of data, as made explicit in the work of Shimizu et al. (2022) «the major challenge is the lack of available labelled datasets… propose… unsupervised deep learning using only healthy normal data». Here the tension between the abundance of *data* and the scarcity of *dataset* labelled datasets highlights a structural limitation, which pushes towards the adoption of unsupervised techniques and adaptive methodological solutions.

The topic expresses the datafication and algorithmisation of medical knowledge: models, algorithms and systems reorganise clinical knowledge into computational forms. *Classification, detection and prediction* indicate a cognitive delegation to automated systems, whilst *accuracy* becomes a normative criterion. Dataset quality, noise and informational limits reveal the material and infrastructural constraints of knowledge production. Overall, "Advanced Models for Health Data Analysis" represents advanced modelling in digital health, in which *deep learning and neural network* redefine diagnosis, management and monitoring of health systems.

The fifth topic designated "Impact and Cost-Effectiveness in Digital Health Implementation"[7] takes shape as a discursive field centred on the experimental evaluation and empirical evidence of digital health interventions, in which technological implementation is analysed through formalised methodological devices oriented towards the measurement of outcomes. The distribution of words as *intervention, trial, randomize, systematic, review, study, protocol, outcome, participant, conduct, report, app, mobile, mHealth, digital, health*, evidences a semantics strongly anchored to the logic of controlled experimentation and the production of standardised evidence.

The textual extracts confirm this configuration. A passage from Van der Horst et al. (2025) «the potential of digital health interventions to optimize healthcare is promising… however… a systematic review… is lacking» signals a tension between expectations of impact and the necessity of empirical validation.

The presence of terms such as *intervention*, *protocol*, *conduct* and *participant* indicates that digital health technologies are treated as experimental objects, subjected to rigorous design and implementation procedures. This emerges implicitly in the cited studies, in which *digital health interventions* are analysed in relation to their *outcome*, both in clinical terms and in terms of health service utilisation. In this framework, the co-occurrence of *report* and *outcome* highlights the centrality of the measurement and formalisation of results as a condition for scientific legitimation.

The applicative dimension is further reinforced by the presence of *app*, *mobile* and *mHealth*, which evoke specific forms of digital intervention, as evidenced in the passage from Morris et al. (2023) «*digital health interventions such as smartphone applications (mHealth) or Internet resources (eHealth)... to improve the management of chronic conditions*». This indicates that the experimentation concerns not abstract technologies, but concrete devices embedded in care practices and in the everyday contexts of users.

From a sociological standpoint, the topic may be interpreted as an expression of an experimental rationality in digital health, in which technological innovation is subjected to validation processes based on standardised methodologies, such as *randomized controlled trials*, *systematic review* and formalised research protocols. *intervention* thus become objects of empirical proof, inserted into an evidence regime that privileges the measurability of *outcome* and the replicability of studies. In this perspective, digital health is constructed as a field of intervention governed by the logics of evidence-based medicine, in which the legitimacy of technologies depends on their capacity to demonstrate efficacy and impact through recognised methodological devices (Greenhalgh, 2017).

The sixth topic, relabelled "Modelling of Patient Admission Processes and Data Protection"[8] takes shape, in a sociologically and methodologically oriented perspective, as a discursive field centred on the modelling of patient pathways and the governance of health data, in which digital health practices are articulated at the intersection between informational integration, data security and the construction of predictive models. The semantics recurring in the elementary contexts as *patient data*, *health data*, *data protection*, *interoperability*, *secure exchange*, *clinical decision support systems*, *modelling*, *prediction*, *admission processes*, *data warehouse*, delineates a discursive domain in which data management represents simultaneously an analytical resource for the production of knowledge and an object of normative and institutional regulation.

The textual extracts articulate this configuration along complementary interpretive axes. The passage from Duguet et al. (2025) «*personal medical data... are isolated in an independent exclusive medical system that respects professional secrecy... not linked to administrative data*» highlights an institutionally sanctioned separation between different types of health data, inscribed within a normative framework of *data protection* that reflects the tension between professional confidentiality and informational integration. This configuration is further specified in the passage «*a digital platform where patients can store and manage access to their personal health data in a fully protected and secure manner*», which introduces a dimension of distributed control and patient agency in the management of their own health information, attributable to the logics of *patient empowerment* that traverse contemporary discourse on digital health (Lupton, 2014; Andreassen & Trondsen, 2010).

The technical-organisational dimension emerges clearly in the passage from Romaniuk et al. (2021), «*digital transformations... aim at creating an interoperable digital healthcare ecosystem... secure exchange of personal medical data... strict compliance with the access levels*», in which *interoperability*» in which interoperability and security protocols are discursively constructed as infrastructural conditions for systems integration. In this perspective, data management is not exhausted in its technical valence, but takes shape as a process regulated by norms, standards and differentiated access levels, which may lead to logics of stratification in access to informational resources and to power dynamics between differently positioned institutional actors (Bowker & Star, 2000).

The adoption of instruments such as *word embedding* for modelling the semantic relations between symptoms, diagnoses and hospitalisations signals a growing sophistication in the computational representation of clinical data and, at the same time, a progressive redefinition of clinical judgement as a hybrid practice, in which professional competences and algorithmic systems stand in a relation of mutual influence (Topol, 2019; Elish & Boyd, 2018).

Overall, the topic "Modelling of Patient Admission Processes and Data Protection" takes shape as a discursive repertoire of health data governance and modelling, in which the adoption of digital health depends on the capacity of institutional actors to construct infrastructures that are simultaneously interoperable, secure and analytically performative. Digital health thus emerges as a sociotechnical space in which data protection and their predictive valorisation are profoundly intertwined, rendering necessary an analysis of the institutional, normative and technological conditions that regulate their access, use and distribution of benefits.

The seventh topic, relabelled "Machine Learning as Predictive Instrument"[9] takes shape as a discursive field focused on the use of machine learning as a predictive device in clinical practice, in which digital health is articulated through the transformation of health data into instruments of risk anticipation and decision support. The dominant semantics in the elementary contexts as *prediction*, *model*, *machine learning*, *clinical features*, *risk*, *data*, *radiomics*, *staging*, delineates an epistemic orientation in which medical knowledge is progressively reformulated in probabilistic and computational terms, signalling a transformation of the modalities through which clinical knowledge is produced, validated and applied (Topol, 2019; Obermeyer & Emanuel, 2016).

The textual extracts articulate this configuration along complementary interpretive axes. The passage from Stark et al. (2019) «*we developed machine learning models that used highly accessible personal health data to predict five-year breast cancer risk*» highlights a transition from traditional statistical models to machine learning models capable of operating on more immediately available personal health data, reducing dependence on costly or invasive diagnostic procedures.

The integrative dimension of the models emerges with clarity in the work of Zhang et al. (2025), «*a model constructed by combining machine learning (ML) with clinical features and ultrasound radiomics in the clinical staging of cervical cancer*» which highlights how prediction is the result of the systematic combination of heterogeneous informational sources. Such integration reflects a growing complexity of modelling apparatuses, in which clinical signals and digital data are articulated to produce classifications and predictions of greater accuracy, according to a logic of hybridisation between medical expertise and algorithmic inference that redefines traditional diagnostic practices (Lupton, 2014; Timmermans & Berg, 2003).

At the interpretive level, the topic may be read as an expression of a predictive rationality in contemporary medicine, in which machine learning operates as a device for the anticipation and stratification of risk. The models do not merely describe existing clinical conditions but produce projections on future health status - *risk prediction, clinical staging* - contributing to redefining diagnostic and decision-making practices according to an anticipatory logic that shifts the focus of medical intervention from the observation of the present to the probabilistic management of the future (Adams, Murphy & Clarke, 2009).

An element of analytical significance is represented by the redefinition of the relationship between technical complexity and data accessibility. If on the one hand machine learning models allow the valorisation of *personal health data* of more immediate availability, on the other they introduce a growing opacity in decision-making processes, connected to the non-interpretable nature of many machine learning algorithms: the so-called problem of the *black box* (Pasquale, 2015). Such opacity raises structural questions concerning transparency, independent validation and accountability in the use of predictive instruments in high-impact clinical contexts, interrogating the boundaries between the professional autonomy of the clinician and algorithmic delegation, and returning to the centre of the debate the question of *explainability* as a requirement that is at once epistemic and ethical (Doshi-Velez & Kim, 2017).

Overall, the topic "Machine Learning as Predictive Instrument" takes shape as a discursive repertoire of algorithmic prediction in health, in which the adoption of digital health manifests through the capacity to transform heterogeneous data into risk estimates and clinical decision support.

The eighth topic, relabelled "Machine Learning as Research Instrument"[10] takes shape as an epistemic device to produce knowledge in digital health contexts, in which artificial intelligence is not merely an applicative or predictive instrument, but a method of inquiry for the identification of patterns, risk factors and latent relations in health data. The more frequent words and textual segments as *machine learning, mental health, risk factors, prediction, data, youth, children, adolescents, well-being, behaviour, health information*, delineate an epistemic orientation in which empirical research is progressively mediated by computational techniques, signalling a transformation of the knowledge infrastructures of contemporary health research (Kitchin, 2014; Lupton, 2014).

The textual extracts articulate this configuration along distinct and complementary interpretive axes. The passage from Ndikumana et al. (2025) «*the study aims to apply machine learning techniques to predict mental health and identify its associated risk factors among Rwandan youth*» highlights how machine learning is employed not only as a predictive instrument in the strict sense, but as an analytical device for the identification of the determinants of mental health, extending the epistemic function of the algorithm from prediction to the exploration of underlying causal structures.

The properly cognitive dimension of machine learning emerges with even greater evidence in the passage from Wang et al. (2022), «*based on machine learning and health information statistics, this paper studies the development of infant health diagnosis and intelligence*». They put computational techniques within a framework of *health information statistics*, highlighting a convergence and progressive hybridisation between traditional statistical approaches and algorithmic methods. In this perspective, machine learning does not replace the established analytical instruments of health research, but constitutes an extension and reformulation thereof, redefining the thresholds of manageable complexity and the modalities of inference production (Obermeyer & Emanuel, 2016).

A further significant analytical axis concerns the capacity of the models to render visible complex and non-linear relations between variables. The passage «*this study aimed to identify key mental health and addictive behaviour factors associated with adolescent SWB through machine learning models*» shows how algorithms are used to identify associations between *mental health, behaviour* and *subjective well-being*, bringing to light patterns that are difficult to detect through linear analytical approaches. The centrality of concepts such as *well-being, quality of life* and *life outcomes* furthermore signals an extension of the analytical object beyond clinical outcomes in the strict sense, towards psycho-social and subjective dimensions that broaden the epistemic perimeter of algorithm-mediated health research, bringing it closer to the traditions of the sociology of health and the life course (Cockerham, 2005).

The topic may thus be read as an expression of an epistemological transformation in health research, in which machine learning progressively assumes the role of a knowledge infrastructure capable of redefining the modalities of knowledge production. The models do not simply operate as instruments for the verification of theoretically grounded hypotheses, but as exploratory devices that contribute to the generation of new analytical categories and the discovery of emergent relations in the data, according to a logic that shifts the research process from hypothetico-deductive approaches towards inductive and *pattern-oriented* modalities (Anderson, 2008).

An element of sociological significance is represented by the specificity of the populations studied, frequently constituted by groups in developmental phases as *youth*, *children*, and *adolescents* which evidences a particular attention to processes of biographical formation and life trajectories as privileged objects of computational inquiry. This orientation suggests that machine learning is mobilised to understand complex and multidimensional phenomena across the life course, integrating biological, psychological and social dimensions into analytical configurations that exceed the capacities of traditional statistical instruments, whilst raising unresolved questions regarding the reducibility of subjective experience to computationally detectable patterns (Lupton, 2016; Ruckenstein & Schüll, 2017).

Overall, the topic "Machine Learning as Research Instrument" takes shape as a discursive repertoire of the computationalization of health research, in which the adoption of digital health manifests through the use of machine learning as an instrument of analysis, exploration and knowledge production. This configuration brings to light how contemporary health research is progressively oriented towards analytical models capable of managing the complexity, heterogeneity and multidimensionality of data, whilst simultaneously redefining the epistemic categories through which the field constructs its own objects of inquiry.

DISCUSSION

The analysis of the topics emerging from the LDA modelling of the corpus allows them to be traced back to four analytical dimensions that structure the discursive field of digital health in a complementary manner (as shown in Figure 4): the dimension of *tools and techniques*, that of *professionalism*, that of *clinical-operative implementations*, and that of *governance and social impact*. In this perspective, the four dimensions do not operate as rigid classificatory categories, but as analytical lenses capable of illuminating different aspects of one and the same transformation process, in keeping with the co-production approach elaborated by Jasanoff (2004), according to which technical order and social order mutually stabilise one another in configurations that cannot be understood by artificially separating the technical dimension from the institutional and normative one.

Figure 4. Visual model of the eight LDA-derived topics organised across four analytical dimensions of digital health as a sociotechnical field (N = 5977 articles; WoS, 2012–2025). (own elaboration)

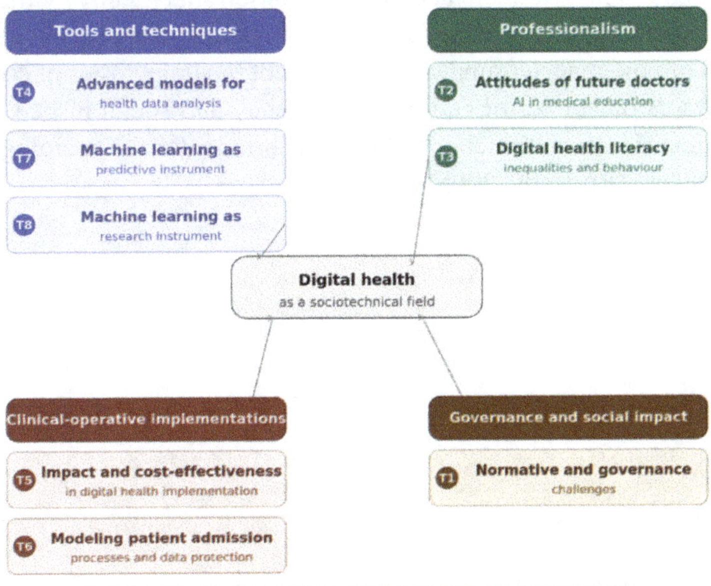

CONCLUSIONS

The analysis maps digital health as a sociotechnical field traversed by epistemic and normative tensions that resist both techno-optimistic readings and critical oversimplifications (Jasanoff, 2004; Lupton, 2017). The most significant result is the progressive digitalisation of medical knowledge as a structural process that redefines the categories through which clinical knowledge is produced, validated and applied, and through which welfare systems organise access to social and health services.

Future perspectives require, in the short term, investment in situated empirical studies on algorithmic implementation in health and welfare contexts, developing analytical instruments capable of capturing the configurations generated by the intersection between digital exclusion, social marginalisation and health literacy deficits through intersectional and longitudinal approaches (Beaunoyer et al., 2020). In the medium to long term, a comparative research agenda on the regimes of algorithmic governance across European welfare systems - in dialogue with law, political economy and political science (Fourcade & Healy, 2017) - is urgently needed.

In conclusion, digital health takes shape as a sociotechnical field in which the fundamental categories of medical knowledge, the material conditions of access to care and the forms of institutional rationality that govern welfare in contemporary societies are redefined. To understand this redefinition analytically (without yielding either to uncritical enthusiasm or to aprioristic pessimism) and to contribute to the construction of governance frameworks that orient the trajectories of computationalisation towards objectives of equity, transparency and social justice, constitutes one of the most significant intellectual responsibilities for the sociology of health in the years ahead (Burawoy, 2005).

REFERENCES

Adams, V., Murphy, M., & Clarke, A. E. (2009). Anticipation: Technoscience, life, affect, temporality. *Subjectivity, 28*(1), 246–265. DOI: 10.1057/sub.2009.18

Amaturo, E., & Punziano, G. (2013). *Content analysis tra comunicazione e politica.* Ledizioni.

Anderson, D. R. (2008). *Model based inference in the life sciences: a primer on evidence.* Springer New York. DOI: 10.1007/978-0-387-74075-1

Andreassen, H. K., & Trondsen, M. (2010). The empowered patient and the sociologist. *Social Theory & Health, 8*(3), 280–287. DOI: 10.1057/sth.2010.9

Arab-Borzu, Z., Keikha, L., & Shahraki-Mohammadi, A. (2025). Knowledge, Readiness, and Perception of Medical Students Toward Medical Artificial Intelligence: A Cross-Sectional Study. *Journal of Medical Education and Curricular Development, 12*, 23821205251407758. Bandura, A. (2004). Health promotion by social cognitive means. *Health Education & Behavior, 31*(2), 143–164.

Beaunoyer, E., Dupéré, S., & Guitton, M. J. (2020). COVID-19 and digital inequalities: Reciprocal impacts and mitigation strategies. *Computers in Human Behavior, 111*, 106424. DOI: 10.1016/j.chb.2020.106424 PMID: 32398890

Blei, D. M., Ng, A. Y., & Jordan, M. I. (2003). Latent dirichlet allocation. *Journal of Machine Learning Research, 3*(Jan), 993–1022.

Bodewitz, H. J. H. W., Buurma, H., & de Vries, G. H. (1987). Regulatory science and the social management of trust in medicine. In Bijker, W. E., Hughes, T. P., & Pinch, T. (Eds.), *The social construction of technological systems* (pp. 243–259). MIT Press.

Boumans, J. W., & Trilling, D. (2018). Taking stock of the toolkit: An overview of relevant automated content analysis approaches and techniques for digital journalism scholars. *Rethinking research methods in an age of digital journalism*, 8-23.

Bowker, G. C., & Star, S. L. (2000). Invisible mediators of action: Classification and the ubiquity of standards. *Mind, Culture, and Activity, 7*(1-2), 147–163. DOI: 10.1080/10749039.2000.9677652

Bramer, W. M., De Jonge, G. B., Rethlefsen, M. L., Mast, F., & Kleijnen, J. (2018). A systematic approach to searching: An efficient and complete method to develop literature searches. *Journal of the Medical Library Association: JMLA, 106*(4), 531. DOI: 10.5195/jmla.2018.283 PMID: 30271302

Burawoy, M. (2005). For public sociology. *American Sociological Review, 70*(1), 4–28. DOI: 10.1177/000312240507000102 PMID: 15926908

Chang, J., Gerrish, S., Wang, C., Boyd-Graber, J., & Blei, D. (2009). Reading tea leaves: How humans interpret topic models. *Advances in Neural Information Processing Systems*, •••, 22.

Chung, Y., Shin, H., Kim, H., & Kim, J. S. (2024). The role of health empowerment on digital health technology literacy by generation. *American Journal of Health Behavior, 48*(4), 967–978. DOI: 10.5993/AJHB.48.4.8

Clarke, A. E., & Shim, J. (2010). Medicalization and biomedicalization revisited: technoscience and transformations of health, illness and American medicine. In *Handbook of the sociology of health, illness, and healing: A blueprint for the 21st century* (pp. 173–199). Springer New York.

Cockerham, W. C. (2005). Health lifestyle theory and the convergence of agency and structure. *Journal of Health and Social Behavior, 46*(1), 51–67. DOI: 10.1177/002214650504600105 PMID: 15869120

Corbetta, (2003). *Social Research Theory, Methods and Techniques*, Londra. *Sage (Atlanta, Ga.).*

D'ignazio, C., & Klein, F., L. (. (2020). Seven intersectional feminist principles for equitable and actionable COVID-19 data. *Big Data & Society, 7*(2), 2053951720942544. DOI: 10.1177/2053951720942544 PMID: 32802347

Damschroder, L. J., Aron, D. C., Keith, R. E., Kirsh, S. R., Alexander, J. A., & Lowery, J. C. (2009). Fostering implementation of health services research findings into practice: A consolidated framework for advancing implementation science. *Implementation Science : IS, 4*(1), 50. DOI: 10.1186/1748-5908-4-50 PMID: 19664226

Doshi-Velez, F., & Kim, B. (2017). Towards a rigorous science of interpretable machine learning. *arXiv preprint arXiv:1702.08608.*

Duan, S., Liu, C., Rong, T., Zhao, Y., & Liu, B. (2025). Integrating AI in medical education: A comprehensive study of medical students' attitudes, concerns, and behavioral intentions. *BMC Medical Education, 25*(1), 599. DOI: 10.1186/s12909-025-07177-9 PMID: 40269824

Duguet, A. M., Dubruel, N., & Sebbag, E. R. (2025). Digital Health, Health Data Base and Artificial Intelligence in France: What Benefits for Patients and Society Interests. *Medicine and Law*, •••, 201. DOI: 10.63776/CHMT7934

Elish, M. C., & Boyd, D. (2018). Situating methods in the magic of Big Data and AI. *Communication Monographs, 85*(1), 57–80. DOI: 10.1080/03637751.2017.1375130

Esping-Andersen, G. (1990). *The three worlds of welfare capitalism.* Polity Press.

Eubanks, V. (2018). *Automating inequality: How high-tech tools profile, police, and punish the poor*. Macmillan+ ORM.

Eurofound (2025). *Europe's Digital Welfare Revolution: Progress at What Price?* European Foundation for the Improvement of Living and Working Conditions.

Evans, R. S. (2016). Electronic health records: then, now, and in the future. *Yearbook of medical informatics, 25*(S 01), S48-S61.

Fourcade, M., & Healy, K. (2017). Classification situations: Life-chances in the neoliberal era. *Historical Social Research. Historische Sozialforschung, 42*(1), 23–51.

Georgantopoulos, A., & Lamnisos, D. (2025). Associations of Health and Digital Health Literacy with Health-Related Quality of Life: A Cross-Sectional Study in Greece and Cyprus. *Journal of Health Literacy, 11*(1), 64–79.

Ghanem, S., Moraleja, M., Gravesande, D., & Rooney, J. (2025). Integrating health equity in artificial intelligence for public health in Canada: A rapid narrative review. *Frontiers in Public Health, 13*, 1524616. DOI: 10.3389/fpubh.2025.1524616 PMID: 40171421

Greenhalgh, T. (2017). *How to implement evidence-based healthcare*. John Wiley & Sons.

Hsieh, H. F., & Shannon, S. E. (2005). Three approaches to qualitative content analysis. *Qualitative Health Research, 15*(9), 1277–1288. DOI: 10.1177/1049732305276687 PMID: 16204405

Huang, B., Gan, W., & Li, Z. (2021). Application of medical material inventory model under deep learning in supply planning of public emergency. *IEEE Access : Practical Innovations, Open Solutions, 9*, 44128–44138. DOI: 10.1109/ACCESS.2021.3057869

Jasanoff, S. (2004). The idiom of co-production. In *States of knowledge* (pp. 1–12). Routledge. DOI: 10.4324/9780203413845-6

Ji, H., Dong, J., Pan, W., & Yu, Y. (2024). Associations between digital literacy, health literacy, and digital health behaviors among rural residents: Evidence from Zhejiang, China. *International Journal for Equity in Health, 23*(1), 68. DOI: 10.1186/s12939-024-02150-2 PMID: 38594723

Kharisma, D. B., Hernoko, A. Y., & Thalib, P. (2026). Artificial intelligence in healthcare: Risk analysis and regulatory issues. *The Theory and Practice of Legislation, 14*(1), 46–62. DOI: 10.1080/20508840.2025.2576415

Kitchin, R. (2014). Big Data, new epistemologies and paradigm shifts. *Big Data & Society, 1*(1), 2053951714528481. DOI: 10.1177/2053951714528481

König, L., Kuhlmey, A., & Suhr, R. (2024). Digital health literacy of the population in Germany and its association with physical health, mental health, life satisfaction, and health behaviors: Nationally representative survey study. *JMIR Public Health and Surveillance, 10*(1), e48685. DOI: 10.2196/48685 PMID: 38381497

Krippendorff, K. (2018). *Content analysis: An introduction to its methodology.* Sage publications.

Kumar, R., Singh, A., Kassar, A. S. A., Humaida, M. I., Joshi, S., & Sharma, M. (2025). Adoption challenges to artificial intelligence literacy in public healthcare: An evidence based study in Saudi Arabia. *Frontiers in Public Health, 13*, 1558772. DOI: 10.3389/fpubh.2025.1558772 PMID: 40371275

Lancia, F. (2004). *Strumenti per l'analisi dei testi.* Franco Angeli.

Lupton, D. (2014). *Digital sociology.* Routledge. DOI: 10.4324/9781315776880

Lupton, D. (2016). *The quantified self.* John Wiley & Sons.

Lupton, D. (2017). *Digital health: Critical and cross-disciplinary perspectives.* Routledge. DOI: 10.4324/9781315648835

Marent, B., & Henwood, F. (2021). Digital health. In *Routledge international handbook of critical issues in health and illness* (pp. 261–275). Routledge. DOI: 10.4324/9781003185215-24

Marent, B., & Henwood, F. (2023). Digital health: A sociomaterial approach. *Sociology of Health & Illness, 45*(1), 37–53. DOI: 10.1111/1467-9566.13538 PMID: 36031756

Meijer, A., & Bolívar, M. P. R. (2016). Governing the smart city: A review of the literature on smart urban governance. *International Review of Administrative Sciences, 82*(2), 392–408. DOI: 10.1177/0020852314564308

Morris, T., Aspinal, F., Ledger, J., Li, K., & Gomes, M. (2023). The impact of digital health interventions for the management of type 2 diabetes on health and social care utilisation and costs: A systematic review. *PharmacoEconomics Open, 7*(2), 163–173. DOI: 10.1007/s41669-022-00377-9 PMID: 36495462

Ndikumana, F., Izabayo, J., Kalisa, J., Nemerimana, M., Nyabyenda, E. C., Muzungu, S. H., Komezusenge, I., Uwase, M., Ndagijimana, S., Twizere, C., & Sezibera, V. (2025). Machine learning-based predictive modelling of mental health in Rwandan Youth. *Scientific Reports, 15*(1), 16032. DOI: 10.1038/s41598-025-00519-z PMID: 40341215

Neittaanmäki, N. (2025, February). Swedish medical students' attitudes toward artificial intelligence and effects on career plans: A survey. [). Frontiers Media SA.]. *Frontiers in Education, 10,* 1517116. DOI: 10.3389/feduc.2025.1517116

Nilsen, P., Svedberg, P., Nygren, J., Frideros, M., Johansson, J., & Schueller, S. (2022). Accelerating the impact of artificial intelligence in mental healthcare through implementation science. *Implementation Research and Practice, 3,* 26334895221112033. DOI: 10.1177/26334895221112033 PMID: 37091110

Ning, L., Zheng, Z., Liu, M., Gao, S., Yang, X., Bi, J., Yu, X., & Yi, D. (2024). Profiles of digital health literacy among university students and its association with mental health during the COVID-19 pandemic: A latent profile analysis. *Digital Health, 10,* 20552076231224596. DOI: 10.1177/20552076231224596 PMID: 38205038

Norman, C. D., & Skinner, H. A. (2006). eHealth literacy: Essential skills for consumer health in a networked world. *Journal of Medical Internet Research, 8*(2), e506. DOI: 10.2196/jmir.8.2.e9 PMID: 16867972

Obermeyer, Z., & Emanuel, E. J. (2016). Predicting the future-big data, machine learning, and clinical medicine. *The New England Journal of Medicine, 375*(13), 1216–1219. DOI: 10.1056/NEJMp1606181 PMID: 27682033

OECD (2023). *Health at a Glance 2023: OECD Indicators.* OECD Publishing. https://doi.org/DOI: 10.1787/7a7afb35-en

Page, M. J., McKenzie, J. E., Bossuyt, P. M., Boutron, I., Hoffmann, T. C., Mulrow, C. D., ... & Moher, D. (2021). The PRISMA 2020 statement: an updated guideline for reporting systematic reviews. *bmj, 372.*

Pasquale, F. (2015). *The black box society: The secret algorithms that control money and information.* Harvard University Press. DOI: 10.4159/harvard.9780674736061

Petersen, A. (2018). *Digital health and technological promise: A sociological inquiry.* Routledge. DOI: 10.4324/9781315200880

Petticrew, M., & Roberts, H. (2008). Systematic reviews–do they 'work' in informing decision-making around health inequalities? *Health Economics, Policy, and Law, 3*(2), 197–211. DOI: 10.1017/S1744133108004453 PMID: 18634627

Prior, L. (2020). *Using documents in social research. Qualitative Research* (5th ed.). Sage.

Roberts, M. E., Stewart, B. M., Tingley, D., Lucas, C., Leder-Luis, J., Gadarian, S. K., Albertson, B., & Rand, D. G. (2014). Structural topic models for open-ended survey responses. *American Journal of Political Science, 58*(4), 1064–1082. DOI: 10.1111/ajps.12103

Romaniuk, O. O., Kozak, L. M., & Kovalenko, O. S. (2021). Formation oF interoperable Digital meDicine inFormation environment: personal meDical Data. *Science and innovation*, (17,N° 5), 50-62.

Ruckenstein, M., & Schüll, N. D. (2017). The datafication of health. *Annual Review of Anthropology, 46*(1), 261–278. DOI: 10.1146/annurev-anthro-102116-041244

Salganik, M. J. (2019). *Bit by bit: Social research in the digital age.* Princeton University Press.

Sharon, T. (2018). When digital health meets digital capitalism, how many common goods are at stake? *Big Data & Society, 5*(2), 2053951718819032. DOI: 10.1177/2053951718819032

Shimizu, M., Perinpanayagam, S., & Namoano, B. (2022). A real-time fault detection framework based on unsupervised deep learning for prognostics and health management of railway assets. *IEEE Access : Practical Innovations, Open Solutions, 10*, 96442–96458. DOI: 10.1109/ACCESS.2022.3205352

Siala, H., & Wang, Y. (2022). SHIFTing artificial intelligence to be responsible in healthcare: A systematic review. *Social Science & Medicine, 296*, 114782. DOI: 10.1016/j.socscimed.2022.114782 PMID: 35152047

SkyQuest Technology Consulting. (2024). *Global digital health market size, share and industry report, 2032*. SkyQuest Technology Consulting.

Srnicek, N. (2017). *Platform capitalism.* John Wiley & Sons.

Stark, G. F., Hart, G. R., Nartowt, B. J., & Deng, J. (2019). Predicting breast cancer risk using personal health data and machine learning models. *PLoS One, 14*(12), e0226765. DOI: 10.1371/journal.pone.0226765 PMID: 31881042

Sun, K., Chen, J., & Viboud, C. (2020). Early epidemiological analysis of the coronavirus disease 2019 outbreak based on crowdsourced data: A population-level observational study. *The Lancet. Digital Health, 2*(4), e201–e208. DOI: 10.1016/S2589-7500(20)30026-1 PMID: 32309796

Timmermans, S., & Berg, M. (2003). The practice of medical technology. *Sociology ofHealth & Illness, 25*(3), 97–114. DOI: 10.1111/1467-9566.00342 PMID: 14498932

Topol, E. J. (2019). High-performance medicine: The convergence of human and artificial intelligence. *Nature Medicine, 25*(1), 44–56. DOI: 10.1038/s41591-018-0300-7 PMID: 30617339

Tung, L. T., Thang, P. N., & Tram, N. H. M. (2025). Impact of technological development on national competitiveness: Empirical evidence from developing countries. *Competitiveness Review*, •••, 1–23.

van der Horst, A. Y., Kelders, S. M., Bohlmeijer, E. T., Schreurs, K. M., & Jukema, J. S. (2025). Digital health interventions for spinal surgery patients: A systematic scoping review. *Digital Health, 11*, 20552076251328549. DOI: 10.1177/20552076251328549 PMID: 40297368

Van Dijk, J. A. (2020). *The network society* (3rd ed.). SAGE Publications. DOI: 10.4135/9781529739114

Wang, S., Li, M., & Ng, S. B. (2022). Research on infant health diagnosis and intelligence development based on machine learning and health information statistics. *Frontiers in Public Health, 10*, 846598. DOI: 10.3389/fpubh.2022.846598 PMID: 35719653

Winner, L. (2017). Do artifacts have politics? In *Computer ethics* (pp. 177–192). Routledge. DOI: 10.4324/9781315259697-21

World Health Organization. (2021). *Global strategy on digital health 2020–2025*. https://iris.who.int/handle/10665/344249

World Health Organization Regional Office for Europe. (2025). *Artificial intelligence is reshaping health systems: State of readiness across the WHO European Region*. https://www.who.int/europe/publications/i/item/WHO-EURO-2025-12707-52481-81028

Zarcadoolas, C., Pleasant, A., & Greer, D. S. (2006). *Advancing health literacy: A framework for understanding and action*. John Wiley & Sons.

Zhang, M., Zhang, Q., Wang, X., Peng, X., Chen, J., & Yang, H. (2025). Prediction of clinical stages of cervical cancer via machine learning integrated with clinical features and ultrasound-based radiomics. *Scientific Reports, 15*(1), 18862. DOI: 10.1038/s41598-025-03170-w PMID: 40442164

Zuboff, S. (2019, January). Surveillance capitalism and the challenge of collective action. [). Sage CA: Los Angeles, CA: Sage Publications.]. *New Labor Forum, 28*(1), 10–29. DOI: 10.1177/1095796018819461

ENDNOTES

1 Summarised in the *Global Strategy on Digital Health 2020–2025* (WHO, 2021), adopted by more than 129 countries, and in the OECD recommendation according to which investments in health digitalisation can generate a return of three dollars for every dollar invested (OECD, 2023)

2 Given the component is so residual as to preclude an evident comparative synthesis of the trend, this research area was not projected on the chart.

3 This topic concentrates 19% of the total information contained in the dataset.

4 This topic concentrates 10% of the total information contained in the dataset.

5 This topic concentrates 13% of the total information contained in the dataset.

6 This topic concentrates 14% of the total information contained in the dataset.

7 This topic concentrates 14% of the total information contained in the dataset.

8 This topic concentrates 7% of the total information contained in the dataset.

9 This topic concentrates 13% of the total information contained in the dataset.

10 This topic concentrates 8% of the total information contained in the dataset.

Chapter 6
Continuous Monitoring, Early Prediction, and Public Health Policy Using IOB

Kathirvel Ayyaswamy
http://orcid.org/0000-0002-5347-9110
Department of Computer Science and Engineering, Saveetha Engineering College, Chennai, India

Naren Kathirvel
http://orcid.org/0009-0003-7581-5482
Anand Institute of Higher Technology, India

ABSTRACT

Internet of Bodies (IoB) technologies are often presented as technical infrastructures for continuous sensing, data analytics, and early risk prediction. This chapter instead treats IoB as a communication system that shapes how health information flows between bodies, devices, clinicians, institutions, and publics. We explore how connected devices on, in, and around the human body transform occasional clinic-based encounters into continuous, everyday exchanges of data, alerts, and recommendations. Building on recent work on IoT, IoMT, and IoB in healthcare, we describe the main categories of IoB devices and the types of physiological, behavioural, and contextual data they generate, but focus especially on how these data are translated into risk messages, decision support, and public-facing narratives. Particular attention is given to public health policy issues, including regulatory communication on privacy and security, institutional accountability for algorithmic decisions, and the risk that IoB-driven monitoring could widen existing inequities.

DOI: 10.4018/979-8-2600-3043-1.ch006

1. INTRODUCTION

The way we consume health is evolving from sporadic and facility-centered treatment to persistent, data-driven healthcare that follows individuals in their everyday lives. Existing IoT services in healthcare are already supported by wearable connected devices, cellphones, and cloud-based systems to support remote monitoring, telehealth, and efficient smart hospital workflows (Singh et al., 2023; Zhu & Zhu, 2023). Following on from this the Internet of Medical Things(IoMT) connects medical devices, wear devices, and health care clinical information systems to build digital health systems to allow efficient and personalized access to health care (Matthew et al., 2025; Huang et al., 2023).

IoB stands for Internet of Bodies. Patient data and health information do not have to be limited to medical reports and traditional methods. It is believed that use of IoB will ensure that the human body will become an IoT device. Thus, healthcare will be able to depend on quite intimate data flow. IoB data will be more intimate and real-time than IoT data and IoMT sensor data. The Internet of Bodies (IoB) is expected to be the next evolution of Healthcare Networks. Sensors that will be either placed on the body or implanted inside will be able to capture data in real-time. These signals will include our heartbeats, blood pressure, and even our movement pattern. Nonetheless, for optimum use of IoB in smart hospitals, integration with Blockchain, Digital Twins and other advanced technologies is essential.

In this context, Blockchain provides a strong security solution, ensuring the integrity of data and immutable audit trails for sensitive health data generated by IoB devices. In addition, experts would have the ability to analyse and simulate critical events with the aid of Digital Twins and IoB devices and systems. Hospital blockchain solutions can provide IoB data to patient-specific digital twins, enabling a real-time and dynamic personalized care ecosystem. Due to this convergence of IoB, blockchain and digital twins, a smart hospital infrastructure will be formed that will be more responsive, secure and data-driven. Boddington (2021) describes the IoB as the blending of our physical and data selves, where bodies become active nodes in digital networks. Technical work on bioelectronic sensor nodes for the IoB emphasizes ultra-low-power sensing, secure communication, and on-body energy harvesting, so that implants and wearables can operate continuously and safely as part of a dense body-centric network (Chatterjee et al., 2022). Recent reviews further argue that the convergence of micro-electro-mechanical systems (MEMS), bio-MEMS, and networked interfaces enables truly personalized medicine when these devices are integrated into IoB architectures (Marinescu et al., 2025; Mazzeo & dos Santos, 2025)

Several forces are pushing healthcare toward such IoB-driven models. The health care systems worldwide are under extreme pressure with chronic illnesses, ageing populations and the work-force scarcity to ensure quality and efficiency of patient care through only the traditional episodic visits (Zhu & Zhu, 2023; Singh et al., 2023). Reviews on IoT and IoMT have consistently found remote patient monitoring, home-based healthcare, and telehealth as the key solutions for reduced hospitalizations, decreased in-patient length of stays and enhanced care continuity in long-term chronic illnesses (Matthew et al., 2025; International Journal of Science and Research Archive (International Journal of Science and Research Archive, 2024). Meanwhile patients also have changed their attitudes towards health care; now expecting proactive, individualized health care related to their real life circumstances and not for their brevity-visit medical appointment.

In addition to the basic IoT/IoMT framework, IoB represents two critical evolutions. The first is an increased coupling between physiological, behavioral and digital data. Wearable and implantable sensors generate granular physiological data streams such as heart rate, respiratory rate, activity rhythms, and sleep patterns, while smartphone and ambient sensors provide context such as location, ambient environment and life rhythms (Taherdoost, 2024; Shajari et al., 2023). Secondly, analyses of data are coming closer to the body. Edge and on-device intelligence allow the near real-time analysis of data for pattern identification and abnormality detection, leading to immediate feedback, alarms and micro-interventions, bypassing lengthy clinic visits and periodic, centralized, batch processing (Chatterjee et al., 2022; Matthew et al., 2025).

There is growing empirical evidence that continuous monitoring can detect deterioration earlier and support safer, more efficient care. A recent hospital study using wearable sensors for continuous vital sign tracking showed that such systems can reliably measure heart rate, respiratory rate, and temperature in acutely unwell patients and support earlier recognition of clinical deterioration and virtual ward models (Joshi et al., 2025). Literature reviews of IoT-based vital sign monitoring similarly report that body-worn and home-based sensors can reduce the gaps between measurements, enable trend analysis, and improve clinician situational awareness, though they also caution about data overload and alarm fatigue (Andrade et al., 2024; Taherdoost, 2024). Remote patient monitoring programs that integrate these data streams into telehealth workflows are already being used to support chronic disease management and post-discharge follow-up and are expected to play a central role in value-based care models (Dubey & Tiwari, 2023; Schultz, 2023).

From a technological viewpoint, the IoT of the body (IoB) is built upon and integrates IoMT, wearable computing, AI and cloud/edge computing. Overviews of IoMT literature (Matthew et al., 2025; Huang et al., 2023) present system architectures that link together body area networks, secure gateways and cloud platforms to acquire and analyze medical data from the home, community and clinical environment, whereas works related to AI in wearable sensors describe how machine learning can convert body signals to meaningful outputs-e.g. Detect arhythmias, changes in gait or the development of respiratory difficulties in a passive manner (Shajari et al., 2023). Orchestrated from an IoB perspective, these component disciplines combine to move away from single device approaches towards predictive monitoring pipelines incorporating sensing, secure data transmission, multimodal data fusion, risk stratification, and timely interventions.

The attributes which are appealing about the IoB for health purposes also present significant new risks and responsibilities. The data in question are uniquely sensitive and intimate: heart rhythm, blood glucose levels, sleep stages, patterns of movement and levels of stress, and even implant telemetry, are able to convey not only states of health but also intimate details about everyday lives and activities. Surveys of the Internet of Things in health consistently flag privacy, security, interoperability and governance as persistent issues (Singh et al., 2023; International Journal of Science and Research Archive, 2024). Reviews of IoMT suggest that without robust security and interpretability mechanisms, widespread medical device networks will become vulnerable to cyber attacks, or trust in digitally delivered health services will diminish (Matthew et al., 2025). A paper by Boddington on the IoB brings to the fore broader ethical concerns around the ownership of body data, bodily autonomy and the potential for 'prediction economies' or new forms of surveillance fed by continuously measured data of all aspects of a body's state (Boddington, 2021).

Existing literature tends to fall into two camps. On one side are highly technical treatments focused on hardware, communication protocols, and low-level optimization of IoMT/IoB components (Chatterjee et al., 2022; Marinescu et al., 2025). On the other are broad IoT/IoMT or IoB conceptual and ethical discussions that describe potential opportunities and risks at a high level (Singh et al., 2023; Zhu & Zhu, 2023; Boddington, 2021). There is comparatively less work aimed at clinicians, health-system leaders, and policy makers that connects the technical capabilities of IoB with concrete care pathways, outcome measures, and practical design choices in a clear, non-technical way.

This article addresses that gap by focusing on IoB-driven healthcare for continuous monitoring, early prediction, and better outcomes, without assuming deep engineering expertise. The purpose of this framework is to: (a) clarify what IoMT and IoB are and how they relate to IoT, (b) show the flow of data for IoB across home, community and clinical settings, (c) connect IoB functionalities to clinical contexts (chronic disease management, acute exacerbation recognition, mental health, etc.) and (d) bring to the forefront the crucial ethical, legal and human factors required for deployment. Unlike previous IoMT (Matthew et al., 2025, Huang et al., 2023, Taherdoost, 2024, Shajari et al., 2023) and wearable monitoring literature, which focuses primarily on detection of critical issues or measurement across a particular domain, the proposed framework explains how IoB is applied to move clinical care "upstream", from reaction to prediction and prevention in a clinical context, whilst keeping real-world limitations in consideration. Rest of paper is divided into sections as follows. Section 2, defined the three concepts, IoT, IoMT and IoB in the health domain and outlined their unique scope and functions. Section 3 proposed a new IoB-driven health architecture and data-flow, which ranged from data sensing to analysis, prediction and intervention. Section 4 shows that this architecture can be used to deliver continuous health monitoring and early predictions in specific clinical use-cases and patient journeys. Section 5 explored the ethical, legal and social aspects in relation to IoB, focusing on privacy, consent, transparency and equality issues. Section 6 discusses future directions and summarizes how IoB-driven healthcare can contribute to better clinical outcomes, stronger patient engagement, and improved well-being when implemented responsibly.

Figure 1. IoB-driven healthcare overview

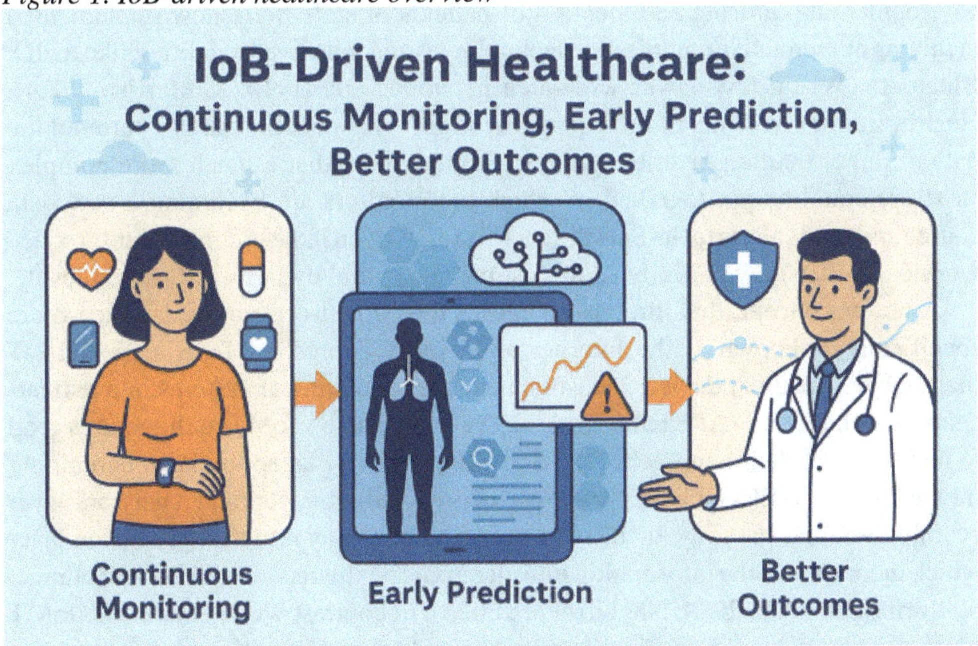

Figure 1. IoB-driven healthcare overview. The illustration shows how continuous monitoring with body-worn and ambient Internet of Bodies (IoB) devices feeds data into cloud and edge analytics for early risk prediction, which in turn supports clinicians in making proactive decisions that improve patient outcomes.

2. BACKGROUND: FROM IOT TO IOB IN HEALTHCARE

The journey from IoT to IoMT to IoB is nothing but a gradual procedure through which different technologies in the digital world are getting more and more submerged into a human body-related affair in the area of health care. When the Internet of Things (IoT) was introduced in the healthcare field, the focus was on securing access to bedside monitors, infusion pumps, and hospital equipment externally, in order that one could easily collect data automatically and share it with information systems. Extensive reviews indicate that the IoT in healthcare has matured into a research field encompassing everything from industrial processes to getting smart wards and monitoring vital signs remotely (Rejeb et al., 2023; Singh, 2023). As a result, these systems have already altered healthcare workflows in continuous data acquisition, resource visibility, and replaced manual data entries.

According to recent studies, equipment in hospitals supporting the locations, environment monitoring and location of patients or staff, were now implemented involving numerous communication technologies and sensitive modalities, like RFID, Bluetooth, Wi-Fi, low-power wide-area networks, etc. (Felix & Martins, 2024). Healthcare IoT, which is in its "first generation," is connecting devices around the patient rather than on or in the patient. Studies show that a much more complex structure could be put together, in which the monitors are becoming a new data source and sends alerts to the Surveillance System. Even if these deployments reduce workloads, they only partially address some contextual dynamics at person level.

A newer concept, that directly addresses the patient-centric needs much more specifically, is known as the Internet of Medical Things. IoMT is a special IoT that includes medical devices, sensors, actuators and clinical systems in a patient-centred architecture (Al Khatib et al., 2024). Reports on IoMT architectures tend to be layered in their approach. This typically entails a perception layer containing medical sensors (ECG, blood pressure, oxygen saturation, etc) and a network layer routing through a gateway. In turn, the data find their way into the application layer which incorporates the information into electronic health records (EHR) and clinical platforms (He et al., 2024; Naghib et al., 2025). In contrast with generic IoT, IoMT must often comply with medical regulations and safety constraints. It has stringent requirements for reliability and latency. Any failure can directly impact a diagnosis or treatment.

The research on IoMT has risen exponentially in the past few years due to the emergence of remote patient monitoring, chronic disease management, telemedicine. Systematic reviews indicate the increasing usage of IoMT for continuous monitoring and management of conditions such as hypertension, diabetes, heart failure, and respiratory disorders (El-deep et al., 2025; Matthew et al., 2025). A lot of these systems use wearable sensors and home monitoring kits linked to the cloud platform. These systems have the ability to automatically measure intelligence. They can analyze for early signs of decompensation. They alert clinicians in advance of impending crises. They also endorse "hospital at home" designs that let stable patients stay home while still under supervision from care teams in parallel. He et al. (2024); Ahmed et al. (2025) state that emerging IoMT applications combine sensor data with AI, as well as machine learning with the aim of providing risk predictions, personalizing treatment plans, or using resources more efficiently.

As IoMT devices get deployed within hospitals, at homes, and even the community settings, their security and privacy requirement become more complex. IoMT environments have less patching and securing of large numbers of heterogeneous mobile ad hoc networks with often resource-constrained devices than classical clinical systems. In a systematic review on intrusion detection in IoMT, a vast range of attacks; device, network and application layer attacks have been discussed. Attacks which include medical devices and data flows comprise eavesdropping, spoofing, denial-of-service and ransomware (Naghib et al., 2025). Due to their sensitive nature and continuous streaming, IoMT data need lighter mechanisms that include cryptography, blockchain-trace audit, AI-based intrusion detection, and other mechanisms to reduce performance impact (El-deep et al., 2025; He et al., 2024). Connecting even more medical devices raises not just technical problems but also governance and trust problems, these issues bring to light.

The Internet of Bodies is the latest advancement of Internet of Things (IoT) and Internet of Medical Things (IoMT). The Internet of Bodies is digital systems applied to and inside the human body. The Internet of Bodies is networks of devices worn on the body, embedded under the skin, or even located inside organs that continuously sense biological signals, and in some cases enable actuation, such as drug delivery or neuromodulation (Datta & Sen, 2023). IoMT refers to medical devices that can physically distance from the patient, such as smart hospital beds and connected imaging equipment. However, IoB pertains to devices that have intimate physical contact with the person, which means being part of the body's extended sensorimotor loop. This covers top-of-the-line wearables including implantable cardiac monitors, neurostimulators, smart prosthetics, and ingestible sensors that send data after they are swallowed.

According to the expert, microelectronics, MEMS, BioMEMS, and flexible electronics will enable the Internet of Body (IoB). Sensors that can distinguish between very subtle changes are now available as soft, skin-conformable patches or as micro scale implants. They are capable of measuring fine physiological details such as multi-lead ECG, intracranial pressure, local biochemical markers and complex motion. This has been stated by Marinescu and others in 2025 as well as Liu and Liu in 2025. At the same time, body-heat thermoelectric generators and motion-energy harvesting to deliver sustainable power with a view to reducing battery dependency to achieve more practical continuous monitoring (Tabaie & Omidvar, 2023).

As a result of these advancements, IoB devices can now function for long periods of time with little user input or interaction while generating dense, personalized data streams for predictive analytics and closed-loop therapies.

In a nutshell, IoB underscores a transition from "around-the-patient" monitoring to "with-the-patient" and "in-the-patient" integration. Until recently, the usual external gadgets such as smartwatches and fitness bands have been implemented in order to obtain simple parameters such as steps or heart beat (Khan & Alam, 2021). IoB goes a step further by making technology used to implant intelligence within the body's devices that augment or restore body functionality like smart prosthetic limbs, biofeedback devices for rehabilitation or implantable pumps or stimulators that adapt therapy in real time (Marinescu et al., 2025). Personalized treatment in medicine can be realized with dynamic titration of drug delivery for Parkinson's, reactive neuromodulation for epilepsy, or adaptive cardiac pacing based on real time physiological input.

Along with these chances, IoB comes with some ethical, legal and social queries that go above and beyond what was debated regarding IoT as well as IoMT. When we incorporate devices into our body or come into very close contact with our body, issues of autonomy, informed consent, and bodily integrity may be more acute. An example of a situation engages debate over rights is that of an implanted cardiac device. Who has the right to access, control, or alter, and under what conditions, the software that drives the device?

Researchers discuss how IoB complicates existing frameworks for privacy, data ownership, and responsibility, as the distinction between person and device becomes blurred (El-Khoury & Arikan, 2021; Datta & Sen, 2023). People also worry that the super-detailed biometrics and behavioral data collected by IoB devices could be used for more than just health care targeting marketing, insurance profiling, even surveillance, unless precautions are set to prevent it.

In summary, the path of development from IoT to IoMT and then IoB in healthcare depicts a gradual trend towards deeper interconnection of digital systems with the human body. The first example of IOT in Healthcare connects environments and equipment. IoMT includes clinical-grade devices that directly connect with patients' data and care pathways. IoB takes this idea a step further, creating devices that actually become part of the body's structure. Every phase along this spectrum provides more comprehensive, detailed information and more potent actions. However, it also raises additional risk layers which include safety, cybersecurity, and ethical concerns (Ahmed et al., 2025; El-deep et al., 2025). Because of this, the need for frameworks that utilize IoB to support continuous monitoring, early prediction, and improved outcomes is underscored while respecting human dignity, privacy, and equity. The remainder of the article discusses this evolution and shows how it is possible to design IoB-driven systems that provide clinically meaningful benefits without overwhelming patients, clinicians or health systems.

3. CONTINUOUS MONITORING IN IOB-DRIVEN HEALTHCARE

Real-time monitoring is what truly makes IoB-based care a practical solution. Instead of only periodically observing an individual's vital signs or behaviors a few times a day, sensor data from wearables, beds, mobile devices, and even home appliances flows almost continuously. This change from a set number of observations to near real-time monitoring is the aspect that facilitates the detection of a slow decline, reinforcement of healthy behavior, and enabling of timely intervention.

3.1 IoB as the Sensory Layer for Healthcare Digital Twins

Digital Twins in health care stand to benefit considerably from IoB data, among the most promising applications. A digital twin is a continuously evolving virtual representation that is updated and modified in real time of the physical and physiological state of a patient. Devices that comprise the Internet of Bodies (IoB)–such as wearables, implants, and ambient sensors–generate continuous streams of physiological and behavioural data to feed a digital twin.

The Internet of Bodies (IoB) acts as the sensory layer for digital twins in healthcare settings, capturing real-time vital signs (like heart rate, blood pressure, and glucose levels) and movement patterns along with activity and sleep patterns. As data streams of IoB feed into a digital twin of an individual patient, the actual patient's health state is updated in the model. Through predictive simulations, health professionals can predict health issues before they happen and identify early warning signs of deterioration for personalized interventions.

An example of this would be a digital twin who uses IoB data to show how a patient's heart condition might evolve based on their current activity, medication, and sleep levels. As arrhythmia or heart failure exacerbation difficulties can be predicted, treatment-related changes could also be recommended by the model. Furthermore, IoB devices provide real-time data feedback which keeps the digital twin updated. This ensures that the digital twin is an accurate representation of the patient's status allowing for timely interventions.

Within hospital wards, continuous monitoring of vital signs is being used to reduce the "critical care gap" between the ICU and general wards. Practices are still based on periodic checks of vital signs every 4-8 hours by nurses, using paper or electronic early warning scores to trigger escalation. These provide large blind spots during which hypoxia, hypotension or arrhythmia can go unobserved. Evidence shows that wearable or contactless monitoring can improve detection of abnormal vitals considerably, and possibly outcomes. One propensity-matched analysis from 2025 found that continuous, wireless, ward-level monitoring was associated with reduced odds of ICU admission and mortality for surgical patients when compared to intermittent monitoring (Rowland et al., 2025). One systematic review and meta-analysis focused on randomised trials similarly found that continuous ward-level monitoring was associated with reduced number of rapid response activations and potential for reduced length of stay with less certainty about mortality impact (Bowles et al., 2024). Both show that a stream of continuous data can potentially alter the course of in-hospital deterioration.

These applications at the ward-level become increasingly feasible with the development of new generations of sensors. Portable wireless systems which can be worn on the arm, chest or finger are already capable of recording heart rate, blood pressure proxies, respiratory rate and oxygen saturation without restricting patient mobility. One BJA Education article from 2025 describes how portable, lightweight, wireless patches and hubs provide almost ICU level surveillance, while also permitting patient mobility, vital for recovery (Hicks et al., 2025). Preliminary studies on wearable, photoplethysmography-based, upper-arm devices have been able to accurately measure heart rate and oxygen saturation in ward patients compared to references, thus showing that devices could be integrated into existing systems safely and could provide a steady stream of information (de Waal et al., 2025). These systems are increasingly viewed by clinicians as a vital first step in minimizing unnoticed deterioration at the ward-level, and even for step-down and telemetry units (Michard & Saugel, 2025).

Contactless sensing goes one step further by providing continuous data without needing to be adhered to the patient directly. By utilizing the micro-vibrations generated by bodily processes when lying down, ballistocardiography sensors integrated into an under-mattress device can estimate heart rate, respiratory rate, and blood pressure proxies. A 2024 study in India involving 706 general-ward patients monitored by a Dozee-EWS system produced data across over 84,000 hours that predicted a 16-hour improvement over the conventional period from initial vital sign abnormality to clinical deterioration. Such contactless monitoring fits perfectly into an IoB structure: passive measurement of physiology and behavior can feed data to the cloud and back to bedside teams in the form of risk scores and alerts.

This concept is being stretched beyond hospital use to include remote monitoring of chronic disease sufferers. Through the use of telemetry and a communications infrastructure health care professionals can monitor their patients remotely via wearable sensors and communications networks. It was noted in the journal Medical Internet Research in 2025, in a viewpoint article, that RPM is essential in managing the most prevalent chronic diseases in the US and, while already widely used in the US, its uptake in patients with heart failure, diabetes, and hypertension is predicted to increase even further (Paul et al., 2025). Wearable devices can also be useful in managing patients with COPD for the identification of exacerbations as the trend of respiratory rate, movement and oxygen saturation is monitored (Coutu et al., 2023). Unlike routine hospital visits, a patients dyspnoea, lower number of steps per day, or high number of respiratory events at night will be a useful indicator of risk through digital readouts.

Continuous monitoring on a larger scale also includes more than just the classic physiological vital signs. Wearable sensors are used to monitor fatigue and functional status which are crucial to understand people suffering chronic diseases,shift workers, and elderly patients. A recent open-access review from Computers in Biology and Medicine summarizes how artificial intelligence can be used in conjunction with multi-modal wearable sensors (such as ECG, EMG, PPG, motion, and sleep monitors) to continuously estimate physical and cognitive fatigue, thereby preventing incidents in safety-critical jobs or monitoring progression in chronic illness (Kakhi et al., 2025). This monitoring fits well into an IoB system because it correlates body signals to behaviour and context, for example, measuring how long someone has been awake and whether their physiological reserve is able to cope.

Figure 2. Continuous monitoring workflow in IoB-driven healthcare

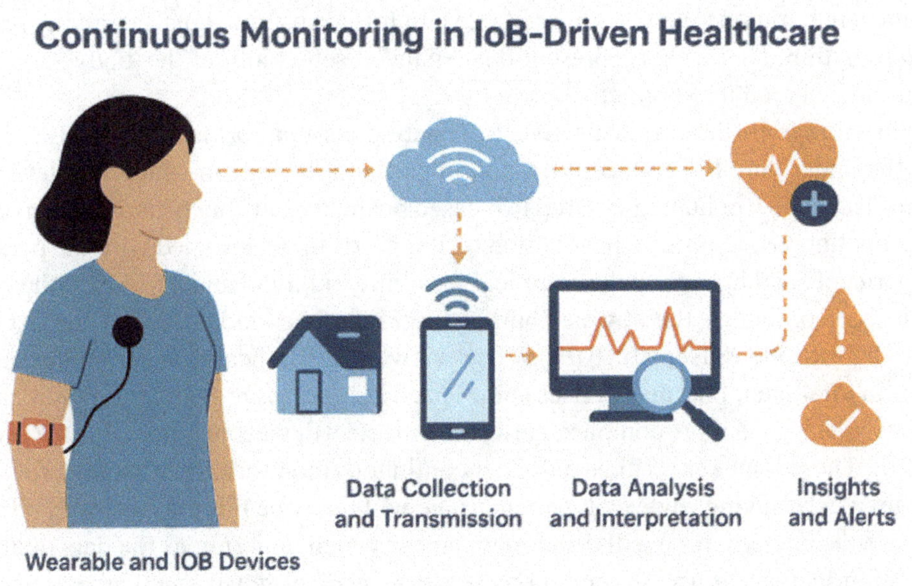

Within IoB, all of these streams-vitals, motion, sleep, social data-are used to create "digital biomarkers" and "digital phenotypes"-algorithmic features more direct in representing health than the raw data. The Artificial Intelligence Review has a 2025 systematic review describing the use of non-invasive, passive sensor data from wearable and smartphones (such as accelerometer, heart rate variability, passive activity traces) combined with machine learning for continuous predictions of CV events, progression of neurodegenerative disorders, stress etc. (Sameh et al., 2025). The paper strongly emphasizes that the continuous, passive nature of sensor data makes it particularly suitable for IoB, because it requires no active input from patients, and because it tracks changes on the time scale of weeks or months, rather than single 'snapshot' measurements.

One particularly strong use case of continuous, IoB-style monitoring is for mental health and behaviors. In contrast to clinic-based questionnaires, mental health researchers are now leveraging phone and wearables passive sensor data-location variability, phone call and text usage patterns, screen time, sleep and activity rhythm-as proxy for mood and symptom trajectories. A 2025 scoping review on J Med Internet Res describes dozens of studies where these signals were analyzed using machine learning to monitor the symptoms of depression, anxiety, psychosis, and stress across real-world conditions (Shen et al., 2025). An accompanying commentary in JAMA Network Open discusses the ability of passive phone sensing to monitor broad dimensions of psychopathology, but also highlights data quality, interpretability, and surveillance concerns, outlining some design principles for clinical integration (Webb & Fisher, 2025). In IoB terms, the signals (walking pace, sleep rhythm, phone use) represent the expanded sensorium of the 'body', and are continuously fed into predictive models.

From a system design perspective, IoB continuous monitoring is extremely reliant on the underlying IoT connectivity, and in particularly, human-centred system design. The review of human-centred IoT-based health monitoring from 2024 suggests that continuous, long-term health monitoring needs to be designed with the patient experience, and not solely the technical feasibility, in mind and highlights the current shortcomings in the way user burden, user interfaces and the social context are handled (Rashid & Nemati, 2024). The review on IoT in healthcare from the same year in Intelligent Pharmacy raises some specific concerns regarding useability and safety when using more complex, networked medical devices at home (Parihar et al., 2024). These issues are critical to IoB: if continuous monitoring is a user-unfriendly or obviously 'spying' endeavor, patient usage will likely be limited, and even if they do use the devices, they will do so in a manner which undermines the data quality.

With increasing use of continuous sensors, medical sensing and analytics will have an increasing role to play. Several reviews of emerging medical sensing technologies explain the combination of AI with new materials such as smart textiles, implantable devices and multi-analyte biosensors to offer real-time, continuous health monitoring for diseases such as cardiovascular disease, diabetes, and infection (Kirubakaran, 2025). These novel sensors can capture signals beyond the range of current wearable sensors (e.g., blood glucose, inflammatory markers, drugs levels) which IoB systems could stream into the physiological-behavioral model. However, ward-based accuracy studies caution that a single signal from any new sensing technology will require significant clinical validation, for example, the reported accuracy of the sensors of wearability-based monitoring for respiration rate was notably worse than for heart rate and oxygen saturation, suggesting that this is an area of further improvement required for early warning scores (de Waal et al., 2025; Hicks et al., 2025). Any benefit derived from continuous, IoB monitoring rests heavily upon the quality of the raw data being captured.

The presence of rich, continuous streams poses challenges for interpreting work processes. Meta-analytic work indicates that continuous monitoring detects more variances and may reduce adverse events. However, the effects on hard outcomes depend on the incorporation of alerts into clinical workflow (Bowles et al., 2024). If continuous monitoring does not come with intelligent alerting, it will generate more false alarms leading to alarm fatigue and staff frustration. According to Michard and Saugel (2025), as clinician-oriented commentaries reveal, the current focus is on evolving from historical threshold-based systems to trend-based, multivariate risk score and AI-enabled early warning systems. This, in turn, would focus on combinations of vital signs, with an eye on their trajectories and the relevant baseline pertinent to the patient. There is a similar issue with issues around home RPM. In a 2025 perspective, it is noted that whether or not metrics can be aligned with reimbursement, staffing models, and follow-up pathways, there are not only technical means to stream more and more numbers from people's homes (Paul et al. 2025).

When constant monitoring shifts to the IoB space, privacy, security, and ethics become critical issues. Constant data collection could be able to bring out sensitive information about routine, mental health and social behaviour. According to recent reviews (Parihar et al., 2024), IoT-based healthcare privacy requires privacy-preserving analytics and secure data transmission as well as user-centric control mechanisms which help in allowing patients in charge of what is collected and how it is used. The articles that focus on mental health issue warning that continuous monitoring of the behaviour is considered intrusive. They also suggest framing clinical deployment as a tool to collaborate but not as surveillance (Webb & Fisher, 2025; Shen et al. 2025). You cannot view these factors as optional. They determine whether continuous IoB systems can be acceptable to patients or clinicians in the first place.

In conclusion, continuous monitoring changes IoB-based healthcare from an archive of visits into a dynamic representation of the physiology and behavior of each individual. In hospital wards it can be used to diagnose deterioration earlier and staff can make better decisions and free up their time. In the home it may be used for management of chronic diseases, tracking fatigue and function and supporting patients with mental illness. Combinations of wearable and non-contact sensors with IoT technology and AI, result in data streams that are translated into digital biomarkers for earlier and more personalized interventions. While the evidence base is still immature and not every deployment is guaranteed to result in improved outcomes, continuous monitoring does provide a source of data that predictive, IoB based systems can draw upon to offer assistance. We will look at how these continuous data streams can be turned into dependable early warnings and targeted behavioural interventions, in the coming sections.

4. EARLY PREDICTION AND PROACTIVE CARE WITH DIGITAL TWIN SIMULATIONS

Predicting early is part of IoB-driven healthcare that enables timely action that can stop or lessen the condition of diseases. Static risk scores cannot predict any stakeholder's individual trajectory relative to other population members. Nonetheless, data from the Internet of Bodies (IoB) can elevate prediction to new heights. How? By processing the data to create a digital twin for each patient. These twins can simulate a patient's health trajectory and predict future outcomes on the basis of data from IoB devices.

Data from IoB sensors like heart rate, activity patterns, medication adherence, and sleep behavior can be connected to the cloud to continuously update a patient-specific digital twin, for example. This latest information allows healthcare providers to run "what-if" scenarios or model how changes in intervention or care plans would affect the patient's health. A digital twin could model what happens if a patient changes their medication dosage, increases their physical activity, or alters their diet so clinicians know what will happen before making a decision.

The utilization of IoB-driven data in conjunction with digital twin simulations provides a powerful tool for personalized care planning. Through simulations, clinicians can trial multiple interventions to assess which one would be the best for a patient that they are managing. Furthermore, it allows healthcare providers to take pre-emptive positive steps in patient care by being able to mitigate health detriments before they take place rather than responding to the effects.

4.1 Digital biomarkers and risk stratification

From a practical perspective, early prediction starts with risk stratification. Instead of seeing every patient with hypertension or heart failure as having the same short-term risk, IoB platforms constantly recompute a probability of deterioration using incoming sensor data and electronic records. Reviews of digital biomarker platforms highlight how combinations of heart-rate variability, sleep architecture, gait stability and self-reported symptoms can be used to cluster patients into low-, medium- and high-risk groups that change dynamically over time.

These risk estimates become more powerful when sophisticated analytics are added. Network meta-analyses of machine-learning models for sepsis prediction, for example, show that neural networks and decision-tree–based methods can outperform traditional scoring systems such as SOFA, qSOFA and NEWS in terms of discrimination. However, the same work also underlines that the prediction window matters: algorithms tend to be more accurate in the short term than when they attempt to forecast events many hours in advance. In other words, early prediction is not magic foresight; it is a careful balance between lead time and reliability.

4.2 Predicting deterioration in acute care

In acute settings, early prediction is often framed in terms of early warning scores. Large comparative studies in hospital wards have evaluated several artificial-intelligence-based scores against simpler, transparent tools such as NEWS and NEWS2. The findings are nuanced. Some machine-learning models, such as eCART, achieve higher accuracy and can identify more patients who will deteriorate within the next day, while triggering fewer false alarms. At the same time, some widely deployed proprietary scores perform worse than open, non-AI tools, reminding clinicians that "AI" in the label does not guarantee better performance.

IoB expands these hospital-based early warning systems by incorporating continuous wearable data that follow patients into and out of the ward. A recent Nature Communications study used deep learning on continuous vital-sign data from clinical-grade wearables to predict ward deterioration several hours in advance. The model learned subtle patterns in respiratory rate, heart-rate dynamics and movement that humans would struggle to recognise, and it updated risk in real time. In an IoB framework, similar models could extend into the home, learning each person's "normal" pattern and flagging deviations that might indicate early pneumonia, arrhythmia or decompensation.

Sepsis prediction illustrates both the promise and the limitations of such systems. Meta-analytic evidence suggests that machine-learning models, on average, outperform traditional sepsis scores when evaluated retrospectively. Yet a prospective evaluation of a widely used commercial sepsis model found that, when the analysis was limited to predictions made before clinicians had already started treatment, performance dropped close to chance. For IoB-driven early prediction, this is an important warning: models must be evaluated in realistic workflows and on truly prospective data, rather than only on historical records where clinicians have already acted.

4.3 Predicting exacerbations in chronic disease

Early prediction is equally important for long-term conditions, where the goal is to avoid slow, cumulative damage and sudden exacerbations. Heart failure is a clear example. Reviews of remote multiparametric monitoring through cardiac implantable electronic devices show that combining several sensor streams—intrathoracic impedance, heart rate, activity level, arrhythmia burden and respiratory patterns—can detect subclinical congestion well before the patient feels short of breath. More recent work on remote monitoring in heart failure reports algorithms that can predict hospitalisation risk weeks in advance, sometimes with average lead times of more than a month, allowing time to adjust medication, reinforce self-care and schedule earlier follow-up.

IoB extends this concept beyond implantable devices. Reviews of chronic-disease monitoring using IoT mobile sensing describe how home blood-pressure monitors, smart scales, spirometers, glucometers and environmental sensors can be linked through cloud platforms and analysed using machine learning to detect early signs of decompensation in cardiovascular disease, chronic lung disease and diabetes. By combining physiological data with behavioural indicators, such as declining step counts, increased phone inactivity or changes in speech, IoB-based predictive models can distinguish a temporary bad day from the beginning of a serious exacerbation.

Recent chronic-disease self-management reviews highlight how artificial intelligence, when wrapped into mobile apps and conversational agents, can give patients personalised recommendations in response to these early warnings. For example, a system might detect that a person with diabetes has had several nights of poor sleep and rising nocturnal glucose variability, and then suggest a tailored plan that combines modifications in evening meals, light activity, stress-reduction techniques and temporary medication adjustment, with an automatic alert to the care team if the trend continues. In this way, prediction becomes a shared decision-making tool, not simply a background algorithm.

4.4 From prediction to proactive care pathways

Early prediction only improves outcomes if it is tightly coupled to action. Studies of digital biomarker platforms stress that predictions should trigger structured care pathways that specify what clinicians, nurses, allied health professionals and patients themselves should do at each risk level. In some heart-failure remote-monitoring programmes, for instance, a rising risk score automatically queues a teleconsultation within a fixed time window, prompts medication titration protocols and activates educational messages to the patient.

In IoB-driven systems, proactive care also reaches beyond individual episodes toward long-term behaviour change. When alerts are framed as coaching rather than warnings, patients often perceive them as supportive nudges rather than surveillance. Evidence from mobile-health interventions suggests that persuasive design features, such as goal-setting, timely feedback and social support, can increase adherence and help people sustain lifestyle modifications that reduce long-term risk.Over time, the same behavioural data that feed the prediction models become a record of progress, helping both patients and clinicians to see the effect of small daily choices on future clinical trajectories.

Figure 3. IoB-enabled patient–clinician interaction

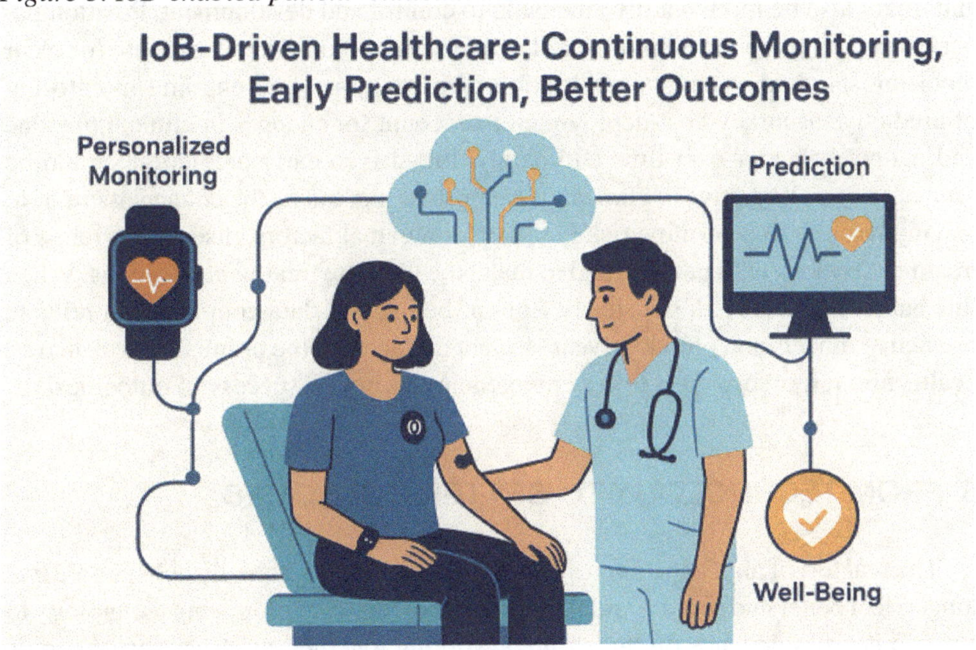

Figure 3 illustrates how IoB-derived predictions can support a collaborative, proactive consultation between patient and clinician

4.5 Challenges, fairness and trust

Despite its potential, IoB-based early prediction raises important challenges. These technical problems, which include data quality, missingness and drift (that a model that performs well on one type of device and set of behaviors might have reduced performance if a patient changes wearable or environment, routine, etc.), mean that the conclusions from a meta-analysis of sepsis and deterioration models are limited by the high heterogeneity in their studies and the limited external validation. A danger that the models look promising on retrospectively collected data but fail when applied to prospectively collected new situations is evident in the papers. The problem of fairness is an important aspect-if training data does not correctly capture the proportions of people from different groups that you find in the general population, the error of a predictive model may disproportionately higher for certain minority groups, making the model widen health inequalities instead of reducing them.

As such, a balance of transparency and clinical control is key. For example, work in the field of comparative analysis of early warning scores has revealed that simpler, more transparent tools can be almost as accurate as more complicated ones, and might also be more readily amenable to control and development. Position papers concerning the development and use of digital biomarkers advocate for clear reporting standards, accurate calibration of predictions, and ongoing monitoring of predictive accuracy post-deployment to account for changes in clinical practice and patient behavior over time.Ultimately, IoB-driven early prediction should be seen not as an alternative to clinical decision-making, but as the enhancement of it, leaving humans to determine risk based on contextual factors, discuss the range of treatment options with patients and to make the ultimate treatment decisions. When this balance is achieved, the steady flow of behavioral data coupled with reliable predictive models and pre-emptive treatment can achieve the promise of IoB-driven healthcare: fewer surprises, fewer emergencies and more successful outcomes.

5. FROM TECHNOLOGY TO BETTER OUTCOMES

The real test of any IoB-driven system is simple: does it actually help people live longer, feel better and avoid avoidable crises. Moving from promising technology to better outcomes depends on three things working together: evidence that the tools improve hard clinical endpoints, designs that genuinely support patients in daily life and health systems that can absorb and act on the extra information.

Large-scale studies of remote patient monitoring offer a clear example of how technology can translate into measurable benefit when it is integrated into care pathways. A recent meta-analysis of non-invasive remote patient monitoring in heart failure pooled data from over 16,000 patients across 41 randomised trials and found that such programmes reduced both mortality and first heart failure hospitalisation compared with usual care. Interventions that paired monitoring with structured self-management and education, and used richer communication such as video calls, achieved the biggest reductions in hospital use. (De Lathauwer et al., 2025).That pattern is very much in line with an IoB perspective: data streams by themselves matter less than how they are tied to human contact, coaching and timely decisions.

Randomised trial evidence now shows that carefully designed, IoB-like programmes can change outcomes even in the high-risk "vulnerable phase" just after hospital discharge. The HERMeS trial in Spain tested a mobile-health platform that combined daily telemonitoring of weight, blood pressure and symptoms with scheduled video visits and nurse-led teleintervention for patients with chronic heart failure. Over six months, the intervention significantly lowered the composite of cardiovascular death or worsening heart failure events compared with usual care, with particularly strong effects on cardiovascular mortality and decompensation episodes (Yun et al., 2025). The key design elements mirror the IoB idea: continuous biometric and behavioural data, integrated into a structured remote-care workflow, with clear rules for how clinicians respond to early signs of deterioration.

Beyond single conditions, digital interventions need to show that they work across a wide range of patients and diseases. An umbrella review in The Lancet Digital Health synthesised 34 meta-analyses covering 235 randomised trials of mobile phone interventions for chronic disease management, including diabetes, hypertension, cardiovascular disease and HIV (Sun et al., 2024). Overall, mobile apps and text messaging produced convincing or highly suggestive benefits for several outcomes, such as HbA1c reduction in type 2 diabetes, blood pressure control in hypertension and medication adherence in cardiovascular disease and HIV. At the same time, about 40% of effects were non-significant, and evidence from low- and middle-income countries remained sparse. For IoB-driven healthcare, this is an important message: digital and behavioural data can help, but impact depends heavily on how interventions are targeted, designed and supported.

Hard outcomes can remain largely unaffected, even if soft but important ones like self-management and Quality of Life can be influenced by a combined approach of monitoring (both via telehealth and clinicians), and behavior change intervention. A systematic review and meta-analysis of telehealth intervention for chronic conditions published in 2023 concludes that daily, long-term monitoring and feedback, and education systems are linked to small but consistent improvements in clinical outcomes and self-rated health across several chronic conditions (Xiao & Han, 2023). Such systems do much more than merely transporting bio-data; in fact it's through giving the patientfeedback and instructions, personal coaching in how to achieve behavior change on the basis of personal bio-data that those systems encourage healthier lifestyle during the daily life in a way similar to the IoB approach, in which prediction is not only used for stratification of risk for clinicians, but also to nudge for healthy behavior.

5.1 Patient experience and engagement

Reduced admissions and mortality are only part of what defines better outcomes-also, can the patient actually live with these technologies? Remote heart failure programmes such as HERMeS show high retention rates and high satisfaction in patients who often liked feeling "watched over" and video calls more than regular visits to the hospital (Yun et al. 2025; De Lathauwer et al. 2025) and studies for systems that monitor mixed chronic-disease patient populations point out increased patient confidence in self-management and increased partnerships with providers (Xiao and Han 2023). From an IoB perspective this is important as you only have long term behavioural data if you keep patients wearing devices, answering prompts and using the apps. When programmes explain to the patient why the prompts are being sent and offer feedback, patients feel like they are working with their providers, rather than being monitored without consultation. If algorithms are unclear, prompts come very frequently but don't provide useful information, or the devices are uncomfortable to use then retention will drop off rapidly.

5.2 Health-system performance and value

In the health system context, remote monitoring and IoB-like interventions are often encouraged for their cost savings and de-escalation of acute hospital resources. De Lathauwer and colleagues' systematic review on telemonitoring for heart failure demonstrated lower heart failure rehospitalisations and in some of these programs, all-cause readmissions, particularly for programs that included education and self-management modules in the service (De Lathauwer et al., 2025). Observational evidence from accountable care systems suggests that post discharge remote monitoring may have associations with lower mortality in selected high-risk populations even with relatively limited reductions in readmissions, indicating downstream economic value related to avoiding acute events and subsequent morbidities. Systematic reviews of chronic disease management via telehealth however indicate that value is not guaranteed. Significant initial capital investment required for device deployment, IT systems and staffing may be necessary and the impacts on utilisation remain disease- and design- dependent (Xiao & Han, 2023). Telemonitoring at times appears to shift exacerbation management toward the earliest possible detection and treatment rather than reducing exacerbations overall, increasing short term costs while perhaps avoiding later, more intense illness. For IoB driven care, economic value relies on both careful risk stratification for each intervention and clear de-escalation procedures.

5.3 Equity, trust and the risk of a widening gap

Arguably the most critical question for "better outcomes" is "better for whom"? A 2024 scoping review was undertaken on the intersection of digital health and health inequities in high income settings (Badr et al., 2024). The authors discovered that most evaluations measured discrepancies in health equity based on access and use on grounds of age, income status, race and location and there was consistent evidence of the older, poorer or digitally excluded using digital services to less avail. Direct measurement of outcome disparities was infrequent but the review warned that in the shift of key services and monitoring to digital channels without rigorous equity protections "existing morbidity and mortality disparities may actually increase".

For IoB-based systems, this risk is even sharper, because predictive models and behavioural nudges depend on large volumes of high-quality data. If disadvantaged patients are less likely to own compatible devices, have reliable connectivity or feel comfortable with apps, they may be missing from the data that train and refine models. That can lead to biased algorithms whose risk scores are less accurate precisely for the groups who already bear a higher burden of disease. The review by Badr and colleagues argues for embedding an explicit equity lens in digital-health strategy, including targeted support for access and literacy, co-design with underserved communities and routine reporting of outcomes by demographic group, not just overall averages (Badr et al., 2024).

5.4 Putting IoB to work

In sum, evidence up to this point indicates that IoB enabling technologies may enhance health when incorporated into well-designed care pathways. Randomised and meta-analytic data indicate that remote monitoring linked with education, self-management support and live contact may decrease morbidity and hospitalisations in heart failure and enhance important risk factors in various chronic conditions (De Lathauwer et al., 2025; Sun et al., 2024; Yun et al., 2025). Telephone management systems maintained over time may provide a small gain in health outcomes that are measured by clinical markers and patient self report in a number of conditions (Xiao & Han, 2023). In parallel, concerns about digital divide and inconsistent adoption maintain that technologies will not inevitably ensure equitable distribution of health gains (Badr et al., 2024).

In IoB-enabled health care, getting that balance right-so we use the wealth of behavioral and physiological data to instigate timely human response, and we create the kinds of devices that individuals are willing and able to use over a period of months and years; we restructure financial incentives so that practitioners receive payment not just for the acute treatment, but also for prevention; and we incorporate equity and transparency into every element-is how we achieve "better outcomes." When all these factors align, the promise of IoB is not about data; it is about avoiding unnecessary crises, about achieving more sustained control of chronic illness, and about creating more caring and proactive humanistic models of care.

6. CHALLENGES, RISKS AND BLOCKCHAIN SOLUTIONS

The IoB-driven healthcare is promising, however, it highlights several challenges and risks which need to be addressed in order to implement it successfully. Concerns around security, privacy, inequity and data breach are some of these issues. With IoB devices generating enormous amounts of sensitive health data, it is essential to ensure its proper use.

Many of these concerns can be resolved or alleviated through blockchain's ability to secure data and ensure transparency. The transmission of IoB data is vulnerable, as is its storage; both are at potential risk. With blockchain, a decentralized method for managing data is created whereby the health data will not be stored in a central one which can easily be accessed and attacked by cybercriminals. Data is not localized which results in it being distributed on the network. Hence, this cannot be compromised on a large scale. Furthermore, because blockchain can't be changed, it offers a system of checks and balances against this kind of activity.

Privacy of the data is another serious concern. Blockchain-powered solutions like self-sovereign identity (SSI) & smart contracts can help patients take control of their own data. With the use of SSI, people can have access to their health information. Similarly, smart contracts give patients the ability to allow and revoke data sharing. This allows patients to sustain confidentiality while also utilizing the benefits of IoB systems.

To prevent unfairness in health care, blockchain can be used for better access and tokenized incentives to participate. Through the establishment of open and verifiable data access, blockchain guarantees that every party, inclusive of underprivileged sectors, will have the same opportunity to profit from care involving the IoB. Tokenized incentives can spur further participation in IoB systems, especially in vulnerable populations. Individuals might be rewarded for their engagement and for sharing data, ensuring they stay in control.

Last, but not least, the use of Blockchain technology will enable access to patient data will provide auditable access logs. The measures are aimed at improving accountability while addressing concerns of surveillance misuses. By implementing these controls, blockchain can considerably mitigate the likelihood of IoB data hacks and other security flaws.

Embedding blockchain in the IoB systems will boost security and privacy while also building trust with the patient and doctor. It allows using IoB technologies in a responsible and ethical way.

6.1 Security, privacy and device safety

The Internet of bodies (IoB) offers new opportunities in personalized healthcare but also brings important security and privacy risks. As IoB devices constantly harvest sensitive biometric data, including heart rate, movement patterns, and stress signatures, ensuring its confidentiality, integrity, and availability is critical. Conventional security measures generally fail in specific situations especially in the contexts of real-time data processed at the edge, the constraint of resources in the end devices, and the exposure of vulnerabilities due to frequent transmission of data.

In this regard, blockchain enhances the security and privacy of IoB systems, which is a step in the right direction. Blockchain technology can deliver tamper-proof audit trails, and all data from the IoB devices cannot be changed or modified after being recorded. This feature is essential for health data integrity, which assures the verifiability and reliability of any medical decision made based on the data.

Also, blockchain can be used to ensure data provenance. This ensures that the origin and lifecycle of every piece of data – whether it is from a wearable sensor or an implantable device – can be traced to the source location, giving assurance to healthcare providers. In addition, the patient-centred governance is secured by tamper-proof consent logs enabled by blockchain technology and allows patients to control data sharing. The use of self-sovereign identity (SSI) models based on blockchain and smart contracts may provide patients with dynamic consent management, allowing for the revision or removal of permissions whenever they like, without third parties.

Incorporating blockchain within IoB's security and privacy framework will aid in developing an efficient system that builds more trust between patients, clinicians as well as healthcare service providers. This is going to solve security vulnerabilities and empower the patients with control over their data, which will add to the ethical governance of IoB systems.

6.2 Autonomy, Consent, and Blockchain for Data Ownership

As IoB systems continue to emerge on the market, there are growing concerns about their ethical implications, particularly interference, consent, and surveillance. Since IoB devices record sensitive personal data like heart rhythms, glucose levels, and everyday activities, ensuring informed consent and respecting people's rights are essential for deploying them responsibly.

Using blockchain technology, self-sovereign identity (SSI) systems were established to help with these issues. Patients in SSI have full control over their data and have the choice of who can access it and when. Smart contracts that activate the execution automatically to act on consent such as granting or revoking access to particular health information can help in this case. The decentralized design of blockchain prohibits any single person or entity from amendment of the blockchain. This implies that not one person or one entity can control patient data in blockchain technology.

Dynamic consent management is enabled by blockchain technology, which allows patients to update their preferences at any time regarding how the data will be used. The system's design enables it to respond to changes. For instance, if a patient agrees to data sharing for one medical procedure and takes it back for another one. Using blockchain for patient-centric data governance enables individuals to take control of their health data while guaranteeing integrity and security of the data.

Upon the integration of the blockchain in the IoB systems, it will ensure data ownership remains with the patient. Hence, patients can control their health data. This also helps in respecting the ethical principles of autonomy, privacy, and informed consent.

6.3 Inequity, exclusion and governance gaps

There is also a significant threat in IoB systems for exacerbating inequalities. Both devices and connections are expensive; literacy and language skills can impact usability of apps and portals, and historical experience and culture influence levels of tolerance for being digitally monitored. If accurate, beneficial IoB systems are mostly taken up by wealthier, urban and more technologically competent communities, the resulting predictive models will be mostly trained on data reflecting their behaviours, and will be largely fine-tuned to these, resulting in greater rates of error for communities that already carry high disease burdens, for instance those lacking stable housing, access to good broadband or physical and learning disabilities that preclude the effective use of standard wearables.

Lastly, governance lags behind IoB innovation: regulatory approaches remain focused on devices, software and data security in silos, despite the ways IoB collapses such categories. The ethical and accountability questions (e.g. If an algorithm incorrectly assessed risk, who is accountable?; how long can raw bodily data be retained and reused?), for instance, are far from settled across many countries. Numerous cybersecurity reviews of health care reiterate that technical solutions are insufficient and that institutional processes, staff training, accountability and cross- sectoral working are critical too (Ewoh & Vartiainen, 2024). In order to design safe, trusted IoB enabled health care systems, security, ethics and equity need to be established as first principles in design rather than added after the technology has already entered our bodies and our homes.

7. A CONCEPTUAL FRAMEWORK FOR IOB-DRIVEN HEALTHCARE

Framework of IoB-driven healthcare use keep together four closely-laboring phases, which are: Monitor, Understand, Act, and Learn. These Phases Are Designed to Enable Continuous Data Flows, Real-Time Monitoring, Predictions, and Personalization.

During the monitoring stage, the data from the patient is collected continuously by IoB devices. This includes aspects such as vital signs, activity levels, and behaviour. However, the data must be trustworthy, which is the function of the blockchain. The role of blockchain technology in the Internet of Behaviours is to offer verified data provenance through which all the data streams are added by IoB devices. It produces a transparent and immutable record of patient data necessary to induce correct clinical decisions.

In the Understand stage, data collected from IoB devices is analysed for the identification of patterns and derivation of useful insights. The data used in this stage will be secure and auditable because of the blockchain technology, which enables trusted collection and analysis of data from heterogeneous devices. In the Act stage, outputs derived from the data is applied. Outputs could be an automatic warning or personalized health plans to clinician or patients, the blockchain smart contract could automatically adjust drug dosage or schedule follow-up appointments based on the real-world data. In the Learn phase, feedback from interventions are used to adapt the care cycle. An immutable log of actions taken and outcomes obtained via blockchain guarantees that the learning is based on a secure patient history, assisting clinicians and system in designing better future plans. By combining blockchain and IoB system the cycle of data driven, secure and trustworthy health delivery cycle of IoB is completed. A better understanding of human behavior and engagement allows the processes of pharmaceutical applications to be better controlled.

It is not uncommon for technology-driven IoB-powered healthcare to become a complex array of devices, applications, and data streams without a logical, patient-centered design to underpin it. This complexity is best navigated through conceptualizing IoB systems as a closed loop of four tightly connected stages: Monitor, Understand, Act, and Learn. This cycle spans across settings (e.g., home, hospital, back to home) and time to convert raw physiological and behavioral signals into improved decisions and, ultimately, better health outcomes. Furthermore, it aligns with the principles of learning health systems and data-driven digital health, where the feedback loop between clinical practice and evidence is crucial for ongoing improvement (Cresswell et al. 2025).

Monitor: The primary function of IoB systems lies in their ability to continuously sense data from, on, and around the body. The applications are diverse, ranging from wearable devices to implantables, ingestible sensors, and room-level devices designed to capture physiological, behavioral, and contextual information. At this stage, critical questions pertain to the selection of parameters to be monitored, the comfort and the breadth of coverage across various aspects of people's lives, and the reliability of the data: are users comfortable with using the technology in the long term, while simultaneously being sufficiently robust to yield meaningful signals? Recent advances in sensing technology and digital biomarkers indicate that even simple signals collected over extended periods can yield reliable insights into health trajectories and disease progression (Smokovski et al. 2024).

Understand: The raw streams of biological and behavioral data acquired by the sensors must be processed into clinically meaningful information. This process involves several steps, such as noise filtering, feature extraction, digital biomarker development, and risk assessment. Clinicians may visualize this interpreted data through graphs illustrating trends, summary statistics, or early warning scores, while patients may receive simplified color-coded dashboards or personalized behavioral recommendations. The main objective at this stage is not solely statistical accuracy, but also contextual interpretability. Research in AI-driven early warning systems and chronic disease management highlights the importance of calibration, explainability, and seamless integration of model outputs into the clinical workflow, rather than simply presenting raw data to clinicians (Edelson et al. 2024; Zhang et al. 2025).

Act: The ultimate goal of monitoring is to enable and trigger clinical actions. These actions encompass a spectrum of interventions, from simple automated medication prompts and self-management advice to nurse-led phone calls and clinical reviews followed by treatment escalation. In an optimally designed IoB pathway, each type of alert or patient state should be directly linked to a specific action, thereby providing clear guidance on what needs to be done and who is responsible. Studies of remotely monitored heart failure programs and mobile health interventions consistently demonstrate that mortality, hospitalization rates, and risk factors are reduced more significantly when remote monitoring is integrated with comprehensive patient education, coaching, and clinical input, rather than being merely an add-on feature (Smokovski et al. 2024; Zhang et al. 2025).

Learn: The final stage of the cycle is the feedback loop where information about alerts, actions, and outcomes is utilized to enhance both models and the care pathway itself. Over time, certain alarm thresholds can be adjusted, and an individual patient's treatment can be tailored to their specific responses and preferences. At scale, this transforms IoB programs into learning health systems, where patient care delivery and knowledge generation occur in parallel (Cresswell et al. 2025). Critically, the learning process should encompass not only model performance metrics but also patient perspectives, equity in access, and potential negative impacts of alarms and workload.

Collectively, the Monitor-Understand-Act-Learn cycle serves as a critical organizing framework for IoB-driven healthcare, shifting the focus from technology alone to patient outcomes. It frames the various technological components of an IoB system not as isolated entities but as interconnected elements within an adaptive process that is integrated into real-world clinical workflows, clearly identifying the points where responsibilities and risks arise: data privacy and safety in monitoring, transparency in understanding, ethics and shared decision-making in acting, and governance and equity in learning. The subsequent sections explore how this framework can guide the development of future IoB systems to ensure they are both technically sound and clinically effective, user-acceptable, and cost-efficient.

8. IOB, BLOCKCHAIN, AND DIGITAL TWINS: A TRIAD FOR SMART HOSPITALS

The IoB, Blockchain, and Digital Twins convergence will create a new paradigm within smart hospitals, especially for patient care through monitoring, data security, and prediction. When combined, these are able to improve healthcare efficacy. Further, they have the ability to reshape healthcare through personalization and security.

Continuous Data Collection by IoB.

The ecosystem is underpinned by The Internet of Bodies (IoB) that enables access to data streams in real time from sensors on or in the body. Wearables collect vital signs, activity, sleep and even behavioral data to create a dynamic and personalized digital twin of each patient. Data from the Internet of Bodies allows for real-time monitoring and prediction of special cases of deterioration of health while also tracking the patient's progress over time.

Utilization of Blockchain for Security, Provenance, and Access Control.

A crucial role of blockchain is to secure the amount of data created by devices of IoB. The secure provenance of every piece of data sourced from the IoB devices is bestowed with immutable audit trails resulting in guaranteed integrity. In addition, the patients can control access to their data using blockchain technology, allowing for better privacy. Using blockchain and smart contracts, self-sovereign identity (SSI) systems can promote dynamic consent management to guarantee access to health data by authorized users only.

Digital twins allow for their simulation, prediction and personalisation.

Digital Twin continues updating a virtual model of the patient with the data coming from IoB devices. The model uses predictive analytics to allow healthcare providers to run simulations for potential health outcomes, test operational ideas and interventions before applying them. Combining IoB data with digital twins enables health care professionals to provide tailored treatment while intervening sooner to avert complications. Digital twins can also be used to improve hospital efficiency by anticipating future patient circumstances and resource needs through real-time data.

A smart hospital system using IoB, Blockchain and Digital Twins helps in building a secure, efficient and responsive smart healthcare system. The combination of these three components will empower patients by focussing them more on wise decision-making. Through the use of these technologies together, smart hosptitals can ensure not only better healthcare but also a more transparent, secure and patient-centered experience.

9. FUTURE DIRECTIONS AND RESEARCH OPPORTUNITIES

With the progression of IoB from isolated trials to a health ecosystem, the next research challenge is no longer how to develop the device or the model but how to build a trusted, interoperable and patient-benefit-driven ecosystem that benefits patients over the course of several years. There are three general directions: more intelligent privacy-preserving data infrastructure, deeper and richer representations of the body with digital twins, and more human-centered and interpretable intelligence on top of the IoB data.

9.1 Smarter and more private data ecosystems

A prominent research challenge is learning across a collection of IoB data without ever bringing all the sensitive records into one place. While FL models training hospitals and vendors have already demonstrated this is possible but the majority of this research has been proofs-of-concept with very few of the models in clinical practice (Teo et al., 2024). Work moving forward must therefore consider what really affects an ML model in a real-world setting: the unreliable networks, the wide disparity in devices, the highly non-uniform distributions of data among the sites, and the inducements for smaller organizations to participate. Further research should aim to provide standardized evaluation mechanisms assessing not only the accuracy of ML models, but their robustness to malicious actors, fairness among subsets and integration with clinical workflow.

For IoB specifically, federated learning and related privacy-preserving methods could be extended down to the edge of the network, so that wearables and implants contribute to population models without exposing raw signals. This raises questions about how to coordinate updates across millions of intermittently connected devices, how to verify that local models are behaving honestly, and how to allow regulators or patient groups to audit behaviour without compromising privacy. Addressing these questions will require joint work between machine-learning researchers, cryptographers, device engineers and health-policy experts.

9.2 From digital biomarkers to digital twins of health

A second direction is to move beyond simple thresholds and risk scores towards richer, personalised models of each person's health state. Digital twin research in healthcare IoT shows how real-time data from sensors can be linked to dynamic virtual replicas that simulate organ function, hospital operations or even whole-population health scenarios (Kabir et al., 2025). For IoB, an obvious extension is the "behavioural and physiological twin" that combines activity patterns, sleep, vital signs, medication use and environmental exposures into a living model that can be probed and updated continuously.

Open questions here include how detailed these twins need to be for specific tasks, how to validate them across different demographics and disease profiles, and how to represent uncertainty so that clinicians do not over-trust simulated trajectories. There is also scope for research on modular twin architectures, where components for heart, lungs, mood, and daily function can be assembled and reused across conditions. Finally, linking individual twins with system-level twins (for wards, clinics or health systems) could support planning for staffing, bed capacity and supply chains based on real-time IoB data rather than static averages.

9.3 Blockchain-Secured Digital Twins for Personalized IoB Care

With the evolution of healthcare systems, personalized treatment could be possible with the coupling of digital twins and blockchain data and IoB. A digital twin is a constantly evolving virtual representation of a person's health, updated by data from

IoB devices. Digital replicas allow alteration within software to allow stimulation and prediction of patient conditions. This predicts health risks and outcomes.

Nevertheless, digital twin data's security and privacy is a concern. In this regard, blockchain can play an important role in ensuring the integrity and privacy of data. By securing digital twin data with blockchain, each patient's digital twin can have an immutable record, ensuring that all health data remains secure and traceable. It is especially important for digital twins that collect large amounts of sensitive data from various IoB devices and blockchain ensures that only authorized parties gain access to and control the data.

Furthermore, leveraging digital twins and blockchain creates the potential for federated learning. Federated learning allows hospitals, clinics, and healthcare providers to train predictive models together without centralizing any health data. The data remains encrypted, local and on-premises that means no sensitive data is uploaded. The process is enabled by blockchain that ensures that the data provenance in each case is verified and that the federated learning ecosystem maintains security compliance with everyone.

Using blockchain to secure digital twin data and enable federated learning allows healthcare to create a more collaborative, privacy-preserving, and personalized IoB ecosystem (Raghavan 2022) The combination enables clinical decision-making while secure sharing of healthcare data among organizations while patients' data being secure.

9.4 Human-centred and explainable IoB intelligence

A third set of opportunities lies in making IoB-driven predictions understandable and actionable for both clinicians and patients. Reviews of explainable and interpretable AI in medicine highlight an explosion of techniques, but also note that many explanations are designed in isolation from real users and rarely evaluated in clinical workflows (Frasca et al., 2024). For IoB, research needs to focus on explanations that fit continuous, multi-modal data: showing how a week of disrupted sleep, missed doses and rising resting heart rate combine to trigger a heart-failure alert, for example, rather than just displaying a single risk number.

There is a rich agenda around co-designing explanation interfaces with clinicians and patients, testing how different visualisations or narratives affect understanding, trust and behaviour change, and exploring how to personalise explanations to literacy levels and cultural context. Studies will also need to examine unintended effects, such as anxiety caused by overly frequent alerts or blame when models highlight "non-adherence." Finally, legal and ethical scholarship must keep pace with these technical advances, clarifying responsibility when semi-autonomous IoB systems contribute to decisions and ensuring that explainability requirements are realistic but robust.

Taken together, these future directions suggest that IoB-driven healthcare is less about inventing ever more exotic sensors, and more about weaving existing and emerging technologies into learning, privacy-aware and human-centred systems. Interdisciplinary collaborations that bring together engineering, data science, clinical practice, social science and law will be essential to turn continuous monitoring and early prediction into durable gains in outcomes and equity.

10. CONCLUSION

As the world of healthcare is rapidly changing, IoB, Blockchain, and Digital Twins are smart ways of smart hospital care. IoB continuously produces real-time data from sensors on and inside the body to continuously paint a dynamic picture of the patient. Unless secured, trusted, and woven into healthcare workflows, the data won't matter much, for all the information will be useless without creating impact. Blockchain plays a crucial role here by helping maintain data integrity, allowing secure access and ensuring patient control and autonomy over their records. The tamper-proof audit history and decentralised governance of blockchain empowers patients to take control of their health data with flexible consent/ privacy management.

Besides, Digital Twins will also create a virtual replica of the patients, which will be constantly updated using IoB data. This digital model can simulate predictions to formulate individual interventions and improve the judgement of healthcare professionals using data. With IoB data integration with Digital Twins, clinicians can now simulate how patients will respond to treatments and test "what-if" scenarios to predict health outcomes.

The combination of IoB, Blockchain and Digital Twins is a triad of innovation that transforms healthcare. Patients can look forward to an increasingly personalized, safer and more transparent journey through the healthcare ecosystem. Clinicians, on their, will be benefitted by enhanced accuracy and real-time insights for better decision-making and fewer errors. With this trio of technologies coming together, smart hospitals will be more efficient and proactive, allowing for better outcomes and greater patient involvement and awareness.

By incorporating responsible technologies, we can integrate them into an ecosystem that facilitates care that is continual, credible, and bespoke. In this manner, we can advance to a better health system.

REFERENCES

Ahmed, S. F., Sharmin, S., Kuldeep, S. A., & Gandomi, A. H. (2025). Transformative impacts of the Internet of Medical Things on modern healthcare. [CoLab]. *Results in Engineering*, *25*, 103787. DOI: 10.1016/j.rineng.2024.103787

Al Khatib, I., Shamayleh, A., & Ndiaye, M. (2024). Healthcare and the Internet of Medical Things: Applications, trends, key challenges, and proposed resolutions. [MDPI]. *Informatics (MDPI)*, *11*(3), 47. DOI: 10.3390/informatics11030047

Andrade, A. N., Cabral, A. T., Bellini, B., Facco Rodrigues, V., da Rosa Righi, R., André da Costa, C., & Barbosa, J. L. V. (2024). IoT-based vital sign monitoring: A literature review. *Smart Health (Amsterdam, Netherlands)*, *32*, 100462. Advance online publication. DOI: 10.1016/j.smhl.2024.100462

Badr, J., Motulsky, A., & Denis, J. (2024). Digital health technologies and inequalities: A scoping review of potential impacts and policy recommendations. *Health Policy (Amsterdam)*, *146*, 105122. DOI: 10.1016/j.healthpol.2024.105122 PMID: 38986333

Boddington, G. (2021). The Internet of Bodies—alive, connected and collective: The virtual physical future of our bodies and our senses. *AI & Society*, *38*(5), 1897–1913. DOI: 10.1007/s00146-020-01137-1 PMID: 33584018

Bowles, T., Trentino, K. M., Lloyd, A., Trentino, L., Jones, G., Murray, K., Thompson, A., Halpin, S., & Waterer, G. (2024). Outcomes in patients receiving continuous monitoring of vital signs on general wards: A systematic review and meta-analysis of randomised controlled trials. *Digital Health*, *10*, 20552076241288826. DOI: 10.1177/20552076241288826 PMID: 39398891

Chatterjee, B., Mohseni, P., & Sen, S. (2022). Bioelectronic sensor nodes for Internet of Bodies. arXiv. https://arxiv.org/abs/2212.11370

Coutu, F.-A., Iorio, O. C., & Ross, B. A. (2023). Remote patient monitoring strategies and wearable technology in chronic obstructive pulmonary disease. *Frontiers in Medicine*, *10*, 1236598. DOI: 10.3389/fmed.2023.1236598 PMID: 37663662

Cresswell, K., Papoutsi, C., Simon, G. E., Bates, D. W., & Sheikh, A. (2025). Advancing learning health systems: Leveraging routine data for improvement and research. *NPJ Digital Medicine*, *8*, 12. DOI: 10.1038/s41746-024-01045-4

Datta, A., & Sen, S. (2023). Invited: IoB: The vision of the Internet of Bodies. *Proceedings of the IEEE Midwest Symposium on Circuits and Systems (MWSCAS)*, 444–448. DBLPDOI: 10.1109/MWSCAS57524.2023.10405903

De Lathauwer, I. L. J., Nieuwenhuys, W. W., Hafkamp, F., Regis, M., Brouwers, R. W. M., Funk, M., & Kemps, H. M. C. (2025). Remote patient monitoring in heart failure: A comprehensive meta-analysis of effective programme components for hospitalization and mortality reduction. *European Journal of Heart Failure*, *27*(9), 1670–1685. Advance online publication. DOI: 10.1002/ejhf.3568 PMID: 39834044

de Waal, C.. (2025). Accuracy of vital sign monitoring using a photoplethysmography upper arm wearable in hospitalised patients. *Journal of Clinical Monitoring and Computing*. Advance online publication. DOI: 10.1007/s10877-025-01358-z

Dubey, R., & Tiwari, A. (2023). Artificial intelligence and remote patient monitoring in US healthcare market: A literature review. *Journal of Market Access & Health Policy*, *11*(1), 2205618. DOI: 10.1080/20016689.2023.2205618 PMID: 37151736

Edelson, D. P., Churpek, M. M., Carey, K. A., Lin, Z., Huang, C., Siner, J. M., Johnson, J., Krumholz, H. M., & Rhodes, D. J. (2024). Early warning scores with and without artificial intelligence. *JAMA Network Open*, *7*(10), e2438986. DOI: 10.1001/jamanetworkopen.2024.38986 PMID: 39405061

El-deep, S. E., Abohany, A. A., Sallam, K. M., & Abd El-Mageed, A. A. (2025). A comprehensive survey on impact of applying various technologies on the Internet of Medical Things. [SpringerLink]. *Artificial Intelligence Review*, *58*(3), 86. DOI: 10.1007/s10462-024-11063-z

El-Khoury, M., & Arikan, C. L. (2021). From the Internet of Things toward the Internet of Bodies: Ethical and legal considerations. Journal of Strategic Contracting and Negotiation, 7(2), 307–314. doi:10.1002/jsc.2411 RSD Journal

Ewoh, P., & Vartiainen, T. (2024). Vulnerability to cyberattacks and sociotechnical solutions for health care systems: Systematic review. Journal of Medical Internet Research, 26, e46904. 10.2196/46904

Felix, F. A. S., & Martins, L. E. G. (2024). IoT devices in use in healthcare applications: A systematic literature review. [SpringerLink]. *Research on Biomedical Engineering*, *40*(3-4), 547–561. DOI: 10.1007/s42600-024-00356-5

Frasca, M., La Torre, D., Pravettoni, G., & Cutica, I. (2024). Explainable and interpretable artificial intelligence in medicine: A systematic bibliometric review. *Discover Artificial Intelligence*, *4*(1), 15. DOI: 10.1007/s44163-024-00114-7

He, P., Huang, D., Wu, D., He, H., Wei, Y., Cui, Y., Wang, R., & Peng, L. (2024). A survey of Internet of Medical Things: Technology, application and future directions. Digital Communications and Networks. Advance online publication. sciencedirect. comDOI: 10.1016/j.dcan.2024.11.013

Hicks, M. H., Tore, M., Michard, F., & Khanna, A. K. (2025). Portable wireless monitoring of vital signs in hospital wards. *BJA Education, 25*(7), 265–272. DOI: 10.1016/j.bjae.2025.04.004 PMID: 40575591

Huang, Y., Wang, J., Wang, S., & Zhang, Y. (2023). Internet of medical things: A systematic review. *Neurocomputing, 557*, 126719. Advance online publication. DOI: 10.1016/j.neucom.2023.126719

Joshi, M., Iqbal, F. M., Sharabiani, M., Ashrafian, H., Arora, S., McAndrew, K., Khan, S., Cooke, G., & Darzi, A. (2025). Performance of continuous digital monitoring of vital signs with a wearable sensor in acute hospital settings. *Sensors (Basel), 25*(9), 2644. DOI: 10.3390/s25092644 PMID: 40363083

Kabir, M. R., Shishir, F. S., Shomaji, S., & Ray, S. (2025). Digital twins in healthcare IoT: A systematic review. *High-Confidence Computing, 5*(3), 100340. DOI: 10.1016/j.hcc.2025.100340

Kakhi, K., Jagatheesaperumal, S. K., Khosravi, A., Alizadehsani, R., & Acharya, U. R. (2025). Fatigue monitoring using wearables and AI: Trends, challenges, and future opportunities. *Computers in Biology and Medicine, 195*, 110461. DOI: 10.1016/j.compbiomed.2025.110461 PMID: 40580618

Khan, S., & Alam, M. (2021). Wearable Internet of Things for personalized healthcare: Study of trends and latent research. In Das, H. (Eds.), *Health informatics: A computational perspective in healthcare* (pp. 43–60). Springer., DOI: 10.1007/978-981-15-9735-0_3

Kirubakaran, D. (2025). Review on emerging frontiers in medical sensing: Innovations shaping the future of healthcare. *Biomedical Materials & Devices, 3*, 385. DOI: 10.1007/s44174-025-00385-3

Liu, J., & Liu, H. (2025). Research on flexible sensors for wearable devices: A review. *Nanomaterials (Basel, Switzerland), 15*(7), 520. DOI: 10.3390/nano15070520 PMID: 40214565

Marinescu, M.-R., Ionescu, O. N., Pachiu, C. I., Dinescu, M. A., Muller, R., & uchea, M. P. (2025). Next-gen healthcare devices: Evolution of MEMS and BioMEMS in the era of the Internet of Bodies for personalized medicine. *Micromachines, 16*(10), 1182. DOI: 10.3390/mi16101182 PMID: 41156428

Matthew, A. J., Dhanalakshmi, R., & Vimal, S. (2025). A systematic review of Internet of Medical Things (IoMT) in healthcare. *Sci, 7*(2), 36. DOI: 10.3390/sci7020036

Matthew, P., Mchale, S., Deng, X., Nakhla, G., Trovati, M., Nnamoko, N., Pereira, E., Zhang, H., & Raza, M. (2025). A review of the state of the art for the Internet of Medical Things. *Sci*, *7*(2), 36. DOI: 10.3390/sci7020036

Mazzeo, A. E. P., & dos Santos, L. W. (2025). Integration of biomedical devices and the internet of bodies revolution. Research. *Social Development*, *14*(5), e48921. DOI: 10.33448/rsd-v14i5.48921

Michard, F., & Saugel, B. (2025). New sensors for the early detection of clinical deterioration on general wards and beyond – A clinician's perspective. *Journal of Clinical Monitoring and Computing*, *39*(2), 435–442. DOI: 10.1007/s10877-024-01235-1 PMID: 39546216

Naghib, M., Chalechale, A., & Gharehchopogh, F. S. (2025). A comprehensive and systematic literature review on intrusion detection systems in the Internet of Medical Things: Current status, challenges, and opportunities. *Artificial Intelligence Review*, *58*(4), 114. Advance online publication. DOI: 10.1007/s10462-024-11101-w

Parihar, A., Prajapati, J. B., Prajapati, B. G., Trambadiya, B., Thakkar, A., & Engineer, P. (2024). Role of IoT in healthcare: Applications, security & privacy concerns. *Intelligent Pharmacy*, *2*(5), 707–714. DOI: 10.1016/j.ipha.2024.01.003

Paul, M. M., Khera, N., Elugunti, P. R., Ruff, K. C., Hommos, M. S., Thomas, L. F., Nagaraja, V., Garrett, A. L., Pantoja-Smith, M., Delafield, N. L., Lizaola-Mayo, B. C., Kresin, M. M., Seetharam, M., Nagarakanti, S. R., & Kaur, M. (2025). The state of remote patient monitoring for chronic disease management in the United States. *Journal of Medical Internet Research*, *27*, e70422. DOI: 10.2196/70422 PMID: 40570326

Rashid, S., & Nemati, A. (2024). Human-centered IoT-based health monitoring in the Healthcare 5.0 era: Literature descriptive analysis and future research guidelines. *Discover Internet of Things*, *4*(1), 26. DOI: 10.1007/s43926-024-00082-5

Rejeb, A., Rejeb, K., Treiblmaier, H., Appolloni, A., Alghamdi, S., Alhasawi, Y., & Iranmanesh, M. (2023). The Internet of Things (IoT) in healthcare: Taking stock and moving forward. *Internet of Things : Engineering Cyber Physical Human Systems*, *22*, 100721. DOI: 10.1016/j.iot.2023.100721

Rowland, B., Saha, A., Motamedi, V., Bundy, R., Winsor, S., McNavish, D., Lippert, W., & Khanna, A. K. (2025). Impact on patient outcomes of continuous vital sign monitoring on medical wards: Propensity-matched analysis. *Journal of Medical Internet Research*, *27*, e66347. DOI: 10.2196/66347 PMID: 40068153

Sameh, A., Rostami, M., Oussalah, M., Korpelainen, R., & Farrahi, V. (2025). Digital phenotypes and digital biomarkers for health and diseases: A systematic review of machine learning approaches utilizing passive non-invasive signals collected via wearable devices and smartphones. *Artificial Intelligence Review*, *58*(2), 66. DOI: 10.1007/s10462-024-11009-5

Schultz, C. (2023). Telehealth and remote patient monitoring innovations in nursing practice: State of the science. Online Journal of Issues in Nursing, 28(2). *Online Journal of Issues in Nursing*, *1*(2). Advance online publication. DOI: 10.3912/OJIN.Vol28No02ST01

Shajari, M., Kuruvinashetti, K., Komeili, A., & Sundararaj, U. (2023). The emergence of AI-based wearable sensors for digital health technology: A review. *Sensors (Basel)*, *23*(23), 9498. DOI: 10.3390/s23239498 PMID: 38067871

Shen, S., Qi, W., Zeng, J., Li, S., Liu, X., Zhu, X., & Lou, X. (2025). Passive sensing for mental health monitoring using machine learning with wearables and smartphones: Scoping review. *Journal of Medical Internet Research*, *27*, e77066. DOI: 10.2196/77066 PMID: 40811794

Singh, B., Lopez, D., & Ramadan, R. (2023). Internet of things in healthcare: A conventional literature review. *Health and Technology*, *13*(5), 699–719. Advance online publication. DOI: 10.1007/s12553-023-00771-1

Singh, B., Lopez, D., & Ramadan, R. (2023). Internet of things in healthcare: A conventional literature review. *Health and Technology*, *13*(5), 699–719. DOI: 10.1007/s12553-023-00771-1

Smokovski, I., Steinle, N., Behnke, A., Bhaskar, S. M. M., Grech, G., Richter, K., Niklewski, G., Birkenbihl, C., Parini, P., Andrews, R. J., Bauchner, H., & Golubnitschaja, O. (2024). Digital biomarkers: 3PM approach revolutionizing chronic disease management—EPMA 2024 position. *The EPMA Journal*, *15*(2), 149–162. DOI: 10.1007/s13167-024-00364-6 PMID: 38841615

Smokovski, I., Steinle, N., Behnke, A., Bhaskar, S. M. M., Grech, G., Richter, K., Niklewski, G., Birkenbihl, C., Parini, P., Andrews, R. J., Bauchner, H., & Golubnitschaja, O. (2024). Digital biomarkers: 3PM approach revolutionizing chronic disease management—EPMA 2024 position. *The EPMA Journal*, *15*(2), 149–162. DOI: 10.1007/s13167-024-00364-6 PMID: 38841615

Sun, S., Simonsson, O., McGarvey, S., Torous, J., & Goldberg, S. B. (2024). Mobile phone interventions to improve health outcomes among patients with chronic diseases: An umbrella review and evidence synthesis from 34 meta-analyses. *The Lancet. Digital Health, 6*(11), e857–e870. DOI: 10.1016/S2589-7500(24)00119-5 PMID: 39332937

Tabaie, Z., & Omidvar, A. (2023). Human body heat-driven thermoelectric generators as a sustainable power supply for wearable electronic devices: Recent advances, challenges, and future perspectives. *Heliyon, 9*(4), e14707. DOI: 10.1016/j.heliyon.2023.e14707 PMID: 37025803

Taherdoost, H. (2024). Wearable healthcare and continuous vital sign monitoring with IoT integration. *Computers, Materials & Continua, 81*(1), 79–104. DOI: 10.32604/cmc.2024.054378

Teo, Z. L., Jin, L., Liu, N., Li, S., Miao, D., Zhang, X., Ng, W. Y., Tan, T. F., Lee, D. M., Chua, K. J., Heng, J., Liu, Y., Goh, R. S. M., & Ting, D. S. W. (2024). Federated machine learning in healthcare: A systematic review on clinical applications and technical architecture. *Cell Reports Medicine, 5*(2), 101419. DOI: 10.1016/j.xcrm.2024.101419 PMID: 38340728

Webb, C. A., & Fisher, H. (2025). Tracking psychopathology dimensions through passive smartphone sensing—Promises, pitfalls, and pathways to clinical integration. *JAMA Network Open, 8*(7), e2519054. DOI: 10.1001/jamanetworkopen.2025.19054 PMID: 40608343

Xiao, Z., & Han, X. (2023). Evaluation of the effectiveness of telehealth chronic disease management system: Systematic review and meta-analysis. *Journal of Medical Internet Research, 25*, e44256. DOI: 10.2196/44256 PMID: 37103993

Yun, S., Comín-Colet, J., Calero-Molina, E., Hidalgo, E., José-Bazán, N., Cobo Marcos, M., Soria, T., Llàcer, P., Fernández, C., García-Pinilla, J. M., Cruzado, C., González-Franco, Á., García-Marina, E. M., Morales-Rull, J. L., Solé, C., García-Romero, E., Núñez, J., Civera, J., Fernández, C., & Fernández, C. (2025). Evaluation of mobile health technology combining telemonitoring and teleintervention versus usual care in vulnerable-phase heart failure management (HERMeS): A multicentre, randomised controlled trial. *The Lancet. Digital Health, 7*(5), 100866. DOI: 10.1016/j.landig.2025.02.006 PMID: 40374486

Zhang, B., Chen, C., Lee, I., Lee, K., & Ong, K.-L. (2025). A survey on security and privacy issues in wearable health monitoring devices. *Computers & Security, 155*, 104453. DOI: 10.1016/j.cose.2025.104453

Zhang, K., Jiang, Y., Xi, K., & Sun, N. (2025). Application of persuasive system design in mobile health interventions for chronic disease management: A mini review. *Frontiers in Public Health, 13*, 1718371. DOI: 10.3389/fpubh.2025.1718371 PMID: 41358248

Zhang, Y., Li, X., Wang, H., & Chen, J. (2025). Advanced applications in chronic disease monitoring using IoT mobile sensing devices. *Frontiers in Public Health, 13*, 1510456. DOI: 10.3389/fpubh.2025.1510456

Zhao, Y., Du, Y., Liu, Y., Deng, C., & Li, X. (2025). Artificial intelligence in chronic disease self-management: Current applications and future directions. *Frontiers in Public Health, 13*, 1689911. DOI: 10.3389/fpubh.2025.1689911 PMID: 41358250

Zhu, Z., & Zhu, M. (2023). The usage of Internet of Things in healthcare: A review of mechanisms, platforms, and opportunities from a new perspective. *Journal of Intelligent & Fuzzy Systems, 45*(1), 1–18. DOI: 10.3233/JIFS-224166

Chapter 7
Beyond Datafication:
Algorithmic Inclusion and Welfare in Low- and Middle-Income Countries

Dario Russo
http://orcid.org/0009-0005-7605-2944
RG3 Digital Consulting, Italy

Piero Demetrio Falorsi
http://orcid.org/0000-0002-4524-8638
University La Sapienza Rome, Italy

Ahmad Hussein
http://orcid.org/0009-0009-1708-6756
Qatar National Planning Council, Qatar

ABSTRACT

The digitalisation of welfare systems is reshaping social protection in low- and middle-income countries, where digital platforms, biometric identification, social registries, and algorithmic tools are increasingly used to expand coverage and manage benefit delivery. This chapter argues that digital welfare is not simply a process of administrative modernisation, but a deeper transformation in how states identify vulnerability, classify populations, allocate entitlements, and mediate access to social rights. It introduces the concept of algorithmic inclusion as a framework for assessing whether data-driven welfare systems can recognise diverse forms of vulnerability, ensure transparency and contestability, and protect rights throughout the decision-making lifecycle. Drawing on cases from East Africa, India, and Latin

DOI: 10.4018/979-8-2600-3043-1.ch007

America, the chapter shows that digital welfare can support inclusion, but may also reproduce exclusion through data gaps, biometric failures, weak grievance mechanisms, and limited institutional capacity.

1. INTRODUCTION

Over the past two decades, welfare systems across the globe have undergone a profound transformation driven by digital technologies, data infrastructures, and algorithmic decision-making tools. Social protection, once mediated primarily through face-to-face administrative procedures, paper-based documentation, and human discretion, is increasingly organized through digital platforms, interoperable registries, biometric identification systems, automated eligibility assessments, and predictive analytics. This transformation has been described in the literature as the emergence of a digital welfare state, in which computational systems do not simply support administrative functions, but actively participate in defining, classifying, and governing social need. As Eubanks (2018) shows, digital welfare systems can reshape the distribution of social rights by embedding decisions about eligibility, risk, and deservingness within technical infrastructures. Similarly, studies on algorithmic regulation and governance have emphasized that automated and data-driven systems reconfigure public decision-making by redistributing authority across institutions, software systems, databases, and private technology providers (Yeung, 2018).

This chapter builds on these debates by focusing on the specific conditions under which digital welfare systems are deployed in low- and middle-income countries (LMICs). The central premise is that digitalisation does not merely accelerate existing welfare procedures. Rather, it reshapes how social risks are identified, how vulnerability is represented, and how rights and entitlements are allocated. This argument draws on the literature on datafication, which has shown that the conversion of social life into quantifiable, machine-readable data is not a neutral technical process, but a transformation in the production of social knowledge (van Dijck, 2014). In welfare systems, datafication affects which individuals and groups become administratively visible, which indicators are used to represent poverty or vulnerability, and which forms of need remain difficult to capture. Taylor and Broeders (2015), in particular, highlight how datafication in the Global South can reproduce asymmetries of power when populations are governed through data systems that are incomplete, externally controlled, or poorly aligned with local realities.

The relevance of these debates is particularly evident in LMICs, where digital welfare systems often emerge in contexts characterized by widespread informality, fragmented civil registration systems, uneven administrative capacity, limited digital access, and dependence on external technological infrastructures. Existing research on digital welfare and digital social protection suggests that the institutional conditions under which digital systems are introduced matter significantly for their social effects. In high-income contexts, digital welfare reforms are often layered onto relatively mature administrative systems, consolidated social insurance mechanisms, and more developed legal and regulatory frameworks, even though they may still reproduce surveillance, exclusion, and rights-based concerns (Eubanks, 2018; Alston, 2019). In LMICs, by contrast, digital welfare infrastructures may develop before equivalent safeguards, administrative routines, and accountability mechanisms are fully established, particularly where informality, incomplete registries, weak data infrastructures, and limited public-sector technical capacity shape welfare delivery (Taylor & Broeders, 2015; Lowe, 2022; Guven, Yeachuri, & Almenfi, 2025; World Bank, 2025).

In such settings, digitalisation can become a constitutive component of state capacity itself: it shapes how states see their populations, how they construct categories of vulnerability, and how they organize access to social protection. This argument builds on scholarship showing that information systems and digital infrastructures do not merely implement public policy, but also reorganize administrative discretion, citizen-state relations, and the operational categories through which public institutions act (Bovens & Zouridis, 2002; Henman, 2010; Yeung, 2018).

The expansion of digital welfare in LMICs has been driven by several overlapping pressures. Fiscal constraints, demographic change, urbanization, climate-related shocks, food insecurity, displacement, and persistent poverty have encouraged governments, development agencies, and international organizations to seek scalable and cost-effective solutions to social protection challenges. Digital social registries, mobile money transfer systems, biometric identification programs, and interoperable welfare platforms are increasingly presented as instruments for expanding coverage, reducing leakage, improving targeting accuracy, and accelerating delivery. In some contexts, the absence of entrenched legacy systems has also been framed as an opportunity for institutional and technological "leapfrogging," allowing governments to adopt digital welfare architectures more rapidly than countries with older administrative infrastructures.

Yet this acceleration conceals deep socio-technical tensions. The literature on algorithmic governance has shown that data-driven systems require more than technical performance: they depend on institutional arrangements capable of ensuring transparency, accountability, contestability, and public oversight (Yeung, 2018). These requirements are especially demanding in welfare systems, where algorithmic errors or administrative misclassifications can affect access to food, income support, pensions, healthcare, or other essential services. In LMICs, the risks are intensified by incomplete datasets, weak grievance mechanisms, uneven legal literacy, limited administrative reach, and constrained capacity to audit proprietary systems. As a result, the same technologies that promise inclusion and efficiency may generate new forms of exclusion that are less visible than traditional administrative failures but equally consequential.

Building on critical scholarship on datafication and algorithmic governance, this chapter argues that understanding digital welfare in LMICs requires moving beyond a narrow focus on datafication and technological efficiency. While datafication has become a defining feature of contemporary welfare governance, existing research shows that the production of more data does not automatically generate more equitable or more accurate systems. Data are produced through institutional categories, measurement practices, infrastructures, and power relations; they may therefore reproduce the exclusions embedded in the social and administrative environments from which they are drawn (van Dijck, 2014; Kitchin, 2014; Taylor & Broeders, 2015). When algorithms operate on incomplete, outdated, or biased datasets, or when they are embedded in weak accountability frameworks, they may reinforce structural disadvantage through what can be described as algorithmic exclusion: the systematic misrecognition, misclassification, or invisibilisation of vulnerable populations within data-driven welfare systems. This exclusion is not reducible to model bias alone. It emerges from the interaction between data infrastructures, institutional capacity, technological design, administrative practices, and pre-existing social inequalities.

To address this problem, the chapter introduces the concept of algorithmic inclusion as both an analytical lens and a policy-oriented framework. Algorithmic inclusion refers to the capacity of digital welfare systems to fairly represent diverse populations, recognize different forms of vulnerability, mitigate exclusionary bias, ensure transparency and contestability, and enable meaningful participation by affected communities. The concept builds on, but also extends, debates on algorithmic bias and fairness. Whereas bias-oriented approaches often concentrate on errors within models or datasets, algorithmic inclusion shifts attention to the broader socio-technical ecosystem in which welfare decisions are produced. It therefore encompasses the full lifecycle of data and decision-making systems, including data collection, registry design, model development, administrative implementation, institutional oversight, and mechanisms of appeal and redress.

The central argument advanced here is that algorithmic inclusion cannot be achieved through technical fixes alone, such as improved model accuracy, better data integration, or bias correction techniques. These measures are important, but insufficient. In LMIC contexts, where welfare systems often serve populations at the margins of formal economies and administrative visibility, inclusive digital welfare requires an integrated approach combining robust data governance, institutional accountability, participatory design, civil society oversight, and sustained capacity building within public administrations. Small design or governance failures — such as inaccessible authentication procedures, outdated registries, opaque targeting criteria, or poorly functioning appeal mechanisms — can translate into severe material consequences for beneficiaries.

Empirically, the chapter adopts a comparative perspective, drawing on documented experiences from three contexts in which digital welfare initiatives have advanced rapidly but along different governance trajectories: East Africa, India, and Latin America. These cases are not treated as exhaustive regional evaluations, nor as internally homogeneous units. Rather, they are used as analytically meaningful configurations of digital welfare governance. East Africa illustrates the rise of platform-based welfare and hybrid governance arrangements involving states, telecom operators, payment providers, donors, and humanitarian actors. India represents a highly centralized model of digital identity and biometric welfare integration, especially through Aadhaar. Latin America offers examples of digital targeting and social registry systems operating within more established, but often institutionally fragmented, welfare traditions. Comparing these configurations makes it possible to identify recurring mechanisms through which digital welfare systems may either expand inclusion or reproduce marginality.

The chapter is structured as follows. Section 2 reviews the relevant literature on digital welfare, datafication, algorithmic governance, algorithmic bias, and digital social protection in LMICs, positioning the chapter within interdisciplinary debates on welfare state transformation and digital public administration. Section 3 examines key mechanisms of algorithmic vulnerability and exclusion, including statistical invisibility, biometric failures, predictive targeting, digital conditionalities, governance gaps, and the environmental and infrastructural costs of digital welfare. Section 4 presents the comparative analysis of East Africa, India, and Latin America as three analytical configurations of digital welfare governance, clarifying the rationale for case selection, the comparative criteria, internal regional variation, and the institutional trade-offs associated with each trajectory. Section 5 develops the algorithmic inclusion framework, articulating its core dimensions and operationalising it through a practical checklist for policymakers and development actors. The concluding section discusses policy implications, limitations, trade-offs, and directions for future research, outlining pathways for designing digital welfare systems that strengthen, rather than undermine, social inclusion.

2. LITERATURE REVIEW AND CONCEPTUAL POSITIONING

The digitalisation of welfare systems has generated a growing interdisciplinary literature across welfare studies, digital sociology, public administration, development studies, data governance, and critical algorithm studies. This literature has progressively moved beyond the idea that digital technologies merely improve the efficiency of public administration. Instead, it increasingly interprets digital welfare as a transformation of how states know, classify, monitor, and intervene upon populations. This section reviews the main strands of scholarship relevant to the chapter and positions the concept of algorithmic inclusion within these debates.

This section does not aim to provide an exhaustive systematic review. Rather, it develops a conceptual literature review focused on the bodies of scholarship that are directly relevant to the chapter's argument: digital welfare and the digital welfare state, datafication and statistical invisibility, algorithmic governance and accountability, algorithmic bias and fairness, and digital social protection in LMICs. This structure is intended to clarify the scientific foundations of the chapter's interpretative model and to show how the concept of algorithmic inclusion builds on, and extends, existing debates.

The review is organized around five areas. First, it examines the literature on digital welfare and the digital welfare state, with particular attention to the transformation of state-citizen relations, access to social rights, and computational forms of administrative classification. Second, it discusses datafication and statistical invisibility as central mechanisms through which social protection systems construct, include, or exclude vulnerable populations. Third, it reviews debates on algorithmic governance, accountability, explainability, contestability, and redress in public decision-making. Fourth, it situates the chapter's contribution in relation to the literature on algorithmic bias, arguing that algorithmic inclusion offers a broader socio-technical lens. Finally, it turns to digital welfare in low- and middle-income countries, where development agendas, infrastructural fragility, and state-capacity constraints shape the effects of digital social protection in distinctive ways.

2.1 Digital Welfare and the Digital Welfare State

The concept of the digital welfare state has become central to critical analyses of welfare transformation. It refers to a configuration in which welfare policy, administration, and service delivery are increasingly mediated by digital infrastructures, automated systems, integrated databases, biometric identification, predictive analytics, and platform-based interactions. The digital welfare state is therefore not simply a welfare state that uses digital tools. It is a welfare state in which digital systems participate in defining eligibility, allocating benefits, monitoring compliance, and shaping the terms through which individuals interact with public authority.

A first strand of literature has emphasized the administrative and institutional transformation produced by digital welfare systems. Henman (2010) showed how information technologies reshape welfare administration by embedding policy rules into software systems and by altering the relationship between discretion, standardization, and control. In this perspective, digital technologies do not only execute policy; they contribute to translating policy objectives into operational categories and administrative routines. Bovens and Zouridis (2002) similarly argued that digital administration transforms street-level bureaucracy into forms of system-level or screen-level bureaucracy, where frontline discretion is increasingly mediated or replaced by information systems.

A second strand has focused on the consequences of digital welfare for social rights and vulnerability. Eubanks (2018), in her analysis of automated welfare systems in the United States, argues that digital tools can intensify surveillance and exclusion among poor and marginalized populations when automated decision-making is embedded in punitive or under-resourced welfare regimes. Although her empirical context is a high-income country, the conceptual contribution is broader: digital welfare systems can reproduce inequality not only through explicit policy choices, but also through the design of databases, scoring mechanisms, fraud detection systems, and administrative interfaces. Alston (2019), in his report on digital welfare states and human rights, similarly warned that digital welfare reforms may undermine rights when efficiency, fraud prevention, and fiscal control are prioritized over due process, transparency, and human dignity.

A third strand has examined digital welfare as a form of social sorting and computational classification. Digital welfare systems transform beneficiaries into data profiles and risk categories. Eligibility, priority, and compliance are increasingly assessed through data points, automated checks, and algorithmic classifications. This reconfiguration changes the epistemic basis of social protection: welfare institutions no longer rely only on caseworker judgment, documentary evidence, or household surveys, but also on interoperable databases, digital identities, machine-readable indicators, and automated inferences. In this sense, digital welfare reshapes how states define social need and how individuals become legible to public institutions.

The literature also suggests that the term "digital welfare state" should be used with conceptual precision. Building on studies of electronic government, automated administration, digital welfare, and algorithmic regulation, the term should not refer to any generic use of digital technology in welfare administration. Rather, it should indicate a deeper institutional transformation in which digital infrastructures become constitutive of welfare governance, decision-making authority, administrative discretion, and citizen-state relations (Bovens & Zouridis, 2002; Henman, 2010; Eubanks, 2018; Alston, 2019; Yeung, 2018). This distinction is important for the present chapter. The focus is not on isolated welfare technologies, but on digital welfare systems as socio-technical arrangements that reorganize visibility, eligibility, accountability, and access to rights.

This literature provides a foundation for the chapter's argument. If digital welfare systems participate in defining vulnerability and allocating social rights, then their effects cannot be assessed only through metrics of efficiency, speed, or cost reduction. They must also be evaluated in terms of representation, accountability, contestability, and inclusion. This is particularly important in low- and middle-income countries, where digital welfare infrastructures are often introduced in contexts where administrative systems, legal safeguards, and institutional oversight remain uneven.

2.2 Datafication, Statistical Invisibility and Social Protection

A second body of literature concerns datafication: the transformation of social phenomena into quantifiable, machine-readable data that can be stored, linked, analysed, and acted upon. Van Dijck (2014) describes datafication as a broader cultural and institutional process through which social life is increasingly translated into data traces and governed through data-driven forms of knowledge. In welfare systems, datafication is especially consequential because it affects how poverty, vulnerability, household composition, employment, disability, migration status, and social risk are represented.

Datafication is often presented as a solution to the informational problems of social policy. Welfare institutions need to identify beneficiaries, target scarce resources, prevent duplication, monitor outcomes, and update eligibility over time. Digital social registries, integrated databases, biometric identification systems, and predictive models promise to improve the accuracy, scalability, and timeliness of these functions. From this perspective, datafication appears to strengthen the administrative capacity of welfare systems by making populations more visible to the state.

Critical scholarship, however, has shown that datafication is not a neutral process of capturing reality. Van Dijck (2014) emphasizes that datafication transforms social life into data traces that become embedded in institutional and ideological forms of knowledge production. Kitchin (2014) similarly argues that data are not simply raw representations of reality, but are produced through specific systems of classification, measurement, infrastructure, and interpretation. Taylor and Broeders (2015) extend this critique to the Global South, showing how development-oriented data systems may create new asymmetries of power when populations are made visible through infrastructures controlled by governments, donors, corporations, or international organizations. In welfare contexts, these insights imply that choices about which data are collected, which categories are used, which indicators are treated as relevant, how often information is updated, and whose forms of vulnerability are made measurable are never merely technical. They reflect institutional priorities, political assumptions, fiscal constraints, and normative ideas about deservingness, risk, and need.

The problem is especially acute in the Global South. Taylor and Broeders (2015) argue that datafication in low- and middle-income countries can produce new power asymmetries when populations are rendered visible through data systems controlled by governments, donors, corporations, or international organizations. Their work highlights the connection between development, data extraction, and governance. Datafication may improve planning and service delivery, but it may also expose vulnerable populations to surveillance, commercial exploitation, or exclusion when data systems are incomplete, externally controlled, or disconnected from local realities.

The concept of statistical invisibility is central here. Statistical invisibility refers to the systematic absence or underrepresentation of individuals or groups within the datasets used to design, implement, and evaluate public policy. In welfare systems, those who are absent from administrative databases may also be absent from eligibility assessments, targeting models, benefit rolls, and policy evaluations. This invisibility can affect informal workers, rural populations, migrants, undocumented persons, Indigenous communities, people without formal identification, women in unpaid or informal labour, and households whose vulnerability changes rapidly due to shocks.

Statistical invisibility differs from simple data error. It is not only a matter of inaccurate records or missing variables. It is a structural condition produced by the unequal capacity of institutions to observe, classify, and update information about different populations. In low- and middle-income countries, incomplete civil registration, fragmented administrative systems, limited survey coverage, weak interoperability, and high levels of informality can all contribute to this condition. When digital welfare systems rely heavily on such incomplete datasets, exclusion may be reproduced through apparently objective technical processes.

This point is important for the chapter's argument because algorithmic exclusion often begins before an algorithm is deployed. If the data infrastructure already underrepresents certain forms of vulnerability, then automated eligibility systems, predictive targeting models, and biometric authentication mechanisms may amplify rather than correct these gaps. Datafication can therefore produce a paradox: the expansion of digital visibility may coexist with the deepening invisibility of those who do not fit the categories, identifiers, or data trails required by the system.

For social protection, this means that inclusion cannot be reduced to data collection alone. More data do not automatically produce more equitable welfare systems. The relevant question is whether data systems are capable of representing the diversity, instability, and informality of social life, especially in contexts where vulnerability is dynamic and often administratively hidden. This is the point at which the literature on datafication connects directly with the chapter's concept of algorithmic inclusion.

2.3 Algorithmic Governance, Accountability and Contestability

A third strand of literature concerns algorithmic governance and the accountability of automated decision-making in the public sector. Algorithmic governance refers to the institutional rules, organizational practices, technical standards, and oversight mechanisms that shape how algorithmic systems are designed, deployed, monitored, and contested. In welfare systems, it includes procurement rules, data governance frameworks, model documentation, eligibility algorithms, audit procedures, human oversight, appeal mechanisms, and the allocation of responsibility between public authorities and private vendors.

Yeung (2018) defines algorithmic regulation as a form of governance in which algorithmic systems are used to monitor, predict, and influence behaviour. Her work is important because it shows that algorithmic systems do not merely process information; they structure the conditions under which decisions are made. In public administration, this raises questions about legality, proportionality, fairness, due process, and democratic control. Algorithmic governance therefore cannot be assessed only through technical performance. It must also be evaluated in relation to the institutional arrangements that determine who can understand, challenge, correct, and oversee algorithmic decisions.

The literature on algorithmic accountability has developed several related concepts. Kroll et al. (2017) argue that accountable algorithms require institutional and technical mechanisms that allow decisions to be examined, tested, and justified. Ananny and Crawford (2018) caution that transparency alone is insufficient if it does not enable meaningful forms of scrutiny and power redistribution. Selbst et al. (2019) show that fairness interventions may fail when they treat algorithmic systems as isolated technical objects rather than as components of broader social and institutional processes. These contributions converge on a key point: accountability is not simply a matter of disclosing code or improving model accuracy; it requires institutional capacity, procedural rights, and mechanisms for contestation.

In welfare systems, explainability and contestability are particularly important. Explainability refers to the ability to provide intelligible reasons for a decision, including the criteria, data, and rules that influenced an outcome. Contestability refers to the ability of affected individuals to challenge, correct, or appeal a decision. Redress refers to the availability of remedies when harm occurs, such as benefit reinstatement, correction of records, compensation, or procedural review. These are not abstract principles. They are practical conditions for maintaining social rights in systems where decisions may be automated, semi-automated, or mediated through complex data infrastructures.

Public-sector algorithmic systems raise specific accountability problems because responsibility is often distributed across multiple actors (Levy, Chasalow, & Riley, 2021).

A welfare decision may involve a ministry, a local office, a database manager, a private software provider, a biometric vendor, a payment platform, and an external donor. When an error occurs, beneficiaries may not know which institution is responsible, frontline staff may not understand how the system generated the decision, and public authorities may lack access to proprietary models or technical documentation. This diffusion of responsibility can make algorithmic errors difficult to identify and even more difficult to contest.

In low- and middle-income countries, these challenges are intensified by capacity constraints. Public administrations may lack specialized expertise in data science, algorithmic auditing, cybersecurity, procurement, and digital rights. Data protection authorities or oversight bodies may be under-resourced. Beneficiaries may face barriers related to literacy, geography, language, connectivity, or legal awareness. As a result, formal accountability mechanisms may exist on paper but remain inaccessible in practice. In welfare contexts, this is especially problematic because the consequences of exclusion can be immediate and severe.

The literature on algorithmic governance therefore supports a central claim of this chapter: inclusive digital welfare requires more than technical safeguards. It requires governance arrangements that make automated and data-driven decisions understandable, challengeable, correctable, and institutionally accountable. Without these arrangements, digital welfare systems risk producing forms of exclusion that are administratively efficient but democratically weak.

2.4 From Algorithmic Bias to Algorithmic Inclusion

The literature on algorithmic bias has been essential in showing that algorithmic systems can produce discriminatory or unequal outcomes. Barocas and Selbst (2016), Noble (2018), Benjamin (2019), and Barocas, Hardt and Narayanan (2019), among others, have demonstrated how data-driven systems may reproduce historical inequalities through biased datasets, problematic proxies, flawed model design, or discriminatory institutional contexts. This literature has been particularly influential in debates on credit scoring, policing, hiring, education, healthcare, and public services.

In welfare systems, bias can arise when datasets underrepresent specific groups, when variables function as proxies for protected characteristics, when historical administrative practices encode unequal treatment, or when models are trained on outcomes shaped by past exclusion. A bias-centered approach is therefore necessary. It provides tools for identifying disparate impacts, testing model performance across groups, and questioning claims of algorithmic neutrality.

However, this chapter argues that the concept of bias is not sufficient to capture the full range of exclusionary dynamics in digital welfare systems, particularly in low- and middle-income countries. Bias often directs attention to the model: its training data, variables, outputs, and statistical performance. Yet many welfare exclusions occur across a wider socio-technical lifecycle. They may arise from the absence of individuals in civil registries, the failure of biometric authentication, the inability to access digital interfaces, the lack of effective grievance procedures, the dependence on private vendors, or the inability of public administrations to audit and adapt systems over time.

For this reason, the chapter proposes a shift from algorithmic bias to algorithmic inclusion. This does not mean abandoning bias analysis. Rather, it means embedding bias within a broader framework that includes representation, procedure, institutions, participation, and technological autonomy. Algorithmic inclusion asks not only whether a model produces statistically unequal outcomes, but whether the entire digital welfare system is capable of recognizing diverse forms of vulnerability, adapting to local conditions, explaining decisions, correcting errors, and involving affected communities in governance.

This shift is especially relevant in LMIC contexts. In settings marked by informality, infrastructural fragility, weak administrative capacity, and external technological dependence, exclusion is rarely produced by a single biased model. It is more often cumulative. An informal worker may be absent from administrative records, lack a stable digital identity, face biometric authentication failure, be unable to access an online grievance mechanism, and have no meaningful channel to contest the resulting exclusion. Each step may appear minor or technical, but together they produce a systemic denial of social protection.

Algorithmic inclusion therefore reframes the problem. The central issue is not only whether algorithms are fair in a narrow statistical sense, but whether digital welfare systems are socially and institutionally capable of sustaining inclusion across the full decision-making lifecycle. This includes the production of data, the design of models, the organization of administrative workflows, the governance of vendors, the accessibility of interfaces, the availability of human review, and the role of civil society in monitoring harms.

The contribution of algorithmic inclusion lies in this broader perspective. It treats exclusion not as a residual defect to be corrected after deployment, but as a foreseeable governance risk that must be addressed from the design stage onward. It also links technical concerns with democratic and social-policy concerns: who is represented, who is heard, who can challenge decisions, who controls the infrastructure, and who bears the consequences of error.

2.5 Digital Welfare in LMICs: Development, Infrastructure and State Capacity

While much of the foundational literature on digital welfare, algorithmic bias, and automated public decision-making has emerged from high-income contexts, a growing body of research examines the distinctive conditions of digital social protection in low- and middle-income countries. This literature shows that LMICs cannot be treated simply as delayed or incomplete versions of high-income welfare states. Digital welfare systems in these contexts often develop under different institutional, infrastructural, and political conditions, including high levels of informality, incomplete civil registration, uneven digital access, donor involvement, public-private delivery arrangements, biometric identification, mobile money infrastructures, and constrained administrative capacity (Taylor & Broeders, 2015; Lowe, 2022; Carswell & De Neve, 2022; Masiero & Shakthi, 2020; Muralidharan, Niehaus, & Sukhtankar, 2022; Guven, Yeachuri, & Almenfi, 2025; World Bank, 2025). This literature is essential for the present chapter because it provides the empirical and policy basis for analysing digital welfare in LMICs as a specific governance problem rather than as a simple extension of welfare digitalisation in high-income settings.

One important strand of research links digital welfare to development policy and state-capacity building. Digital identification systems, social registries, mobile money transfers, and interoperable databases are frequently promoted by governments, donors, and international organizations as instruments for expanding coverage, improving targeting, reducing leakage, and responding rapidly to crises. In contexts where administrative capacity is limited and populations are difficult to reach through traditional bureaucratic channels, digital tools can indeed expand the operational reach of social protection.

At the same time, empirical research and policy evaluations on digital social protection have documented that digitalization can also compound exclusion. Studies of biometric authentication, electronic payments, digital identity systems, and registry-based targeting show that vulnerable populations may face exclusion at multiple stages of the welfare delivery chain: registration, identification, eligibility assessment, authentication, payment, information updating, and grievance resolution. Lowe (2022), for example, notes that digital approaches to social protection can entrench exclusion when vulnerable groups are least likely to have access to the devices, networks, documents, and institutional support required by digital delivery systems. Carswell and De Neve (2022), Masiero and Shakthi (2020), and Muralidharan, Niehaus, and Sukhtankar (2022) show, in different ways, how Aadhaar-linked and biometric welfare infrastructures in India can create new forms of mediation, dependency, authentication failure, and exclusion when technological requirements are not matched by robust fallback mechanisms. Research and technical work on social registries similarly highlight that registry coverage, updating cycles, interoperability, and administrative capacity are decisive for whether digital targeting expands or restricts access to social protection (Guven, Yeachuri, & Almenfi, 2025; World Bank, 2025).

A second strand focuses on infrastructure. Digital welfare depends on material systems: connectivity, electricity, servers, biometric devices, payment networks, cloud infrastructures, cybersecurity arrangements, and maintenance capacity. In

LMICs, these infrastructures are often unevenly distributed across urban and rural areas and may be vulnerable to outages, environmental conditions, fiscal constraints, or dependence on external providers. This means that the reliability of welfare delivery is tied not only to policy design, but also to the stability and governance of technological infrastructures. A biometric system, for example, may work well in administrative centres but fail in remote areas because of connectivity problems, device malfunction, or limited technical support.

A third strand concerns the political economy of digital welfare. Digital social protection systems are often built through partnerships involving states, international organizations, humanitarian agencies, telecom operators, fintech companies, biometric vendors, and cloud providers. These arrangements can accelerate deployment and bring technical expertise, but they may also create dependencies and accountability gaps. Public authorities may lack full control over critical infrastructures, may be constrained by proprietary systems, or may struggle to negotiate contracts that preserve auditability, interoperability, and public ownership of data. Taylor and Broeders' analysis of datafication in the Global South is particularly relevant here because it highlights how development-oriented data systems can shift power toward actors that collect, process, and control data infrastructures.

A fourth strand examines crisis-driven digital welfare. The COVID-19 pandemic, climate shocks, food crises, and displacement have accelerated the use of digital systems for emergency cash transfers and social assistance. Digital infrastructures can support rapid scalability, but crisis conditions may also intensify the trade-off between speed and inclusion. Systems deployed quickly may rely on existing registries that exclude informal or newly vulnerable populations. Emergency digital payments may reach those already connected to mobile or banking infrastructures while missing those outside formal systems. In this sense, speed is not only an operational advantage; it can become a source of exclusion when rapid deployment relies on incomplete data and weak feedback mechanisms.

A fifth strand concerns regional variation. In East Africa, mobile money and platform-based welfare have created opportunities for rapid and flexible transfer systems, but also raise questions about platform dependence, data sharing, and hybrid public-private governance. In India, Aadhaar-linked welfare illustrates the power and risks of centralized digital identity, including the potential for scale and integration as well as the systemic consequences of biometric failure or data mismatch. In Latin America, long-standing traditions of targeted social assistance and social registries provide a different trajectory, where relatively mature administrative datasets coexist with institutional fragmentation, political discontinuity, and uneven local implementation capacity.

This literature suggests that digital welfare in LMICs must be analysed through the interaction of development objectives, infrastructural conditions, institutional capacity, and governance arrangements. Digital systems may expand welfare access, but they may also create new thresholds for inclusion: possession of identity documents, biometric legibility, mobile connectivity, digital literacy, administrative visibility, and the ability to navigate grievance procedures. The key question is therefore not whether digital welfare is beneficial or harmful in itself, but under what governance conditions it strengthens social protection and under what conditions it reproduces exclusion.

The concept of algorithmic inclusion developed in this chapter responds to this question. It brings together insights from digital welfare studies, datafication, algorithmic governance, bias research, and development scholarship. Its purpose is to provide a framework for assessing whether digital welfare systems in LMICs are capable of recognizing vulnerability, sustaining rights, and correcting exclusion across the full data and decision-making lifecycle. In this sense, algorithmic inclusion is both an analytical concept and a policy-oriented tool: it helps identify where exclusion is produced, which institutional capacities are required, and how digital welfare systems can be designed to support rather than undermine social protection.

3. ALGORITHMIC VULNERABILITY AND EXCLUSION IN LOW- AND MIDDLE-INCOME COUNTRIES

The introduction of data-driven and algorithmic systems into welfare governance has reshaped not only how benefits are delivered, but also how vulnerability itself is defined, classified, and operationalized. In low- and middle-income countries (LMICs), these transformations intersect with deep-rooted structural inequalities, often producing forms of exclusion that are less visible than traditional administrative failures yet equally consequential. Algorithmic vulnerability emerges when individuals or groups are disadvantaged not by explicit policy choices, but by the interaction between data limitations, technological design, and institutional constraints embedded in digital welfare systems.

This section examines the principal mechanisms through which algorithmic systems may generate or exacerbate exclusion in LMIC welfare contexts. Rather than treating these mechanisms in isolation, the analysis emphasizes their interdependence and cumulative effects, highlighting how multiple sources of vulnerability can reinforce one another over time.

3.1 Informational Gaps and Statistical Invisibility

One of the most pervasive sources of algorithmic exclusion in LMIC welfare systems lies in the uneven availability, quality, and timeliness of data. Digital welfare infrastructures rely on administrative records, surveys, and digital traces to construct representations of social reality. However, these data sources often systematically underrepresent precisely those populations most in need of social protection.

Rural communities, informal workers, seasonal migrants, Indigenous groups, and individuals without formal identification are frequently absent or inconsistently recorded in digital registries.

Empirical studies on digital social protection show that these forms of invisibility are particularly consequential when welfare systems rely on pre-existing administrative databases or social registries to identify beneficiaries. Informal workers may not appear in tax, employment, or social insurance records; seasonal migrants may be registered in one locality while residing or working in another; rural households may be underrepresented because of weak civil registration coverage, distance from administrative offices, or irregular data updating; and individuals without formal identification may be excluded before eligibility is even assessed. In such cases, exclusion is produced not at the moment of algorithmic classification alone, but earlier, through the data infrastructure that determines who can be seen by the welfare system in the first place. Digitalisation can therefore accelerate delivery for those already administratively visible while leaving statistically invisible groups outside the scope of automated targeting and enrolment.

Informality, which characterizes a substantial share of economic activity in many LMICs, complicates the use of income-based or employment-based indicators that underpin many targeting models. As a result, welfare systems that rely heavily on data-driven eligibility assessments risk excluding individuals whose livelihoods and vulnerabilities do not conform to standardized administrative categories.

Statistical invisibility does not necessarily result from deliberate neglect. Rather, it reflects structural asymmetries in data production, administrative reach, and state capacity. When algorithmic systems operate on such incomplete representations, exclusion becomes embedded in the technical functioning of welfare delivery. Importantly, once embedded, this form of exclusion is difficult to detect through conventional policy evaluation tools, as those excluded are often absent from the very datasets used to assess programme performance.

This problem becomes especially acute in crisis contexts. During pandemics, climate-related shocks, food crises, or sudden displacement, vulnerability may expand rapidly among groups that were not previously registered as poor or eligible for assistance. If emergency programmes rely on outdated registries or narrowly defined administrative categories, newly vulnerable households may remain outside the system. The empirical lesson from crisis-oriented digital social protection is therefore ambivalent: digital registries and payment systems can enable faster response, but speed may come at the cost of inclusion when the underlying data do not reflect rapidly changing social conditions. In this sense, statistical invisibility is not only a static problem of missing populations; it is also a dynamic problem of delayed recognition.

3.2 Biometric Identification and Verification Failures

Biometric identification systems are widely promoted as tools to enhance efficiency, reduce fraud, and ensure accurate beneficiary identification. In LMICs, large-scale biometric programs are often integrated into welfare delivery, linking authentication processes directly to access to cash transfers, food subsidies, healthcare, or pensions.

Despite their promise, biometric systems introduce specific vulnerabilities that are often underestimated at the design stage. False negatives, device malfunction, poor connectivity, and inadequate maintenance can prevent successful authentication, leading to denial or interruption of benefits. These risks are exacerbated in contexts characterized by unreliable infrastructure, harsh environmental conditions, and limited technical support capacity.

Certain populations - such as older adults, manual labourers, agricultural workers, or persons with disabilities - may experience disproportionately high rates of biometric failure due to worn fingerprints or physical conditions.

Evidence from Aadhaar-linked welfare delivery in India illustrates how biometric failures can become mechanisms of exclusion when authentication is made a condition for accessing essential benefits (Carswell & De Neve, 2022; Masiero & Shakthi, 2020; Muralidharan, Niehaus, & Sukhtankar, 2022). Studies of biometric and digital mediation in welfare programmes have documented cases in which fingerprint mismatch, connectivity failure, device malfunction, or data inconsistency delayed or prevented access to food rations, pensions, wages, or other entitlements. These failures are not evenly distributed. Elderly beneficiaries, manual workers, agricultural labourers, persons with disabilities, and people living in areas with weak connectivity are more likely to encounter authentication problems and less likely to have the resources needed to resolve them. The result is a shift from administrative discretion to binary technical verification: when authentication fails, the beneficiary may be treated as ineligible or absent, even when the underlying entitlement remains valid.

This illustrates a broader feature of biometric welfare systems: when authentication is directly tied to entitlement delivery, technical failure can have immediate distributive consequences.

When fallback mechanisms are weak or poorly communicated, biometric errors can translate directly into material deprivation.

The empirical issue is therefore not simply whether biometric systems generate errors, but whether welfare systems are designed to absorb and correct those errors. Where fallback mechanisms are available, well communicated, and accepted by frontline administrators, authentication failure may be treated as a procedural problem rather than as a ground for exclusion. Where such mechanisms are absent, discretionary, or poorly implemented, the burden of correction shifts to beneficiaries. They may be required to travel repeatedly to service points, update records, provide additional documents, or navigate opaque administrative channels. For households dependent on welfare benefits, even temporary delays can have serious consequences. Biometric inclusion therefore depends on the institutional design surrounding the technology, not only on the technical reliability of the biometric device.

Over time, repeated authentication failures may discourage beneficiaries from engaging with welfare systems altogether, producing forms of self-exclusion that are difficult to reverse.

3.3 Predictive Bias, Model Design, and Contextual Misalignment

Beyond identification and registration, many digital welfare systems increasingly rely on predictive and classificatory models to assess vulnerability, rank beneficiaries, or detect potential fraud. These models are typically trained on historical data and statistical correlations that reflect existing administrative practices and social hierarchies.

In LMICs, predictive bias frequently arises from contextual misalignment. Models developed using data from one region, population, or policy environment are often transferred to different socio-economic contexts with limited adaptation. Indicators that function as reliable proxies for poverty or risk in one setting may be weak, misleading, or even inversely correlated with vulnerability in another.

Proxy means testing and registry-based targeting provide concrete examples of this problem. In many social protection systems, household welfare is estimated through observable indicators such as dwelling characteristics, asset ownership, household composition, education, employment status, or geographic location. These indicators can be useful when income data are unavailable or unreliable, but they may also misclassify households whose vulnerability is temporary, informal, seasonal, or difficult to observe through standardized variables. A household may appear non-poor because it owns a durable asset, while still experiencing food insecurity, unstable income, debt, disability-related costs, or climate-related loss. Conversely, a model calibrated on historical poverty profiles may fail to detect new forms of vulnerability generated by urban informal work, displacement, or economic shocks. Predictive targeting therefore depends critically on the validity of the proxies used and on the frequency with which registries are updated.

Predictive bias is further compounded when models are embedded in rigid administrative workflows. Even when misclassification is recognised, institutional constraints may limit the ability to override algorithmic outputs. Unlike explicit exclusion criteria, algorithmic misclassification often operates silently, affecting eligibility probabilities or benefit levels without clear explanation to beneficiaries or frontline staff.

These risks are intensified when beneficiaries cannot understand or contest the classification assigned to them. In registry-based or proxy-based systems, households may not know which variables contributed to their exclusion, whether the data used are outdated, or how to correct the underlying information. The classification may appear as an administrative fact rather than as the result of a model or scoring rule. This creates a specific form of algorithmic vulnerability: people are governed by categories that are difficult to see, interpret, or challenge. Empirical evaluations of targeting systems therefore need to examine not only statistical accuracy at the aggregate level, but also the availability of household-level correction, appeal, and updating mechanisms.

Individuals repeatedly misclassified as low priority may experience delayed access, reduced benefits, or exclusion from complementary programmes, reinforcing pre-existing inequalities.

3.4 Digital Conditionalities and Unequal Access

Digital welfare systems frequently introduce implicit conditionalities that shape access to social protection. While eligibility rules may remain formally unchanged, participation increasingly requires access to digital devices, connectivity, and basic digital competencies. These requirements function as de facto conditions for inclusion.

In LMICs, disparities in access to smartphones, stable internet connections, and digital skills are pronounced along lines of gender, age, income, and geography. Women, older adults, rural populations, and persons with limited literacy are disproportionately affected.

Empirical work on digital social protection shows that these barriers often operate cumulatively. A beneficiary may need a mobile phone, a registered SIM card, network coverage, the ability to read digital messages, access to a payment agent, knowledge of programme rules, and the confidence to interact with digital or semi-digital interfaces. Gender inequalities can affect phone ownership and control over mobile money accounts. Age and literacy can shape the ability to interpret SMS notifications, use applications, or complete digital forms. Rural residence can increase the distance from service points and reduce the reliability of connectivity. In such circumstances, digital access is not a neutral delivery channel; it becomes a practical condition for exercising social rights.

When welfare services are primarily delivered through online platforms or mobile applications, these groups may face additional hurdles in registration, information updates, or error resolution.

Digital conditionalities also interact with language and literacy constraints. Interfaces designed without attention to local languages or low-literacy users can further marginalize vulnerable populations. In such cases, exclusion arises not from explicit policy intent, but from design choices that privilege administratively visible and digitally connected users.

Where beneficiaries cannot navigate digital interfaces independently, access to welfare may become mediated by informal or semi-formal intermediaries, including family members, local brokers, payment agents, NGO staff, or frontline administrators. Such mediation can be inclusionary when it helps beneficiaries overcome digital barriers, but it can also create dependency, information asymmetry, transaction costs, or opportunities for abuse. This is particularly relevant in low-literacy or rural contexts, where beneficiaries may not be able to verify whether payments have been received, whether deductions are legitimate, or whether records have been correctly updated. Digital conditionalities therefore reshape not only access to welfare, but also the social relationships through which welfare is accessed.

3.5 Limited Institutional Capacity and Governance Gaps

Underlying many forms of algorithmic exclusion in LMIC welfare systems is limited institutional capacity. Governing complex digital infrastructures requires expertise in data governance, cybersecurity, ethical assessment, and algorithmic auditing. Many public administrations lack these capabilities at scale, constraining their ability to oversee system design, implementation, and long-term operation.

Capacity limitations also affect relationships with external technology providers.

In practice, governance gaps often become visible through procurement and vendor-management arrangements. Digital welfare systems may depend on proprietary software, biometric devices, cloud services, payment platforms, or data analytics tools supplied by private firms or external partners. When contracts do not guarantee access to documentation, audit rights, interoperability standards, data portability, or source-code inspection where appropriate, public authorities may become dependent on vendors for the operation and modification of core welfare infrastructures. This dependency can limit the state's ability to investigate exclusionary effects, adapt eligibility rules, correct system failures, or transfer knowledge to public institutions. Vendor lock-in is therefore not merely a procurement problem; in welfare systems it can become a constraint on accountability and social rights. In such cases, procurement and vendor-management arrangements become central to algorithmic accountability, because they determine whether public authorities can inspect, modify, audit, and correct the systems through which welfare decisions are implemented.

Grievance and redress mechanisms are often underdeveloped or weakly integrated into digital workflows. Even when formal appeal processes exist, they may be inaccessible due to bureaucratic complexity, geographic distance, or lack of awareness. Without effective channels for contestation, algorithmic errors risk becoming normalized features of welfare delivery.

The capacity to audit digital welfare systems is unevenly distributed. Some public agencies may have formal responsibility for oversight but lack the technical expertise, budget, legal authority, or organizational routines required to examine models, databases, authentication logs, or payment failures. Frontline administrators may observe exclusionary effects but have limited ability to modify system rules or escalate technical problems. Oversight bodies may focus on legal compliance without sufficient access to operational data. As a result, implementation failures can persist even when policy objectives are inclusive. This gap between formal design and operational capacity is one of the central reasons why algorithmic inclusion must be understood as an institutional problem rather than a purely technical one.

3.6 Environmental and Infrastructural Costs of Digital Welfare

A further dimension of algorithmic vulnerability concerns the material and environmental costs of digital welfare infrastructures. Digital social protection is often discussed in terms of efficiency, scalability, targeting accuracy, and administrative modernization, but these systems also depend on physical infrastructures that are unevenly distributed and environmentally consequential. Data centres, cloud services, biometric devices, mobile networks, payment terminals, electricity supply, cooling systems, maintenance chains, and electronic waste all form part of the material basis of digital welfare.

In low- and middle-income countries, these infrastructural conditions are especially relevant. Digital welfare systems may operate in areas affected by unstable electricity grids, limited connectivity, weak maintenance capacity, and high dependence on imported hardware or externally managed cloud infrastructures. Biometric devices require repair, replacement, calibration, and secure operation. Mobile-based welfare delivery depends on network coverage, agent liquidity, device ownership, and energy availability. Data-intensive welfare systems may increase demand for storage, processing capacity, and cybersecurity infrastructure. These requirements can generate hidden costs that are not always visible in policy narratives focused on leapfrogging and digital efficiency.

The environmental implications are also important. Expanding digital welfare infrastructures may contribute to energy consumption, hardware turnover, and e-waste, particularly where procurement cycles are short and maintenance systems are weak. These costs do not negate the potential benefits of digital social protection, but they suggest that algorithmic inclusion should be evaluated alongside infrastructural sustainability. A welfare system that expands digital access while relying on fragile, externally dependent, or environmentally unsustainable infrastructures may create new vulnerabilities over time. For this reason, the assessment of digital welfare in LMICs should include not only social and institutional dimensions, but also the material conditions that allow digital systems to function reliably and sustainably.

3.7 Cumulative and Systemic Dimensions of Algorithmic Vulnerability

Taken together, these dynamics suggest that algorithmic exclusion in LMICs should not be understood as a series of isolated technical failures. Rather, it constitutes a cumulative and systemic condition arising from the interaction between data gaps, technological design, and institutional fragility.

For example, statistical invisibility may lead to misclassification, which in turn increases reliance on biometric verification, amplifying the consequences of authentication failure. Digital conditionalities may further restrict access to grievance mechanisms, preventing correction of errors. Over time, these feedback loops can entrench exclusion in ways that are difficult to detect through conventional monitoring and evaluation frameworks.

Recognizing algorithmic vulnerability as systemic has important implications for governance. It underscores the need for integrated approaches that address data quality, institutional capacity, and participatory design simultaneously. This perspective also highlights the limits of purely technical solutions and reinforces the relevance of the algorithmic inclusion framework developed in the following section.

4. COMPARATIVE INTERNATIONAL ANALYSIS: DIGITAL WELFARE TRAJECTORIES IN LMICS

4.1 Case Selection and Comparative Criteria

The comparative analysis developed in this section does not treat East Africa, India, and Latin America as fully representative of all low- and middle-income countries, nor as internally homogeneous regional units. Rather, these cases are selected as three analytically meaningful configurations of digital welfare governance. Each configuration illustrates a distinct trajectory through which digital infrastructures, institutional arrangements, and social protection objectives interact in contexts marked by inequality, informality, and uneven state capacity. The purpose of the comparison is therefore not to produce an exhaustive regional mapping, but to identify recurrent governance patterns, inclusionary potentials, and exclusionary risks that are relevant to the broader framework of algorithmic inclusion.

The first configuration, East Africa, is selected as an example of **platform-based welfare and hybrid governance**. In several East African contexts, digital social protection has developed through the use of mobile money systems, digital payment infrastructures, humanitarian cash transfers, and partnerships involving governments, telecom operators, financial service providers, NGOs, and international development agencies. This trajectory is analytically relevant because it shows how welfare delivery can expand rapidly through private or semi-private digital platforms, especially in contexts where traditional banking and administrative infrastructures are limited. At the same time, it raises questions about public oversight, data sharing, platform dependence, contractual accountability, and the role of non-state actors in welfare governance.

The second configuration, India, is selected as an example of **centralized digital identity and biometric welfare integration**. India's Aadhaar infrastructure represents one of the largest digital identity systems in the world and has been progressively linked to welfare delivery, social protection schemes, food subsidies, pensions, financial inclusion initiatives, and other public services. This trajectory is analytically relevant because it illustrates the benefits and risks of scale, interoperability, and centralization. Centralized digital identity can strengthen administrative integration and reduce duplication, but it can also amplify systemic vulnerabilities when biometric authentication fails, data mismatches occur, or grievance mechanisms are inaccessible to marginalized populations.

The third configuration, Latin America, is selected as an example of **digital targeting and fragmented institutional control**. Many Latin American countries have long-standing traditions of targeted social assistance, conditional cash transfers, household registries, and poverty assessment tools. Digitalization has strengthened data integration, beneficiary identification, and programme coordination in some contexts. However, these systems often operate within institutionally fragmented welfare architectures, where responsibilities are distributed across national, regional, and municipal levels, and where political discontinuity may affect policy implementation and system maintenance. This configuration is analytically useful because it shows how relatively developed social registries and targeting instruments may coexist with uneven administrative capacity, fragmented accountability, and variable local implementation.

These three configurations are comparable because they all involve the use of digital infrastructures to identify, classify, prioritize, authenticate, or reach welfare beneficiaries. They also share a common policy context: the attempt to expand or improve social protection under conditions of resource constraint, social inequality, and administrative complexity. However, they differ in the institutional form through which digital welfare is organized. East Africa foregrounds platform mediation and hybrid public-private governance; India foregrounds centralized identity infrastructure and biometric authentication; Latin America foregrounds social registries, targeting systems, and multi-level institutional coordination. These differences make comparison analytically productive because they allow the chapter to examine how distinct governance arrangements generate different inclusionary and exclusionary dynamics. Table 1 summarizes the analytical logic of the case selection.

Table 1. Case configurations and comparative rationale

Case Configuration	Dominant Trajectory	Rationale for Selection	Main Inclusion/ Exclusion Issue
East Africa	Platform-based welfare and hybrid governance	Selected to examine digital welfare systems mediated by mobile money, telecom operators, payment providers, NGOs, humanitarian agencies, and public-private partnerships. This configuration illustrates how social protection can expand rapidly through platform infrastructures where traditional banking or administrative systems are limited.	Platform dependence; fragmented accountability; payment failures; unclear allocation of responsibility among public authorities, private providers, and humanitarian actors.
India	Centralized digital identity and biometric welfare integration	Selected to examine the welfare implications of a large-scale national digital identity infrastructure. Aadhaar illustrates how centralized identification and biometric authentication can support administrative integration and scale, while also amplifying the consequences of authentication failure or data mismatch.	Biometric authentication failure; exclusion from essential services; weak fallback procedures; systemic risk generated by the coupling of digital identity with welfare entitlements.
Latin America	Digital targeting and fragmented institutional control	Selected to examine registry-based targeting in welfare systems with longer traditions of social assistance and conditional cash transfers. This configuration illustrates how relatively mature social registries can coexist with institutional fragmentation, political discontinuity, and uneven local implementation capacity.	Outdated or incomplete registries; targeting errors; uneven municipal capacity; weak coordination across national, regional, and local welfare institutions.

The three configurations are not intended to represent homogeneous regional models, but to capture different governance arrangements through which digital welfare systems are designed, implemented, and contested in LMIC contexts.

The comparison is structured around seven criteria. The first is the **degree of centralization of digital infrastructure**, which concerns whether welfare systems rely on centralized identity or registry architectures, decentralized platforms, or fragmented institutional databases. The second is the **role of private and international**

actors, including telecom operators, payment providers, technology vendors, donors, humanitarian agencies, and international organizations. The third is the **quality and integration of social data**, including the completeness, timeliness, interoperability, and representativeness of civil registries, social registries, administrative datasets, and beneficiary records.

The fourth criterion is **institutional and administrative capacity**, understood as the ability of public authorities to manage digital welfare infrastructures, oversee vendors, update data, maintain systems, and adapt programmes to changing social conditions. The fifth criterion is the presence and effectiveness of **accountability and redress mechanisms**, including transparency obligations, appeal procedures, human review, grievance channels, and independent oversight. The sixth criterion concerns the **observable forms of algorithmic or digital exclusion**, such as statistical invisibility, biometric authentication failure, misclassification, digital access barriers, payment exclusion, or inability to contest automated decisions. The seventh criterion is the **role of civil society and external auditing**, including community monitoring, social audits, advocacy organizations, local research institutions, legal aid networks, and civic technology initiatives.

By applying these criteria, the comparison seeks to avoid two risks. The first is technological determinism: the assumption that digital welfare systems produce inclusion or exclusion simply because of the technologies they use. The second is regional generalization: the tendency to describe broad regions as if they were internally uniform. Instead, the analysis focuses on governance configurations and institutional mechanisms. The chapter therefore treats East Africa, India, and Latin America not as fixed geographic categories, but as cases that illuminate different ways in which digital welfare systems can be organized, governed, and contested.

This methodological approach supports the broader argument of the chapter. Algorithmic inclusion is not a universal technical property that can be measured independently of context. It is a governance outcome shaped by the interaction between data infrastructures, institutional capacity, technological design, public accountability, and social participation. The comparative analysis that follows uses the three configurations to identify how these dimensions operate in practice and how they may either mitigate or reproduce exclusion in digital welfare systems.

References to East Africa, India, and Latin America in the following analysis do not imply internal homogeneity. Each configuration contains significant variation across countries, states, municipalities, welfare programmes, administrative capacities, and political economies. The purpose of the comparison is not to generalize uniformly across these regions, but to identify governance patterns that recur in documented digital welfare initiatives. For this reason, the analysis uses regional labels as analytical entry points rather than as comprehensive descriptions of internally uniform welfare systems. Where relevant, the discussion points to subnational, national, or programme-level differences in order to avoid treating regional trajectories as monolithic.

4.2 East Africa: Platform-Based Welfare and Hybrid Governance

East Africa represents one of the most dynamic regions globally in terms of digital welfare experimentation, particularly through the integration of mobile money platforms into social protection systems. Governments, humanitarian agencies, and development partners have leveraged widespread mobile phone adoption to deliver cash transfers, emergency relief, and targeted assistance directly to beneficiaries, often bypassing traditional banking infrastructures.

This trajectory, however, should not be read as a uniform regional model. Digital welfare initiatives in East Africa vary considerably across national and local contexts. Kenya is often associated with a more mature mobile money ecosystem and a relatively advanced use of digital payment rails in social assistance and humanitarian transfers. Uganda and Tanzania present different combinations of mobile connectivity, donor involvement, administrative capacity, and regulatory oversight. In refugee-hosting or humanitarian settings, digital cash transfers may be organized through partnerships between international agencies, NGOs, payment providers, and host governments, producing governance arrangements that differ from nationally administered social protection programmes. East Africa is therefore used here as an analytical configuration of platform-mediated welfare, not as a homogeneous regional welfare regime.

From an inclusion perspective, platform-based welfare delivery has produced tangible benefits. Mobile money–enabled transfers have expanded geographic reach, reduced transaction costs, and increased the speed and flexibility of support, especially in rural and underserved areas. For populations exposed to climate shocks, food insecurity, or displacement, digital platforms have enabled rapid scaling and adaptive responses that would be difficult to achieve through conventional administrative channels.

A more localized reading illustrates this diversity. In Kenya, the diffusion of mobile money has created favourable conditions for using digital payment systems in cash transfer programmes and emergency assistance. The welfare function is mediated by an existing commercial and financial infrastructure that can be repurposed for social protection delivery. In humanitarian contexts, by contrast, digital cash transfers often depend on temporary or programme-specific arrangements among international organizations, NGOs, telecom operators, and payment providers. These arrangements can improve speed and reach, but they also raise distinct accountability questions: beneficiaries may interact with a chain of intermediaries rather than with a clearly identifiable public welfare authority. The inclusionary potential of platform-based welfare therefore depends not only on mobile access, but also on the governance of the institutional ecosystem through which transfers are delivered.

However, the reliance on platforms introduces hybrid governance arrangements that blur the boundaries between public authority and private infrastructure. Beneficiary identification and targeting often depend on fragmented datasets assembled from multiple actors, including government agencies, NGOs, telecom operators, and payment service providers. Data quality, interoperability, and update cycles vary widely, increasing the risk of duplication, exclusion, or inconsistent eligibility determinations.

Moreover, algorithmic processes embedded in payment platforms—such as automated enrolment rules or fraud detection mechanisms—are frequently opaque to public authorities. Oversight and accountability mechanisms remain limited, and grievance procedures are often mediated through intermediaries rather than directly accessible to beneficiaries. As a result, while East African digital welfare systems demonstrate high levels of operational innovation, their capacity to ensure algorithmic inclusion depends heavily on external actors and informal governance practices.

An empirical illustration helps clarify this configuration. Mobile money–based cash transfers in Kenya have shown how existing payment infrastructures can be used to deliver assistance rapidly and flexibly, particularly in emergency or humanitarian settings. Early experiences with M-PESA-based transfers and humanitarian e-payments demonstrated the operational advantages of bulk digital payments, including speed, reduced travel costs, and improved reach in areas where banking infrastructure was limited (CALP Network, 2012).

However, these same arrangements also reveal the governance complexity of platform-based welfare. Beneficiaries may depend on telecom operators, payment agents, NGOs, humanitarian organizations, and public agencies at the same time. When payments fail, accounts are blocked, identification data are inconsistent, or agents are unavailable, responsibility may be difficult to assign. The empirical lesson is therefore twofold: platform-based welfare can expand access, but only if payment infrastructures are matched by clear accountability, accessible grievance channels, and public oversight of private intermediaries.

4.3 India: Centralized Digital Identity and Systemic Risk

India's Aadhaar system constitutes one of the most ambitious digital identification infrastructures globally and occupies a central position within the country's welfare architecture. By linking biometric identification to a wide range of social programmes—including food subsidies, cash transfers, pensions, and healthcare—

Aadhaar seeks to streamline delivery, reduce leakage, and enhance administrative control.

India is particularly useful for the purposes of this chapter because it combines a highly centralized digital identity infrastructure with substantial subnational variation in welfare implementation. Aadhaar provides a national layer of identification and authentication, but its effects depend on state-level administrative capacity, local welfare institutions, connectivity, grievance mechanisms, and the specific design of individual programmes. The experience of digital welfare in a state with stronger administrative capacity and higher levels of social development, such as Kerala, may differ significantly from implementation in poorer, more rural, or administratively constrained settings such as Bihar. For this reason, India should not be interpreted as a single homogeneous case, but as a centralized identity architecture whose welfare implications vary across territories, programmes, and administrative contexts.

From a state capacity perspective, Aadhaar has enabled unprecedented integration of welfare databases and facilitated the consolidation of beneficiary records across programmes and jurisdictions. Centralized digital identity has reduced certain forms of duplication and improved the government's ability to monitor expenditure and compliance. These features align with efficiency-driven narratives of digital welfare reform.

The effects of Aadhaar-linked welfare also vary across programmes. Authentication requirements may operate differently in food distribution systems, pension schemes, health insurance programmes, employment-related benefits, or direct benefit transfers. In urban contexts, connectivity, access to service points, and administrative alternatives may reduce the consequences of authentication failure. In rural or remote areas, by contrast, biometric failure, poor connectivity, limited awareness of appeal procedures, and the distance from administrative offices can make exclusion more difficult to correct. The same national infrastructure may therefore produce different welfare outcomes depending on the density of local institutions, the availability of fallback mechanisms, and the capacity of frontline administrators to exercise discretion when digital verification fails.

At the same time, Aadhaar illustrates the systemic risks associated with centralized algorithmic governance. Biometric authentication failures, connectivity constraints, and data mismatches have resulted in documented cases of exclusion from essential services. The binary logic of biometric verification - authentication success or failure - leaves limited scope for contextual discretion, particularly in remote or resource-constrained settings.

Governance concerns extend beyond technical reliability. Aadhaar concentrates significant power over data and decision-making within a limited set of institutions, amplifying the consequences of design flaws or governance failures. While formal grievance mechanisms exist, their accessibility and effectiveness vary widely, especially for marginalized populations with limited administrative literacy. India's experience thus highlights a central trade-off of digital welfare: centralization can enhance control and scalability, but it also amplifies the impact of algorithmic error and weakens individual agency when safeguards are insufficient.

An empirical illustration of this trade-off can be found in Aadhaar-linked welfare delivery, particularly in programmes where biometric authentication is required to access food subsidies, pensions, wages, or cash transfers. Research on India's digital welfare architecture shows that Aadhaar can improve beneficiary identification and reduce certain forms of duplication, but it can also create exclusionary risks when authentication becomes a mandatory gateway to entitlements. In the Public Distribution System, for instance, fingerprint mismatch, connectivity failure, seeding errors, or discrepancies between identity and ration databases may prevent eligible households from receiving subsidized food (Carswell & De Neve, 2022; Muralidharan, Niehaus, & Sukhtankar, 2022). The problem is not simply biometric error in isolation, but the coupling of biometric verification with essential welfare access. Where fallback mechanisms, human discretion, and appeal procedures are weak, a technical failure can become a denial of social rights. India therefore illustrates the systemic risk of centralized digital identity: scale magnifies both administrative efficiency and the consequences of failure.

4.4 Latin America: Digital Targeting and Fragmented Institutional Control

Latin American welfare systems have a long tradition of targeted social assistance, supported by integrated social registries and conditional cash transfer programs. In recent years, these systems have increasingly incorporated digital platforms, data integration tools, and, in some cases, predictive analytics to refine targeting, improve coordination, and monitor programme performance.

Latin America, however, should also be understood as an internally differentiated configuration. Countries in the region vary significantly in the maturity of their social registries, the institutional stability of conditional cash transfer programmes, the degree of interoperability among welfare databases, and the strength of subnational implementation capacity. Some countries have developed relatively sophisticated household registries and targeting systems over several decades, while others face greater fragmentation, uneven data quality, or discontinuity across political cycles. Moreover, even within countries, digital targeting may operate differently across national ministries, municipalities, rural areas, urban peripheries, and Indigenous territories. The regional label is therefore used here to capture a broad trajectory of digital targeting and registry-based welfare, not to imply uniformity across Latin American welfare systems.

Compared to other LMIC regions, Latin America benefits from relatively mature administrative datasets and established social policy institutions. Digital tools have enhanced interoperability across agencies and improved the identification of households eligible for multiple programmes. In some cases, data-driven approaches have supported more nuanced assessments of vulnerability that go beyond income-based measures.

A localized perspective shows that the maturity of social registries does not automatically translate into uniform inclusion. Registry-based systems may perform relatively well where household information is regularly updated, municipal administrations are capable of supporting enrolment, and beneficiaries can access channels for correction or appeal. In more fragmented settings, however, outdated household data, weak coordination between national and local authorities, or limited outreach to rural and Indigenous communities can produce exclusion even when the formal targeting architecture appears advanced. This suggests that the key variable is not only the existence of a digital registry, but the institutional capacity to maintain it, update it, contest it, and connect it to actual welfare delivery.

Nevertheless, institutional fragmentation remains a defining challenge. Welfare responsibilities are often distributed across national, regional, and municipal levels, resulting in heterogeneous implementation capacities and inconsistent data standards. Predictive models used for targeting or prioritization are rarely subject to independent evaluation, and their decision logic is often opaque to both administrators and beneficiaries.

Political volatility further complicates governance. Shifts in government priorities can disrupt digital welfare initiatives, undermining continuity and institutional learning. As a result, algorithmic systems may persist without adequate updating or oversight, increasing the risk of outdated classifications and cumulative exclusion. Latin America thus illustrates a scenario in which relatively advanced data infrastructures coexist with governance gaps that constrain algorithmic inclusion.

An empirical illustration can be drawn from the evolution of social registries in Latin America and the Caribbean (World Bank, 2025; Guven, Yeachuri, & Almenfi, 2025). Countries such as Chile and Brazil have developed relatively mature registry-based systems that support multiple programmes and allow household information to be used across social protection, health, education, employment, or economic inclusion policies.

These systems show the inclusionary potential of integrated registries when data are regularly updated, linked to programme delivery, and supported by intersectoral coordination. At the same time, regional experience also shows that the existence of a registry is not sufficient to guarantee inclusion. Where household data are outdated, municipal capacity is weak, data-sharing arrangements are fragmented, or political cycles interrupt system maintenance, targeting errors and exclusion may persist. Latin

America therefore illustrates a distinctive governance challenge: digital targeting can improve coordination and shock response, but only if registry quality, local implementation capacity, and mechanisms for correction are continuously sustained.

4.5 Cross-Regional Comparison: Patterns and Trade-Offs

The comparison that follows should be read in light of this internal variation. The three configurations do not correspond to uniform regional models, but to dominant governance patterns that appear differently across countries, programmes, and administrative levels. The purpose of comparison is therefore to identify recurrent governance trade-offs without erasing contextual heterogeneity.

A comparative reading of the three regions reveals several cross-cutting patterns. First, digital welfare systems across LMICs tend to prioritize efficiency, scalability, and control, often at the expense of transparency and contestability. Second, algorithmic exclusion rarely stems from explicit policy intent; rather, it emerges from the interaction between data limitations, technological design, and institutional constraints.

At the same time, the regions differ markedly in how risks are distributed. In East Africa, exclusion risks are often linked to platform dependence and fragmented public oversight. In India, risks arise from the concentration of authority and the systemic consequences of centralized failure. In Latin America, exclusion is more likely to result from institutional fragmentation and weak coordination rather than from technological sophistication per se.

These differences suggest that algorithmic inclusion cannot be achieved through a one-size-fits-all model.

A cross-cutting empirical trade-off concerns the tension between speed and inclusion. Digital welfare systems are often valued because they can scale rapidly, especially during emergencies. Mobile money transfers can reach beneficiaries faster than conventional payment mechanisms; centralized identity systems can accelerate verification; social registries can support rapid targeting when shocks occur. Yet speed often depends on pre-existing infrastructures, datasets, and administrative classifications. Populations already registered, connected, identified, and banked are easier to reach quickly, while those outside these systems may remain excluded. This suggests that speed is not merely an operational feature of digital welfare; it is also a distributional variable. The faster a programme relies on existing digital infrastructures without additional outreach, correction, or fallback mechanisms, the greater the risk that rapid delivery will reproduce prior patterns of administrative visibility and invisibility.

Another cross-cutting empirical issue concerns the role of civil society, local researchers, legal aid organizations, and civic technology actors in detecting exclusion. Digital welfare failures are often first observed not through formal audits, but through complaints, field reports, litigation, social audits, journalistic investigations, or community monitoring. In platform-based systems, civil society may identify payment failures or abusive intermediation. In identity-based systems, it may document authentication failures, denial of entitlements, or the absence of effective alternatives. In registry-based systems, it may reveal outdated classifications, exclusion of informal settlements, or barriers faced by Indigenous and rural communities. These forms of external scrutiny are not substitutes for public accountability, but they can act as early warning mechanisms and help translate individual grievances into systemic evidence. For this reason, algorithmic inclusion should include the capacity of welfare systems to receive, process, and respond to evidence generated outside the state.

Governance strategies must be tailored to specific institutional configurations. Where platforms dominate, strengthening public oversight and contractual accountability becomes critical. Where centralization prevails, safeguards for redress and human discretion are essential. Where fragmentation persists, coordination and standard-setting should be prioritized.

4.6 Implications for Algorithmic Inclusion

The comparative analysis reinforces the argument that algorithmic inclusion is fundamentally a governance challenge. Technological tools can support welfare expansion, but only when embedded within institutional arrangements that ensure representation, accountability, and participation. Across all three regions, governance capacity—not technological novelty—emerges as the decisive factor shaping inclusionary outcomes.

These insights inform the framework developed in the following section by illustrating how the dimensions of algorithmic inclusion manifest differently across contexts. The comparative perspective thus serves as a bridge between empirical observation and conceptual generalization, grounding the framework in real-world welfare trajectories.

At the same time, the comparison also shows that algorithmic inclusion cannot be operationalized through a context-blind template. The same governance principle may require different institutional solutions depending on the configuration in which it is applied. In platform-based systems, inclusion may depend primarily on public oversight of private intermediaries, contractual accountability, and accessible payment grievance mechanisms. In centralized identity systems, it may require robust fallback procedures, human discretion, and safeguards against systemic authentication failure. In registry-based targeting systems, it may depend on data updating, local administrative capacity, and coordination across levels of government. Recognizing internal variation is therefore not a limitation of the comparative approach, but a condition for making algorithmic inclusion analytically and operationally meaningful.

The empirical illustrations discussed in this section reinforce the need for a framework that can connect technical design with institutional practice. Mobile money transfers, biometric identity systems, and social registries differ in architecture and policy purpose, but they reveal a common pattern: exclusion is produced across the delivery chain, not only at the point of algorithmic classification. It may occur when people are absent from datasets, when authentication fails, when registries are outdated, when payment systems depend on inaccessible intermediaries, or when grievance mechanisms are too weak to correct errors. The algorithmic inclusion framework developed in the next section is intended to capture precisely this lifecycle dimension of digital welfare governance.

5. THE ALGORITHMIC INCLUSION FRAMEWORK

The analysis developed so far highlights a central paradox of digital welfare in low- and middle-income countries (LMICs): the same technologies that promise expanded coverage, efficiency, and precision can also generate new and less visible forms of exclusion. Digital platforms, biometric identification systems, and predictive analytics are often introduced as neutral tools for improving welfare delivery, yet their social effects depend critically on how they are embedded within data infrastructures, institutional arrangements, and governance regimes.

Addressing this paradox requires moving beyond fragmented or technology-centric interventions and adopting a holistic framework capable of integrating technical design, institutional governance, and social participation. This section introduces algorithmic inclusion as such a framework. Algorithmic inclusion is not conceived as a purely technical attribute of algorithms, nor as a generic normative aspiration. Rather, it is defined as the capacity of digital welfare systems to equitably recognise, process, and respond to social vulnerability across the entire data and decision-making lifecycle, while ensuring transparency, accountability, and meaningful avenues for redress.

In LMIC contexts, algorithmic inclusion provides a particularly useful lens because welfare systems often operate under conditions of scarcity, informality, and administrative fragility. Under these conditions, even minor design choices can have disproportionate distributive effects. The framework articulated here is therefore explicitly context-sensitive and intended to function both as an analytical tool for evaluating existing systems and as a normative guide for future policy design.

The algorithmic inclusion framework is structured around five core dimensions — data representation, transparency and explainability, accountability and redress, participatory governance, and institutional capacity and technological autonomy — complemented by a cross-cutting concern with infrastructural sustainability and data sovereignty. While analytically distinct, these dimensions are deeply interconnected and mutually reinforcing.

5.1 Data Representation and Inclusivity

At the foundation of algorithmic inclusion lies the question of who is represented in data and how. Digital welfare systems rely on data infrastructures that convert lived social conditions into standardized categories and variables. These representations shape how vulnerability is defined, measured, and prioritized. When data are incomplete, outdated, or biased, exclusion becomes embedded at the earliest stage of the algorithmic pipeline.

In LMICs, representational exclusion often reflects structural characteristics of the social and economic environment. High levels of informality, internal migration, seasonal employment, and weak civil registration systems limit the ability of administrative data to capture dynamic forms of vulnerability. As a result, welfare databases may overrepresent populations that are already administratively visible while systematically underrepresenting those at the margins.

Enhancing representational inclusion therefore requires more than expanding data coverage. It involves critical reflection on the categories and indicators used to model vulnerability. Periodic audits of social registries can help identify under-represented groups, inconsistencies across datasets, and systematic biases in data collection practices. Such audits should not be treated as one-off technical exercises, but as ongoing governance processes integrated into welfare administration.

Algorithmic inclusion also implies methodological pluralism. Complementing administrative data with alternative sources - such as community-based surveys, participatory mapping, qualitative assessments, and grievance data - can mitigate statistical invisibility. These approaches recognise that vulnerability is relational and context-dependent, and that not all relevant dimensions of social risk can be captured through standardized quantitative indicators alone.

5.2 Transparency and Explainability

Transparency is a core component of algorithmic inclusion, yet it is frequently interpreted in narrow technical terms. Within digital welfare systems, transparency must instead be understood as the capacity of diverse stakeholders - administrators, beneficiaries, oversight bodies, and civil society -to understand how decisions are made and on what basis.

Algorithmic inclusion requires systematic documentation of model objectives, input variables, decision rules, performance metrics, and known limitations. Such documentation supports internal learning within public administrations and enables external scrutiny. However, transparency cannot be limited to technical disclosure aimed at experts alone. Explainability mechanisms must be tailored to different audiences and levels of digital literacy.

For beneficiaries, explanations should focus on practical intelligibility: why a decision was taken, which factors were considered, and what steps can be taken to challenge or correct an outcome. In LMIC contexts, where literacy and language diversity are significant factors, explainability also depends on interface design, communication strategies, and the availability of human intermediaries.

Transparency further extends to institutional processes surrounding data use and decision-making. Clear communication regarding eligibility criteria, data sharing arrangements, and system updates helps demystify welfare systems and reduces perceptions of arbitrariness. Without such transparency, digital welfare risks undermining trust and legitimacy, particularly among populations already sceptical of state institutions.

5.3 Accountability and Redress Mechanisms

Algorithmic inclusion cannot be achieved without effective accountability structures. In welfare systems, accountability entails the ability to identify responsibility for decisions, correct errors, and provide remedies when harm occurs. Automated and semi-automated decision-making complicates these processes by diffusing responsibility across technical systems, administrative units, and private vendors.

In LMICs, accountability gaps are often exacerbated by limited institutional capacity and fragmented governance. Beneficiaries who experience exclusion due to algorithmic errors may face significant barriers in seeking redress, including geographic distance, bureaucratic complexity, and lack of information. When grievance mechanisms exist, they are frequently under-resourced or poorly integrated into digital welfare workflows.

Algorithmic inclusion requires that grievance and redress mechanisms be accessible, timely, and effective. This includes clearly defined institutional responsibilities, standardized procedures for human review of automated decisions, and fallback options when digital systems fail. Importantly, redress mechanisms should be designed with the assumption that errors will occur, rather than treating them as exceptional anomalies.

Beyond individual cases, accountability also requires systemic oversight. Independent audit institutions, ombudspersons, and data protection authorities play a critical role in monitoring algorithmic welfare systems, identifying patterns of exclusion, and recommending corrective action. Embedding digital welfare within broader legal and institutional frameworks is therefore essential for sustaining algorithmic inclusion over time.

5.4 Participatory and Contextual Governance

A defining feature of algorithmic inclusion is the recognition that technical systems are embedded in social and cultural contexts. Participatory governance mechanisms enable welfare systems to adapt to local realities and to incorporate forms of knowledge that are not readily captured by data-driven models.

Involving communities, civil society organizations, and beneficiary groups in the design, implementation, and evaluation of digital welfare systems can surface contextual insights regarding social norms, informal coping strategies, and local perceptions of vulnerability. Participation can take multiple forms, including co-design workshops, feedback loops, social audits, and community monitoring initiatives.

The role of civil society and local technology ecosystems is particularly important in this regard. In many digital welfare systems, exclusionary effects are first detected not through formal government audits, but through the work of NGOs, legal aid organizations, community groups, journalists, local researchers, civic technology initiatives, data justice organizations, and beneficiary associations. These actors can document authentication failures, payment interruptions, outdated registry classifications, exclusion of informal workers, barriers faced by rural or Indigenous communities, and weaknesses in grievance mechanisms. Their contribution is especially valuable in LMIC contexts, where public oversight bodies may lack sufficient resources or technical expertise to monitor complex digital welfare systems continuously.

Participatory governance should therefore extend beyond consultation at the design stage. It should include institutionalized mechanisms for external scrutiny, community monitoring, social audits, participatory evaluation, and independent reporting of harms. Local civic tech actors and research institutions can help translate individual complaints into systemic evidence, identify patterns of exclusion across territories or social groups, and test whether official explanations correspond to beneficiaries' lived experiences. Legal aid organizations can support contestability by helping affected individuals challenge erroneous classifications or denial of benefits. NGOs and community-based organizations can act as intermediaries between vulnerable populations and public administrations, especially where literacy, language, geography, or digital access create barriers to direct engagement.

However, the involvement of civil society should not be treated as a substitute for state responsibility. Algorithmic inclusion requires public institutions to create formal channels through which evidence generated by civil society, local researchers, beneficiary associations, legal aid organizations, and civic technology actors can influence system redesign, data updating, procurement requirements, audit priorities, and redress procedures. This is particularly important in LMICs, where digital welfare systems are often introduced through top-down processes driven by external funding, technological expertise, or emergency implementation needs, and where affected populations may perceive digitalisation as imposed rather than enabling if they are excluded from decision-making.

For this reason, participation should not be reduced to symbolic consultation. It should become an institutional mechanism through which local knowledge, beneficiary experience, civil society evidence, and independent monitoring can influence system design, implementation, and correction over time. Without such channels, participation risks remaining external to the actual governance of welfare infrastructures. A more inclusive model of digital welfare should therefore combine state accountability with civic oversight, allowing local knowledge and independent monitoring to become part of the institutional learning process.

5.5 Institutional Capacity and Technological Autonomy

The final dimension of algorithmic inclusion concerns institutional capacity and technological autonomy. Governing complex digital welfare systems requires sustained investment in human capital, organizational learning, and regulatory capability. Without such capacity, even well-designed systems risk becoming rigid, opaque, or dependent on external actors.

In LMICs, capacity building should encompass data governance, cybersecurity, ethical assessment, and algorithmic auditing. Strengthening internal expertise enhances the ability of public administrations to oversee vendors, negotiate contractual arrangements, and adapt systems over time. Technological autonomy does not imply rejecting private-sector collaboration, but rather ensuring that public institutions retain strategic control over welfare infrastructures.

In LMIC contexts, technological autonomy also has a geopolitical dimension. Digital welfare systems increasingly depend on cloud infrastructures, biometric technologies, payment platforms, data analytics tools, cybersecurity services, and software architectures that may be supplied by foreign technology providers. In many cases, these providers are embedded in broader geopolitical ecosystems dominated by major technological powers, including the United States, China, and other advanced digital economies. This dependence does not necessarily make digital welfare systems exclusionary, but it raises important questions about data sovereignty, public control, long-term adaptability, and democratic accountability.

Geopolitical data sovereignty refers here to the capacity of public authorities to determine how welfare data are collected, stored, processed, transferred, audited, and governed, without losing strategic control over critical infrastructures. This is particularly important when social protection systems process sensitive information on poverty, identity, household composition, health, migration status, disability, or financial vulnerability. If core components of welfare infrastructure are outsourced through opaque contracts, proprietary platforms, or externally controlled cloud environments, public authorities may face constraints in auditing systems, enforcing data protection standards, modifying eligibility rules, or ensuring continuity of service.

For this reason, technological autonomy should be understood as a governance condition for algorithmic inclusion. It requires procurement strategies that preserve audit rights, data portability, interoperability, open standards, cybersecurity requirements, and public ownership or effective public control over critical data infrastructures. It also requires capacity transfer from vendors and development partners to domestic institutions, so that public administrations are not permanently dependent on external actors for the operation, maintenance, and adaptation of welfare systems. Algorithmic inclusion therefore depends not only on whether digital welfare tools work in the short term, but also on whether states retain the institutional and technological capacity to govern them over time.

Adopting open standards, promoting interoperability, and avoiding excessive vendor lock-in are key strategies for sustaining algorithmic inclusion. These measures translate technological autonomy from an abstract policy aspiration into a concrete condition for accountable and adaptable digital welfare governance.

5.6 Integrating the Framework

Taken together, these five dimensions illustrate that algorithmic inclusion is not a single intervention or checklist. It is a governance orientation that requires coordination across technical, institutional, and social domains. Weaknesses in any single dimension—such as poor data quality, lack of accountability, or limited participation—can undermine the inclusionary potential of digital welfare systems as a whole.

In LMIC contexts, where welfare systems operate under conditions of scarcity and inequality, such coordination is particularly challenging but also particularly consequential. The algorithmic inclusion framework developed here provides a structured way to assess trade-offs, identify governance gaps, and prioritize interventions. It sets the stage for the concluding discussion by linking conceptual analysis to concrete policy implications and pathways for reform.

5.7 Operationalizing Algorithmic Inclusion: A Starter Kit for Policymakers

Beyond its analytical and normative value, algorithmic inclusion can be operationalized as a practical evaluation and policy tool for assessing digital welfare systems throughout their lifecycle. Treating algorithmic inclusion as an operational framework allows policymakers, welfare administrators, development actors, and oversight bodies to move from general principles to concrete governance questions. This is particularly important in low- and middle-income countries, where digital welfare initiatives are often introduced under conditions of limited administrative capacity, fiscal pressure, infrastructural constraint, and urgent demand for rapid scaling.

From an ex-ante perspective, the framework can be used before implementation to identify potential exclusionary risks. At this stage, policymakers should interrogate the assumptions embedded in data sources, eligibility models, authentication procedures, payment systems, procurement choices, and grievance mechanisms. The key question is not simply whether a digital welfare system can deliver benefits more efficiently, but whether it can recognize diverse forms of vulnerability, avoid reproducing administrative invisibility, and preserve meaningful avenues for correction and appeal.

From an ex-post perspective, algorithmic inclusion can be used to evaluate existing digital welfare systems. Each dimension of the framework can be translated into operational questions, indicators, and corrective actions. This allows evaluators to examine not only aggregate performance, such as number of beneficiaries reached or payment speed, but also the distribution of errors, the accessibility of explanations, the effectiveness of redress mechanisms, the role of affected communities, the degree of public control over infrastructure, and the sustainability of the underlying digital architecture.

Table 2 provides a practical starting point for operationalizing algorithmic inclusion in policy design, implementation, monitoring, and evaluation.

Table 2. Operationalizing Algorithmic Inclusion: A Starter Kit for Policymakers

Dimension	Guiding Question	Possible Indicators	Priority Actions
Data representation	Who remains invisible in the data?	Coverage gaps; frequency of data updates; error rates by group, territory, gender, age, disability, migration status, or rural/urban location; share of beneficiaries without formal identification; mismatch between registry data and local evidence	Conduct periodic audits of social registries; integrate community-based data and local verification; update records continuously; use complementary qualitative assessments; identify underrepresented groups before deployment
Transparency	Do beneficiaries understand the decision?	Availability of explanations; clarity of eligibility criteria; documentation of model objectives, variables and decision rules; availability of information in local languages; accessibility for low-literacy users; existence of public model cards or system documentation	Provide simplified communications; publish non-technical explanations; develop public-facing model cards; train frontline intermediaries; use local languages and accessible formats; disclose data-sharing and eligibility rules
Redress	Can an error be contested and corrected?	Number and type of appeals; resolution times; reversal rates; accessibility of grievance channels; availability of physical and digital appeal options; existence of human review; use of fallback procedures when authentication or payment fails	Establish clear appeal mechanisms; guarantee human review of automated or semi-automated decisions; create manual fallback procedures; monitor unresolved complaints; make grievance channels accessible through local offices, mobile units, community organizations, and digital tools
Participation	Do affected communities influence the system?	Number and quality of consultations; existence of social audits; feedback loops from beneficiaries; involvement of NGOs, civic tech actors, local researchers, legal aid organizations and community groups; evidence of system changes following participatory inputs	Introduce co-design processes; institutionalize civic auditing; support community monitoring; involve civil society in evaluation; create channels for external evidence to influence system redesign; include vulnerable groups in testing and review

continued on following page

Table 2. Continued

Dimension	Guiding Question	Possible Indicators	Priority Actions
Institutional capacity	Does the state effectively control the infrastructure?	Availability of internal technical expertise; capacity to audit models, databases and vendors; degree of dependence on external providers; contractual access to documentation and audit rights; interoperability of systems; existence of data governance teams	Invest in public-sector capacity building; include audit clauses in procurement contracts; require open standards and interoperability; avoid excessive vendor lock-in; build internal data governance and algorithmic oversight units; transfer knowledge from vendors to public institutions
Sustainability and sovereignty	Is the system sustainable and technologically autonomous?	Energy and maintenance costs; dependence on foreign cloud or platform providers; hardware replacement cycles; e-waste management; cybersecurity resilience; data localization or data transfer arrangements; continuity risks linked to vendor or donor dependence	Include environmental and infrastructural assessments in digital welfare projects; adopt sustainable procurement strategies; strengthen data sovereignty safeguards; promote interoperability and data portability; assess cloud and platform dependencies; plan for long-term maintenance and institutional ownership

This checklist is not intended to function as a rigid compliance template. Rather, it provides a diagnostic tool for identifying where exclusionary risks may arise and which governance interventions may be required. Its value lies in connecting technical design choices with institutional responsibilities and social consequences. For example, a biometric authentication system should not be assessed only in terms of technical accuracy, but also in terms of fallback options, human discretion, appeal channels, maintenance capacity, and the social groups most exposed to authentication failure. Similarly, a social registry should not be assessed only by the number of households included, but also by the frequency of updates, the visibility of informal and mobile populations, and the ability of households to correct outdated information.

The checklist can also support comparative evaluation across programmes and jurisdictions. By applying the same dimensions to different welfare systems, policymakers and development actors can identify recurring weaknesses, such as poor registry updating, limited contestability, excessive dependence on vendors, or weak civil society involvement. This comparative use is particularly relevant in LMIC contexts, where digital welfare initiatives are often developed through donor-funded projects, public-private partnerships, or crisis-driven interventions that may not be fully coordinated with long-term social protection strategies.

Operationalizing algorithmic inclusion also requires attention to timing. Some questions must be addressed before deployment, such as whether the data used to target beneficiaries are representative, whether procurement contracts preserve public audit rights, and whether fallback procedures exist. Other questions require continuous monitoring after implementation, such as whether certain groups experience higher error rates, whether appeals are resolved within reasonable timeframes, and whether digital infrastructures remain sustainable and secure. Inclusion should therefore be understood as an ongoing governance process, not as a one-time design objective.

For governments, the framework can guide the design of digital welfare reforms and help prioritize investments in data quality, administrative capacity, and accountability. For international organizations and development partners, it can inform funding criteria and technical assistance by shifting attention from technological deployment to institutional sustainability. For civil society and oversight bodies, it can provide a structured vocabulary for identifying harms, documenting exclusion, and demanding corrective action.

In this sense, algorithmic inclusion becomes both an evaluative lens and a practical governance instrument. It translates the chapter's central argument into a set of operational questions: who is represented, who understands the decision, who can contest an error, who participates in system design, who controls the infrastructure, and whether the system can be sustained over time. These questions are essential if digital welfare systems are to strengthen social protection rather than reproduce old forms of exclusion through new technological means.

6. DISCUSSION, POLICY IMPLICATIONS, AND CONCLUSIONS

6.1 Discussion: Rethinking Digital Welfare Through Algorithmic Inclusion

The analysis developed in this chapter highlights that digital welfare systems in low- and middle-income countries (LMICs) cannot be adequately assessed through narrow metrics of efficiency, coverage, or fraud reduction alone. While data-driven tools and algorithmic processes have expanded the operational reach of social protection in many contexts, they have also introduced new mechanisms through which exclusion and vulnerability are produced.

A key insight emerging from the comparative analysis is that algorithmic exclusion is rarely accidental or purely technical. Rather, it reflects the interaction between data infrastructures, institutional capacity, governance arrangements, and structural inequality. Informational gaps, biometric failures, predictive bias, and digital conditionalities do not operate independently; they reinforce one another within socio-technical systems that often lack effective oversight and contestability.

The concept of algorithmic inclusion developed in this chapter responds to these dynamics by reframing digital welfare as a governance challenge rather than a technological one. It shifts analytical attention away from isolated algorithmic artifacts toward the broader institutional ecosystems in which they are embedded. In doing so, it aligns with emerging perspectives that view digital transformation as a contested and politically consequential process, particularly in settings where welfare systems are central to social survival.

Importantly, the framework does not imply that algorithmic systems are inherently exclusionary. Instead, it underscores that inclusion is contingent: it depends on design choices, data practices, institutional safeguards, and participatory mechanisms. In LMIC contexts, where margins of error can have severe material consequences, these contingencies acquire heightened significance.

This discussion sets the stage for the policy implications outlined in the following section.

6.2 Policy Implications

Building on the discussion above, the findings of this chapter translate into a set of policy-relevant implications for governments, international organizations, and development partners engaged in digital welfare initiatives.

First, data governance must be treated as a core component of social policy, not as a technical back-office function. Investments in digital welfare should prioritize data quality, representativeness, and update cycles, with explicit strategies to identify and address underrepresented populations. Periodic audits of social registries and eligibility models should become standard practice.

Second, algorithmic transparency and accountability require institutionalization. Governments should establish clear governance frameworks defining responsibility for algorithmic decisions, including mechanisms for human oversight and accessible redress. In LMICs, simplified and locally accessible grievance procedures are essential to prevent automated exclusion from becoming irreversible.

Third, capacity building within public administrations is critical. Without internal expertise in data governance and algorithmic assessment, states risk becoming dependent on external vendors and donors for core welfare functions. Capacity-building initiatives should be long-term, integrated into civil service development, and aligned with national regulatory frameworks.

Fourth, participatory governance should be recognised as a functional necessity, not merely a normative ideal. Engaging communities, civil society organizations, and beneficiaries in the design and evaluation of digital welfare systems enhances contextual relevance and legitimacy. Participatory mechanisms can also act as early warning systems, identifying exclusionary effects before they become systemic.

Fifth, digital welfare strategies should incorporate infrastructural sustainability and data sovereignty from the outset. Governments and development partners should assess the long-term costs of cloud dependence, biometric hardware, connectivity, energy use, maintenance, cybersecurity, and e-waste. Procurement strategies should preserve public audit rights, interoperability, data portability, and capacity transfer, so that welfare infrastructures remain adaptable, accountable, and under effective public control.

Finally, international development actors should reconsider prevailing narratives of technological leapfrogging. While digital tools can accelerate welfare delivery, speed without governance risks entrenching exclusion. Algorithmic inclusion provides a framework for aligning innovation with social protection objectives and rights-based approaches.

6.3 Limitations, Trade-Offs, and Directions for Future Research

While the framework of algorithmic inclusion developed in this chapter provides a structured lens for analysing digital welfare systems in low- and middle-income countries (LMICs), it is important to acknowledge its limitations and the trade-offs inherent in its application. Explicitly addressing these boundaries is essential both to avoid normative overreach and to identify productive avenues for future research.

First, the framework adopts a **governance-centred perspective** that prioritizes institutional arrangements, accountability mechanisms, and participatory processes over detailed technical assessments of algorithmic performance. While this choice is deliberate and aligned with the chapter's objectives, it implies that some model-level dynamics—such as specific optimisation techniques or statistical properties—are not examined in depth. Future research could complement this approach by integrating technical audits with governance analysis, thereby strengthening the empirical grounding of algorithmic inclusion assessments.

Second, algorithmic inclusion inevitably involves trade-offs between competing policy objectives. Enhancing representational inclusion by expanding data collection may increase administrative complexity or raise privacy concerns. Introducing fallback mechanisms and human review can improve fairness but may reduce efficiency and scalability. Similarly, participatory governance processes can enhance legitimacy but require time, resources, and institutional openness that may be difficult to sustain in resource-constrained environments. Recognising these trade-offs is crucial to avoid treating algorithmic inclusion as a cost-free or universally optimal solution.

Third, the framework is sensitive to contextual variation, yet it cannot fully capture the diversity of political economies, legal traditions, and social norms across LMICs. Digital welfare systems are shaped by historical legacies, power relations, and external dependencies that vary widely across regions and countries. As such, algorithmic inclusion should be understood as a heuristic rather than a prescriptive blueprint. Comparative empirical research is needed to refine the framework across different institutional settings and to identify which governance dimensions are most critical under specific conditions.

Fourth, the analysis presented in this chapter is primarily based on secondary evidence and documented experiences. While this is appropriate for a conceptual and comparative contribution, future research would benefit from micro-level empirical studies examining how beneficiaries experience algorithmic welfare systems in practice. Ethnographic research, user-centred evaluations, and participatory methods could shed light on how algorithmic decisions are interpreted, contested, or internalized by affected populations.

Finally, the rapid evolution of digital technologies poses challenges for any static analytical framework. Advances in artificial intelligence, biometric systems, and data integration will continue to reshape welfare governance in ways that are difficult to anticipate. This underscores the importance of treating algorithmic inclusion as a dynamic and adaptive governance orientation, rather than a fixed set of criteria. Future research should therefore focus on mechanisms of institutional learning, adaptive regulation, and long-term capacity building that enable welfare systems to evolve in socially responsive ways.

By explicitly engaging with these limitations and trade-offs, the chapter positions algorithmic inclusion not as a definitive solution, but as a starting point for sustained analytical and policy-oriented inquiry into the social consequences of digital welfare transformation.

6.4 Conclusions

Digital welfare in low- and middle-income countries should be understood not merely as a tool for efficiency or control, but as a contested socio-technical space. Digital platforms, biometric identification, and predictive analytics can expand coverage, improve administrative coordination, and support more dynamic responses to social risk. At the same time, when deployed in contexts marked by inequality, informality, infrastructural fragility, and limited institutional capacity, these same technologies can produce new and less visible forms of exclusion. The central challenge is therefore not whether digital welfare should be adopted, but under what governance conditions it can strengthen rather than undermine social protection.

This chapter has argued that understanding and governing this ambivalence requires moving beyond datafication as a descriptive concept and toward algorithmic inclusion as an evaluative and operational framework. Algorithmic inclusion foregrounds the conditions under which digital welfare systems recognise vulnerability, enable accountability, and sustain social rights. It emphasizes that inclusion is not a property of algorithms themselves, but of the socio-technical systems within which they operate.

By integrating theoretical insights with comparative evidence from East Africa, India, and Latin America, the chapter contributes to ongoing debates on digital welfare and algorithmic governance from a Global South perspective. It demonstrates that the future of digital welfare in LMICs will be shaped less by technological sophistication than by the capacity of institutions to govern technology in socially responsive ways.

Algorithmic inclusion offers a promising pathway for reimagining digital welfare not as a mechanism of control or efficiency alone, but as a tool for strengthening social protection, democratic accountability, and distributive justice in an increasingly data-driven world.

REFERENCES

Alston, P. (2019). *Digital welfare states and human rights: Report of the Special Rapporteur on extreme poverty and human rights* (A/74/493). United Nations General Assembly.

Ananny, M., & Crawford, K. (2018). Seeing without knowing: Limitations of the transparency ideal and its application to algorithmic accountability. *New Media & Society*, *20*(3), 973–989. DOI: 10.1177/1461444816676645

Barocas, S., Hardt, M., & Narayanan, A. (2019). *Fairness and Machine Learning: Limitations and Opportunities*. fairmlbook.org.

Barocas, S., & Selbst, A. D. (2016). Big data's disparate impact. *California Law Review*, *104*(3), 671–732.

Benjamin, R. (2019). Race After Technology: Abolitionist Tools for the New Jim Code. *Polity*.

Bovens, M., & Zouridis, S. (2002). From street-level to system-level bureaucracies: How information and communication technology is transforming administrative discretion and constitutional control. *Public Administration Review*, *62*(2), 174–184. DOI: 10.1111/0033-3352.00168

CALP Network. (2012). *E-payments in Emergency Cash Transfer Programming*. CALP Network.

Carswell, G., & De Neve, G. (2022). Transparency, exclusion and mediation: How digital and biometric technologies are transforming social protection in Tamil Nadu, India. *Oxford Development Studies*, *50*(2), 126–141. DOI: 10.1080/13600818.2021.1904866

Eubanks, V. (2018). *Automating Inequality: How High-Tech Tools Profile, Police, and Punish the Poor*. St. Martin's Press.

Guven, M., Yeachuri, A., & Almenfi, M. (2025). *Global Insights on Social Registries: Coverage and Beyond*. World Bank. DOI: 10.1596/43585

Henman, P. (2010). *Governing Electronically: E-Government and the Reconfiguration of Public Administration, Policy and Power*. Palgrave Macmillan. DOI: 10.1057/9780230248496

Kitchin, R. (2014). The Data Revolution: Big Data, Open Data, Data Infrastructures and Their Consequences. *Sage (Atlanta, Ga.)*. Advance online publication. DOI: 10.4135/9781473909472

Kroll, J. A., Huey, J., Barocas, S., Felten, E. W., Reidenberg, J. R., Robinson, D. G., & Yu, H. (2017). Accountable algorithms. *University of Pennsylvania Law Review, 165*(3), 633–705.

Levy, K., Chasalow, K. E., & Riley, S. (2021). Algorithms and decision-making in the public sector. *Annual Review of Law and Social Science, 17*(1), 309–334. DOI: 10.1146/annurev-lawsocsci-041221-023808

Lowe, C. (2022). *The Digitalisation of Social Protection Before and Since the Onset of COVID-19: Opportunities, Challenges and Lessons.* ODI Working Paper. ODI.

Masiero, S., & Shakthi, S. (2020). Grappling with Aadhaar: Biometrics, social identity and the Indian state. *South Asia Multidisciplinary Academic Journal, 23*(23). Advance online publication. DOI: 10.4000/samaj.6279

Muralidharan, K., Niehaus, P., & Sukhtankar, S. (2022). Integrating biometric authentication in India's welfare programs: Lessons from a decade of reforms. *India Policy Forum : [Papers]. India Policy Forum. Conference, 18*(1), 139–172.

Noble, S. U. (2018). *Algorithms of Oppression: How Search Engines Reinforce Racism.* New York University Press. DOI: 10.18574/nyu/9781479833641.001.0001

Selbst, A. D., Boyd, D., Friedler, S. A., Venkatasubramanian, S., & Vertesi, J. (2019). Fairness and abstraction in sociotechnical systems. In *Proceedings of the Conference on Fairness, Accountability, and Transparency* (pp. 59–68). Association for Computing Machinery. DOI: 10.1145/3287560.3287598

Taylor, L., & Broeders, D. (2015). In the name of development: Power, profit and the datafication of the Global South. *Geoforum, 64*, 229–237. DOI: 10.1016/j.geoforum.2015.07.002

van Dijck, J. (2014). Datafication, dataism and dataveillance: Big data between scientific paradigm and ideology. *Surveillance & Society, 12*(2), 197–208. DOI: 10.24908/ss.v12i2.4776

World Bank. (2025). *State of the Art of Social Registries in Latin America and the Caribbean.* World Bank.

Yeung, K. (2018). Algorithmic regulation: A critical interrogation. *Regulation & Governance, 12*(4), 505–523. DOI: 10.1111/rego.12158

KEY TERMS AND DEFINITIONS

Algorithmic Inclusion:

The capacity of digital welfare systems to equitably recognize: process, and respond to social vulnerability across the entire data and decision-making lifecycle. It requires representative data, transparent decisions, effective accountability, accessible redress, participatory governance, and sufficient institutional capacity.

Algorithmic Governance:

The set of institutional rules: technical standards, organizational practices, and oversight mechanisms that shape how algorithmic systems are designed, deployed, monitored, audited, and contested in public decision-making.

Datafication:

The process through which social phenomena: behaviours, identities, needs, and vulnerabilities are transformed into quantifiable and machine-readable data used for monitoring, prediction, classification, and decision-making.

Digital Welfare Systems:

Welfare architectures that rely on digital platforms: integrated databases, biometric identification, social registries, automated processes, or algorithmic tools to administer benefits, deliver services, and manage access to social protection.

Statistical Invisibility:

The systematic underrepresentation or absence of specific individuals or groups within administrative: statistical, or digital datasets, which can lead to their exclusion from data-driven welfare policies, eligibility assessments, or social protection programmes.

Biometric Identification:

The use of physiological or behavioural characteristics: such as fingerprints, facial features, or iris scans, to verify identity in digital systems. In welfare contexts, biometric identification may improve authentication but can also generate exclusion when verification fails or fallback mechanisms are weak.

Predictive Targeting:

The use of statistical or machine-learning models to estimate vulnerability: eligibility, risk, or priority for welfare programmes based on observed data patterns, proxy indicators, or historical administrative records.

Redress Mechanisms:

Procedures through which individuals can challenge: correct, or appeal decisions made by digital or algorithmic welfare systems. Effective redress requires accessible grievance channels, human review, timely correction of errors, and remedies when exclusion or harm occurs.

Digital Conditionalities:

Implicit or explicit requirements created by digital welfare systems: such as access to mobile phones, connectivity, digital literacy, biometric authentication, or online interfaces. These conditions may become barriers to social protection for digitally excluded groups.

Technological Autonomy:

The capacity of public institutions to retain effective control over digital welfare infrastructures: including data, software, procurement, audit rights, interoperability, vendor relationships, and long-term system maintenance.

Chapter 8
Digital Welfare and Digital Competence:
Inequality and Exclusion in Digitally Mediated Welfare Systems in Italy

Caterina Ambrosio
http://orcid.org/0009-0009-0313-9781
University of Naples Federico II, Italy

Ciro Clemente De Falco
University of Naples Federico II, Italy

Giulia De Florio
http://orcid.org/0009-0009-7291-872X
University of Naples Federico II, Italy

ABSTRACT

This article examines how the digitalisation of welfare systems reshapes access to social rights, focusing on digital competences as a key condition of social citizenship. As public services are increasingly delivered through digital platforms, the ability to navigate online environments and interact with administrative procedures becomes crucial for accessing welfare. While digital welfare is often framed as a process of administrative modernisation that enhances efficiency and inclusion, it may also generate new forms of inequality. Focusing on the Italian case, the article highlights how digital welfare has developed within a fragmented institutional context characterised by territorial disparities and uneven levels of digital inclusion. Using secondary data on digital skills, the study identifies which social groups are more likely to access digitalised welfare services and which are more exposed to

DOI: 10.4018/979-8-2600-3043-1.ch008

exclusion. The findings show that digital competences act as a stratifying resource, shaping unequal access to welfare and challenging the universalistic principles of social rights.

1. INTRODUCTION

In recent decades, the digitalisation of public administration has significantly reshaped the organisation and delivery of social protection. Welfare systems, historically designed to guarantee social rights and mitigate risks associated with illness, unemployment, and poverty, are increasingly mediated through digital infrastructures. Access to a growing range of services, including pensions, healthcare, and income support, now depends on the ability to interact with online platforms, manage digital identities, and navigate administrative procedures in digital environments. In this context, digital technologies not only enhance administrative efficiency but also constitute a structural component of contemporary welfare systems. This transformation raises important questions regarding the conditions under which social rights can be effectively exercised. While digital welfare is often framed within policy and institutional discourses as a process of modernization capable of improving efficiency and expanding inclusion, existing research has highlighted its potential to generate new forms of inequality. In particular, the uneven distribution of digital skills across the population introduces differentiated capacities to access and use welfare services. Consequently, the universalistic principles underpinning welfare systems may be weakened in practice, insofar as access to social rights becomes contingent upon individuals' digital competencies.

This chapter addresses these issues by focusing on the Italian case, in which the digitalisation of welfare has developed within a broader trajectory of administrative reform and technological innovation. Despite substantial investments and the implementation of national digital infrastructures, the Italian system remains characterized by institutional fragmentation, territorial disparities, and uneven levels of digital inclusion. These features make Italy a particularly relevant case for examining how processes of digital transformation intersect with pre-existing social and regional inequalities, potentially shaping differentiated patterns of access to welfare.

Against this background, this study analysed the distribution of digital competencies within the Italian population and assessed how such a distribution affects the capacity to access digitalised welfare services. More specifically, it investigated which social groups possessed the competencies required to engage with digital public services and which were more exposed to the risks of exclusion. Digital competence is conceptualised not merely as a technical skill but as a key enabling condition for the effective exercise of social rights in digitally mediated welfare systems.

The chapter is structured as follows. The next section provides a historical and theoretical overview of the welfare state and its subsequent digital transformation, with particular attention to the implications of digitalisation for access to social rights and the emergence of new forms of inequality. The third section examines the Italian case by reconstructing the trajectory of welfare digitalisation and analysing its institutional configuration and territorial differentiation. The fourth section outlines the research design, data sources, and indicators employed in the empirical analysis. The fifth section presents the results, focusing on both Italy's position within the European context and the internal distribution of digital skills and access to welfare services. The final section concludes by discussing the implications of the findings and reflecting on the challenges that digitalisation poses for the effective realisation of social rights.

2. FROM WELFARE STATE TO DIGITAL WELFARE

2.1 A Historical Overview of the Emergence and Consolidation of the Welfare State

The Welfare State emerged in response to the profound social and economic transformations brought about by industrialization and the spread of wage labour (Polanyi, 1944; Esping-Andersen, 1990). Between the eighteenth and nineteenth centuries, the shift from rural communities to urban industrial societies led individuals to become increasingly dependent on wages, thereby weakening traditional forms of social support. In this context, workers were largely unprotected in cases of illness, unemployment, or old age, which contributed to the rise of labour movements, trade unions, and socialist demands for better conditions. State intervention in social protection developed partly as a response to these tensions, as governments sought to contain social conflict and strengthen political legitimacy, especially with the expansion of suffrage. The origins of modern welfare are often traced back to the late nineteenth century, and the reforms introduced by Otto von Bismarck, who established the first compulsory social insurance schemes for workers. These reforms were driven not only by social concerns but also by political motivations, particularly the need to counter the growing influence of socialist movements.

From an economic perspective, the Welfare State performs key functions such as stabilizing demand, supporting the reproduction of the labour force, and reducing social conflict (Gough, 1979). After the Second World War, welfare systems became more institutionalized and expanded significantly across Western democracies, incorporating policies related to healthcare, pensions, education, and income support. A defining feature of the Welfare State is its inclusiveness: social rights are, in principle, guaranteed to all citizens, regardless of individual characteristics. As Marshall (1950) argued, these rights enable full participation in social life and include access to essential services, such as education and healthcare. Over time, welfare systems have also developed a more preventive orientation, aiming not only to address social risks but also to anticipate and mitigate them.

2.2 The Digital Transformation of Welfare: From Administrative Modernization to New Forms of Exclusion

In recent decades, the evolution of welfare systems has been driven by the advent of digitalization. The ways in which states deliver social services have undergone a profound transformation. With the introduction of Information and Communication Technologies (ICT), an increasing number of services are being provided through digital platforms that citizens can access via electronic devices. This phenomenon is often referred to as Digital Welfare, meaning the use of online platforms, databases, and automated systems for the management and delivery of social protection services. This process is often presented in political and institutional discourse as a natural form of modernization, capable of ensuring greater efficiency and social inclusion. However, this narrative tends to overlook the real consequences resulting from digitally mediated access to social services, particularly when access is highly automated (Eder & Sjøvaag, 2024). What is often overlooked is that accessing digital services requires a certain level of digital skills, which represents a fundamental prerequisite. As not all individuals possess these skills to the same degree, some may encounter difficulties or be excluded from access to certain services. Consequently, the digitalization of welfare cannot be considered a neutral process, as it can potentially generate the exclusion of part of the population from social rights based on the digital competencies they possess. In practice, citizens are recognized as such and deemed entitled to their rights only if they are able to interact with digital infrastructures; those who are not risk being marginalized (Goswami, 2025).

The consequences of this transformation become even more evident when the digitalization of welfare is examined considering the different national trajectories of integration between social policies and technologies. There is no uniform path; the effectiveness and impact of digital systems depend on the institutional capacities, infrastructure development, and political priorities of each country. In some contexts, digitalization has been accompanied by strong public investments; technological infrastructure is widespread and citizens possess broadly diffused digital skills. In such cases, online platforms can indeed simplify access to services and reduce bureaucratic delays. However, this situation does not represent the norm. In many countries, the diffusion of technologies is uneven, and digital skills are distributed unequally across social groups, territories, and generations. The use of digital platforms presupposes the availability of an internet connection, adequate devices, and basic digital skills. Not all citizens possess these resources. Elderly individuals, people with low levels of education, or those living in peripheral areas often encounter greater difficulties when interacting with fully digitalized systems. This phenomenon is often discussed in relation to the so-called digital divide, which is not merely technological; it becomes a form of social and civic marginalization, where access to essential services-ranging from healthcare to bureaucracy-turns into a privilege rather than a universal right. This perspective aligns with the literature on digital inequalities, which has moved beyond a simple distinction between access and non-access. As argued by Jan van Dijk (2005, 2020), digital divides tend to deepen over time, as initial inequalities in access are reproduced and amplified in terms of skills and outcomes. Similarly, Pippa Norris (2001) distinguishes between different layers of inequality, including a "democratic divide" that concerns unequal participation in public and institutional processes. More recently, Ellen Helsper has emphasised how inequalities in digital access and skills translate into unequal outcomes, particularly in relation to the use of online services and access to opportunities.

The difficulty or impossibility of accessing certain services does not depend solely on the individual, who may lack appropriate devices or skills, but also on political and administrative decisions regarding digitalization, as well as the rigidity and opacity of the implemented digital systems. Therefore, digital exclusion emerges as the result of a dialectical relationship between gaps in individual skills, institutional design choices, and the dynamics of algorithmic mediation. Beyond issues of access, digital welfare also reshapes the underlying mechanisms through which individuals are recognised and evaluated within social protection systems.

Within this scenario, digital competence is not limited to the technical ability to use devices or complete online forms, but also includes access to material resources and the ability to engage critically with digital information. Ilana Snyder et al. (2005) in the chapter "Using Information and Communication Technologies in Adult Literacy Education, " highlight how literacy and technology are now intertwined, since every new mode of communication brings with it new tools and codes to decode. Literacy is no longer just reading and writing; using the Internet, educational software, or online platforms requires adapting one's skills, understanding different contexts, and recognizing reliable sources. In other words, technology redefines what it means to be "literate."

The authors also stress a crucial point: if digital skills are not distributed equitably, the divide between those who can fully participate in digital society and those who are excluded tends to widen. This is not only a technical issue but also one that affects the ability to exercise rights, access essential information, and participate in public life. These skills are unevenly distributed across social groups and are closely correlated with age, education level, income, and place of residence. By shaping the competencies required of citizens, institutions implicitly shift the responsibility for access onto individuals, while simultaneously masking potential governance failures (Rebergen et al., 2025).

3. THE DIGITALISATION OF WELFARE IN ITALY

3.1 The Evolution of Welfare Digitalisation in Italy

The emergence of welfare digitalisation in Italy should be situated within a trajectory that began between the late 1990s and the early 2000s, as part of the broader process of public administration digitalisation. The most important regulatory turning point was the Digital Administration Code (2005), which institutionalised the right to use digital technologies in interactions with the public administration and consolidated the transition towards digital public services. The digitalisation of the Italian welfare system, therefore, did not originate as an autonomous policy domain, but rather as a sectoral articulation of the broader process of administrative modernisation. In the initial phase of development, digitalization in Italy focused primarily on basic administrative services and documentary and informational infrastructures, rather than fully integrated welfare services. Simultaneously, the first institutional websites of the public administration were created, and information and administrative forms began to be published online (Civitarese Matteucci, 2016).

A major early impulse toward the digital transformation of Italian public administration can be traced back to the Public Administration Reorganisation Act (Law No. 124/2015). Civitarese Matteucci, (2016) argues that this reform marked a significant shift in the role of digitalisation within administrative reform processes, placing digital technologies at the centre of the reorganisation of public administration. In this context, digitalisation was presented as one of the main instruments for transforming the functioning of the state: *"Digitalisation is the means to change the State at long last and not simply one among many others. This is why it represents the heart of the reform"* (Civitarese Matteucci, 2016).

This process was soon followed by a more operational stage of implementation. As observed by Battisti (2020), starting in 2016, the Italian government sought to accelerate the digital transformation of the public sector through the establishment of the Digital Transformation Team and the introduction of the Three-Year Plan for Digital Transformation in Public Administration, which became the main strategic framework guiding the development of digital public services and technological infrastructures. During this period, a set of national enabling platforms was created to serve as a common infrastructure for accessing public services. These include

SPID[1], CIE[2], pagoPA[3], ANPR[4], and the IO app[5]. This transition marked a change from a merely documentary form of digitalisation to a more genuinely transactional and interoperable digitalisation of social citizenship.

Regarding welfare-related services, the INPS[6] digital ecosystem represents a particularly illustrative example. In the early 2000s, the portal allowed users to consult their contribution records and access some pension-related services through authentication via a personal PIN. In subsequent years, access through digital identity systems was introduced, the PIN system was gradually phased out, and services such as the management of benefits and social transfers were progressively made available online. The COVID-19 pandemic in 2020 represented a major turning point in accelerating the digitalisation of several welfare services. Electronic health records were implemented across all Italian regions and now operate as an interconnected digital repository containing vaccination data and other health-related information.

However, the digitalisation of Italian public administration and, by extension, the welfare system, cannot be understood as a linear or purely incremental process. Rather, it consists of multiple layers and different modes of interaction between the administration and citizens. First, the digitalisation of public and welfare services in Italy is not distributed uniformly across the national territory. While the state defines national infrastructures and general guidelines, regions and local authorities retain a certain degree of autonomy in organising and delivering services. The Three-Year Plan for ICT in Public Administration itself emphasises that service design must take into account the diverse needs of different territories, thereby highlighting the role of local specificities in the implementation of digital services (AgID, 2024).

Table 1. Timeline of Welfare Digitalisation in Italy

Period / Year	Accelerator / Driver	Policy / Instrument	Main Outputs
Late 1990s – early 2000s	Public administration digitalisation	(General e-government development)	- Digitalisation focused on administrative services - Development of documentary and informational infrastructures - Creation of institutional websites - Online publication of information and administrative forms
Early 2000s (INPS)	Sectoral implementation (welfare)	INPS digital portal	- Access to contribution records - Pension-related services via PIN
2005	Regulatory turning point	Digital Administration Code	- Institutionalisation of the right to use digital technologies - Consolidation of digital public services
2015	Administrative reform	The Public Administration Reorganisation Act (Law No. 124/2015)	- Digitalisation placed at the centre of administrative reform - Digital technologies as main instrument of state transformation
From 2016	Acceleration of digital transformation	Digital Transformation Team + Three-Year Plan for Digital Transformation in PA	- Development of digital public services and infrastructures - Creation of enabling platforms (SPID, CIE, pagoPA, ANPR, IO app) - Transition to transactional and interoperable digitalisation
2020	COVID-19 pandemic	(Emergency-driven acceleration)	- Acceleration of welfare digitalisation - Implementation of Electronic Health Records across regions
Present	Multi-level governance	Three-Year Plan for ICT in PA (AgID, 2024) National Recovery and Resilience Plan (PNRR, Mission 1 – M1C1)	- €9.74 billion for digital transformation of public administration

Another limitation of the Italian case is the absence of a fully integrated digital welfare ecosystem. Within the comparative European framework of the EUROSHIP project ((European Commission, 2022), Italy is described as a relatively lagging country, characterised by slow development, institutional fragmentation, and incomplete coordination between levels of government, technological infrastructures, and support actors. From this perspective, the issue is not simply the extent of digitalisation, but rather the fact that it has not yet translated into a coherent, interoperable, and coordinated ecosystem linking the state, territorial authorities, technological platforms, and organisations that mediate access to welfare services.

To date, there has been no unified and separate quantification of investments devoted exclusively to the digitalisation of welfare in the strict sense. The main source of investment remains the National Recovery and Resilience Plan[7] (PNRR), which finances the overall infrastructure of digital transformation in public administration and, indirectly, the digitalisation of welfare services. On the official Italia Domani portal, Mission 1 (Digitalisation, Innovation, Competitiveness, Culture, and Tourism) represents the main container for digital investments. Within this mission, Component M1C1 (Digitalisation, Innovation, and Security in Public Administration) amounts to approximately €9.74 billion in PNRR funding.

Despite these investments, the issue of citizens' digital skills remains crucial, as in Italy they are still relatively weak and highly unevenly distributed. Building on these considerations, this study aims to systematically examine the social distribution of digital skills among the Italian population. If access to welfare benefits increasingly depends on the ability to navigate digital platforms, understand administrative procedures, and produce data that can be processed by public administrations, it becomes essential to determine which social groups possess these competencies and which are more exposed to the risks of digital exclusion from welfare. In this sense, digital skills do not represent a secondary or optional resource but rather a genuine condition for accessing social citizenship.

3.2 Territorial Inequalities and Fragmentation in the Italian Digital Welfare

As discussed in the previous section, a limitation of the Italian case concerns the absence of a fully integrated digital welfare ecosystem. Within the comparative European framework of the EUROSHIP project, Italy is described as a relatively lagging country, characterised by slow development, institutional fragmentation, and incomplete coordination between levels of government, technological infrastructures, and support actors. From this perspective, the issue is not simply the extent of digitalisation, but rather the fact that it has not yet translated into a coherent, interoperable, and coordinated ecosystem linking the state, territorial authorities, technological platforms, and organisations that mediate access to welfare services.

To better understand this fragmentation, the Italian digital welfare system can be conceptualised as a multi-layered structure composed of at least three interconnected levels. The first is an infrastructural layer, consisting of national enabling platforms such as digital identity systems, payment infrastructures, and data exchange mechanisms, which are designed to standardise access to public services across the country. The second is an organizational layer, largely corresponding to regional and intermediary authorities, which retain significant autonomy in the design, coordination, and implementation of welfare-related services, particularly in key sectors such as healthcare and labour policies. The third is a service delivery layer, primarily located at the local level, where municipalities and territorial administrations are responsible for the provision of services and interaction with users.

Table 2. Multi-Level Architecture of Digital Welfare in Italy

Level	Description	Main functions	Examples	Key issue
Infrastructural (national)	National enabling platforms providing the technical backbone of digital public services	Standard access, authentication, payments, and data exchange across the country	SPID / CIE (digital identity); pagoPA (payments); IO app (service interface); PDND (data interoperability)	Uniform at the national level, but does not ensure homogeneous service quality
Organisational (regional/ intermediate)	Regional and intermediary authorities responsible for coordinating and structuring welfare services	Design, coordination, and integration of services (especially healthcare, labour, social policies)	Regional healthcare systems (for example, Fascicolo Sanitario Elettronico); regional labour platforms; regional welfare portals	High variability across regions in capacity, integration, and service design
Service delivery (local)	Local administrations (municipalities) providing concrete access to services and interacting with users	Service provision, user interface, administrative procedures, local welfare delivery	Municipal platforms for benefits, social assistance services, local portals for applications and requests	Strong fragmentation due to differences in resources, skills, and organisational capacity

However, these layers do not operate as a fully integrated system. On the contrary, institutional reports on the digitalisation of public administration highlight significant variations in implementation capacity across local contexts, despite the widespread adoption of national platforms and the near-universal participation of municipalities in digital transformation programmes (AgID, 2024; DTD & ANCI, 2025). The analysis of the *Three-Year Plan for ICT in the Public Administration 2024–2026 – 2026 Update* highlights how territorial inequalities represent a structural dimension in the digital transformation of public services and, more specifically, in the provision of welfare. The first line of division concerns administrative capacity between large and small municipalities, closely linked to the availability of financial resources, technical expertise, and qualified personnel. The Plan implicitly acknowledges this asymmetry, emphasising that smaller municipalities–particularly those with fewer than 5,000 inhabitants–are not able to autonomously sustain digital innovation processes and must rely on forms of inter-municipal cooperation and centralisation. This gap translates into a differentiated ability to implement digital welfare services: while large municipalities are better equipped to develop integrated, interoperable services oriented toward the personalisation of interventions, smaller entities tend to offer more fragmented services, often still based on analogue procedures and with limited possibilities for system integration. The second dimension concerns the infrastructural divide across territories, which manifests in uneven access to broadband and ultra-broadband connectivity, cloud infrastructures, and basic digital services. The Plan underscores that strengthening such infrastructures constitutes an enabling condition for the uniform provision of digital public services, in line with the objectives of the European *Digital Decade*, which aim to ensure universal coverage with connectivity of at least 1 Gbps by 2030. In this framework, investments financed through the National Recovery and Resilience Plan (NRRP)–particularly those targeting ultra-broadband and public sector cloud infrastructures–are intended to bridge existing gaps, with dedicated funding for so-called "white" and "grey" areas, that is, territories affected by market failure. A further critical element concerns the level of data and information system interoperability, which represents a fundamental prerequisite for the development of advanced forms of digital welfare. The Plan indicates that only 40% of national key datasets are expected to comply with technical standards by 2026, pointing to a still partial process of integration. This limitation results in significant territorial differentiation: more structured entities–typically large municipalities or more advanced regions–are better able to integrate diverse datasets (e.g., demographic, social assistance, and health data), enabling forms of "proactive" welfare based on the automatic identification of needs and beneficiaries. Conversely, in less equipped contexts, information systems tend to remain isolated and poorly interconnected, leading to predominantly "reactive" welfare, dependent on citizens' initiative and characterised by higher administrative burdens. Finally, although the Plan maintains a formally neutral stance, indirect indicators reveal broader territorial inequalities between Northern and Southern regions, as well as between central and peripheral areas. The need to activate support mechanisms, aggregation models, and territorial communities (22 already operational in 2024) points to an uneven distribution of administrative innovation capacities.

The report *"Mappa dei Comuni Digitali 2025"* provides empirical evidence that further clarifies the structural nature of territorial inequalities in the digitalisation of local public services. First, a theoretically significant finding emerges: 70% of Italian municipalities have fewer than 5,000 inhabitants, indicating that the administrative system is predominantly composed of small entities, typically characterised by limited financial resources, weaker technical expertise, and reduced organizational capacity. This configuration is not a marginal aspect but rather a systemic condition that contributes to the production and reproduction of territorial inequalities in the digital transition. Such structural fragility is also reflected at the infrastructural level: the availability of service continuity solutions (backup systems) exceeds 80%

in municipalities with more than 100,000 inhabitants but drops to approximately 43% in those with fewer than 5,000 inhabitants, highlighting a marked disparity in digital resilience. Even more relevant for welfare provision is the significant divide in data interoperability. Integration with external databases, such as those of INPS, is reported in only 21% of social services and 7% of educational services, with differences exceeding 60 percentage points between small and large municipalities. This suggests that the capacity to develop integrated and proactive forms of digital welfare is unevenly distributed and concentrated in more administratively structured contexts. Consistently, the welfare sector emerges as one of the least advanced areas in the digitalisation process: more than half of the municipalities report that they have not digitalised services related to social assistance and disability, in contrast to other domains, such as civil registry or urban planning, which show higher levels of digital maturity. Finally, these inequalities are further reinforced by differences in administrative capacity and governance structures. Overall, 75% of municipalities rely on external providers for ICT service management, and in municipalities with fewer than 5,000 inhabitants, in 66% of cases, the role of information systems manager is held by personnel with an administrative rather than a technical background. Taken together, these elements depict a scenario in which the digital transformation of local public administration and welfare, in particular, is deeply stratified along territorial and demographic lines, with direct implications for equity in access to public services.

These elements suggest that digital welfare in Italy cannot be understood as a unified and coherent system but rather as a territorially differentiated and unevenly integrated assemblage of infrastructure, institutions, and practices. The coexistence of advanced national platforms with fragmented local implementation produces a stratified landscape in which the quality, accessibility, and effectiveness of welfare services vary significantly across contexts. In this scenario, digitalisation does not simply reorganise service delivery, but actively reshapes the conditions of access to social rights, making them increasingly dependent on both territorial factors and the administrative and technological capacities of local systems.

4. RESEARCH STRATEGY, SOURCES, AND INDICATORS

The institutional configuration outlined in the previous section highlights a structurally fragmented and unevenly integrated digital welfare system, in which access to services depends not only on formal entitlements but also on the interaction between technological infrastructures, administrative arrangements, and territorial disparities. In such a context, the analysis of digital welfare cannot be limited to the supply side alone, as the effectiveness of digitalisation ultimately depends on citizens' capacity to access and navigate these systems. Against this background, the present study adopts a demand-side perspective, focusing on the distribution of digital competencies and their role in shaping differential access to welfare services.

The aim of this work is to describe the digital skills of Italian citizens as a component of the digitalisation of welfare on the demand side, that is, the ability to access and use digital services and procedures. To this end, indicators of digital skills are analysed, along with contextual measures and the use of online services. Digital skills are considered a (non-exclusive) prerequisite for the use of digitised welfare services, and their distribution within the population is measured. The research objective is pursued through a secondary analysis of statistical data produced by national and supranational institutions; no original survey was conducted, and the empirical material consists entirely of indicators derived from harmonised sample surveys available in the Eurostat and ISTAT databases. A secondary analysis is appropriate for the aims of this work for three reasons. First, the harmonised Eurostat and ISTAT surveys provide coverage of the resident population and statistical representativeness that no ad hoc survey could replicate. Second, the harmonised nature of the data ensures cross-country and over-time comparability, which is necessary to place the Italian case within the European context. Third, the available variables (access, Internet use, digital practices, and use of public administration services) correspond directly to the analytical dimensions relevant for describing the demand for digitalised welfare.

4.1 The conceptual framework: the DigComp framework

The European Union's conceptual framework for defining citizens' digital competences is the Digital Competence Framework for Citizens (DigComp), developed by the European Commission's Joint Research Centre (Vuorikari et al., 2022). DigComp uses a five-dimensional structure, making it suitable for both design and assessment purposes. Dimension 1 identifies the five competence areas (information and data literacy, communication and collaboration, digital content creation, safety, and problem solving), while Dimension 2 breaks these areas down into 21 competencies. Dimension 3 defines eight proficiency levels (from Foundation to Highly Specialised), in line with a progression logic comparable to and inspired by European qualification frameworks. Dimensions 4 and 5 complete the structure with examples of knowledge/skills/attitudes and use cases (learning and work contexts), making explicit "how" a competence manifests operationally. It is precisely this flexibility that has allowed the framework to evolve in its most recent versions (DigComp 2.1 and 2.2), integrating the conscious use of artificial intelligence as a key competence for understanding how algorithms influence information and digital interaction. DigComp stands out for its transversal and interconnected vision: the 21 competences are described as complementary rather than isolated areas, reflecting the complexity of digital practices in which a single activity can simultaneously require technical skills and critical awareness. This structure is organised into eight proficiency levels, which qualify competence not only based on technical difficulty but also in terms of autonomy and contextual complexity: moving from the guided support of basic levels to the operational independence of intermediate levels, up to the ability to tackle complex problems and support or lead other users, typical of the advanced levels. Finally, the framework integrates attitudinal and awareness dimensions, shifting the emphasis from simply "knowing how to do" to "knowing how to be." From this perspective, a critical and responsible attitude assumes a central role: being competent means not only using digital tools and services but also evaluating the reliability of information and understanding the impact of one's online behaviour. Thus, DigComp is not a statistical indicator but an operational reference that supports the design of curricula, assessment tools, and digital inclusion initiatives. From this standpoint, the framework highlights how failing to achieve minimum proficiency levels today represents a critical factor of exclusion from essential services and the exercise of active citizenship.

4.2 From theoretical definition to measurement: DSI, DESI, and the Digital Decade

The transition from the theoretical definition of DigComp to the empirical measurement of digital skills occurs through the construction of harmonised European-level statistical indicators, which are then used in the Commission's main benchmarking tools. In this context, the DESI (Digital Economy and Society Index) serves as a comparative tool that has historically enabled the annual monitoring of digital performance in Member States and, today, has been integrated into the Digital Decade framework through the State of the Digital Decade. While DigComp provides the "grammar" of skills, DESI (and the current Digital Decade dashboard) offers a comparative "report card" on the progress of countries toward the 2030 targets. Since 2023, DESI has been integrated into the governance framework of the Digital Decade: the "Digital Decade Policy Programme 2030" Decision sets out goals and targets (including those on digital skills), and the "State of the Digital Decade" monitors their annual progress at both the EU level and for each Member State. From an empirical perspective, however, the informational basis does not originate from a test dedicated to DigComp, but rather from a general and harmonised statistical survey: the European survey "ICT usage in households and by individuals," coordinated by Eurostat and conducted annually by national institutes (for Italy, ISTAT). This survey collects microdata on access to and use of digital technologies (including the Internet, online services, e-government, and security). The data from this survey, once harmonised and published by Eurostat, feed the indicators used by DESI and, today, by the Digital Decade monitoring. The architecture of DESI is structured around four main axes (human capital, connectivity, integration of digital technologies, and digital public services). In particular, the human capital pillar includes indicators on the population's digital skills and advanced human capital (e.g., ICT specialists), enabling member states to be compared on this profile. In this area, the component measuring the population's digital skills is captured through the digital skills indicator (DSI), a proxy indicator derived from the microdata of the European survey on ICT use and organised into areas consistent with the DigComp framework. The correspondence between the conceptual areas of DigComp and the statistical indicators of the DSI is, however, not one-to-one. For each of the five areas, the DSI detects whether an individual has carried out at least one of the associated activities, distinguishing between a basic and an advanced level: an operationalisation that captures the presence or absence of digital practices, but not the depth or quality of the underlying competence. The transition from theoretical definition to sample measurement inevitably involves a simplification that must be taken into account when interpreting the results: the indicators describe distributions and comparisons, not individual abilities in the strict sense. Operationally, the DSI classifies the population aged 16–74 into summary levels (e.g., "none/insufficient," "at least basic," "above basic") based on the combination of activities associated with the various competence areas; in this work, these categories are used to describe the distribution of digital skills in Italy and to compare it with the European picture (2021–2024). In this way, the data collected at the national level by individual statistical institutes (for Italy, ISTAT) are harmonised and made comparable at the European level, enabling the quantification of the share of the population with at least basic, above basic, or insufficient digital skills.

4.3 The sources and indicators used

The work jointly employs two data sources that follow a complementary logic: Eurostat ensures cross-country comparability, whereas ISTAT allows for a detailed focus on the Italian case, with breakdowns not available in international comparative datasets. For the European comparison, three Eurostat indicators are used, extracted from the tables isoc_sk_dskl_i21 and isoc_ciegi_ac, updated in February 2026. The choice of these three indicators follows the logic of the study: the basic DSI and the advanced DSI cover the two levels of the skills distribution relevant for describing both the country's structural lag and its catch-up trajectories; the e-government indicator completes the picture by measuring the actual demand for digital public administration services, allowing verification of whether and to what extent digital skills translate into concrete use of digitalised welfare. The time frame covers the period 2021–2025, a methodologically consistent series since the introduction of the current DSI version. For the in-depth analysis of the Italian case, tables from the ISTAT survey "Citizens and ICT" (2024) are used. The selection of tables follows a two-level logic consistent with the analytical framework of the study: the tables on internet access and use (1.1, 1.2, 1.3, 1.4) measure the structural conditions that make interaction with digital services possible or impossible–availability of connection, frequency of use, and socio-demographic and territorial barriers; the tables on e-government (3.1 and 3.2) measure the outcome of that chain, that is, the share of the population that actually ends up using the public administration's digital services. Together, the two groups of indicators allow us to distinguish those excluded due to lack of access from those who, even with access, are unable or unwilling to use digitalised welfare.

Some relevant dimensions of digital welfare could not be empirically investigated due to the lack of available harmonised data. Aspects related to the supply side of digital welfare, such as platform usability, accessibility, institutional design, and the role of intermediary actors, are not captured by any adequately available datasets. For this reason, these elements are addressed only at a theoretical level and considered in the interpretation of the findings, rather than being included in the empirical analysis.

5. DIGITAL SKILLS AND ACCESS TO WELFARE SERVICES: THE ITALIAN CASE AMIDST EUROPEAN GAPS AND INTERNAL INEQUALITIES

This section analyzes Italians' ability to access and use digital welfare services, focusing on the demand side. It first places Italy in a European context using the Eurostat Digital Skills Indicator (DSI) and e-government usage data for 2021–2025, aligning with Digital Decade targets. The second part uses ISTAT's 2024 "Citizens and ICT" survey to map internal digital inequalities by region, age, gender, and education. The digital divide is presented as a range of capabilities leading to varied access to welfare rights.

5.1 The digital skills of Italians in the European comparison

In 2025, the percentage of Italians aged 16 to 74 years with at least basic digital skills reached 54.3%, a significant recovery compared to 45.6% in 2021 and 45.8% in 2023. The progress recorded in the last two years is the most notable of the entire observation period; however, it is still insufficient to bridge the gap with the European average. The EU-27 average is 60.4% in 2025, increasing from 53.9% in

2021. The gap between Italy and the European average, about 8 percentage points in 2021 and 2023, has narrowed to 6.1 percentage points in 2025, indicating a partial recovery that, however, does not represent structural convergence.

Italy ranks in the lower-middle tier of the European distribution, surpassing only the countries with the most critical performances (Romania, Bulgaria, and Greece) and remaining significantly below the leaders. The Netherlands (83.6%), Finland (81.0%), Ireland (82.8%), and Denmark (81.5%) have already reached or surpassed the Digital Decade target by 2025, whereas Italy still lags approximately 26 percentage points behind the goal. The comparison with the major countries of Western Europe is particularly revealing: Germany, which was in a position similar to Italy in 2021 (48.9%), has seen sustained progress, reaching 59.5% in 2025 and surpassing the EU average. Spain stands at 66.5% and France at 65.7%. Only Greece (51.0%) was in a position comparable to Italy. Italy is the only major Western European country not to have crossed the 55% threshold in 2025, with an estimated delay of four to six years compared to the Nordic countries and two to three years compared to the European average.

Table 3. Individuals with at least basic digital skills (% of population aged 16-74).

Country	*2021*	*2023*	*2025*
EU-27	53,9%	55,6%	60,4%
Ireland	70,5%	72,9%	82,8%
Finland	79,2%	82,0%	81,0%
Netherlands	78,9%	82,7%	83,6%
Denmark	68,7%	69,6%	81,5%
Spain	64,2%	66,2%	66,5%
France	62,0%	59,7%	65,7%
Greece	52,5%	52,4%	51,0%
Germany	48,9%	52,2%	59,5%
Italy	**45,6%**	**45,8%**	**54,3%**
Bulgaria	31,2%	35,5%	38,3%
Romania	27,8%	27,7%	31,8%

Source: Eurostat, isoc_sk_dskl_i21.

The share of Italians with digital skills above the basic level (above basic) was 22.5% in 2021 and 22.2% in 2023, essentially stagnant throughout the two-year period. In 2025, there is a significant jump to 31.5%, a figure that surpasses the European average (31.4%) for the first time. This is the most encouraging data point of the entire analysis: Italy's recent progress is mainly concentrated in the higher range of skills, with a growing share of users being able to carry out complex activities in all five DigComp areas. The EU-27 average rose from 26.5% in 2021 to 31.4% in 2025, with a more gradual trend. Among the countries with the highest performance are the Netherlands (55.6%), Finland (54.9%), Ireland (54.4%), and Denmark (53.0%), which have shares of advanced skills nearly double the European average and Italy's 2021-2023 figures. Conversely, Bulgaria (11.8%), Romania (11.1%), and North Macedonia (6.1%) had the lowest values. The sudden leap for Italy in 2025 should be interpreted with caution: since the DSI is measured every two years and the data are based on self-reported activities, it is not possible to rule out effects due to sample composition or changes in what is classified as "advanced" in the latest version of the questionnaire.

Table 4. Individuals with digital skills above the basic level (% of population aged 16-74).

Country	*2021*	*2023*	*2025*
EU-27	26,5%	27,3%	31,4%
Ireland	39,7%	43,8%	54,4%
Finland	48,1%	53,6%	54,9%
Netherlands	51,8%	54,5%	55,6%
Denmark	37,4%	39,4%	53,0%
Spain	38,1%	38,6%	38,9%
France	31,3%	30,6%	35,0%
Greece	21,7%	20,0%	27,5%
Germany	18,8%	19,8%	24,2%
Italy	**22,5%**	**22,2%**	**31,5%**
Bulgaria	7,8%	7,7%	11,8%
Romania	8,7%	9,0%	11,1%

Source: Eurostat, isoc_sk_dskl_i21.

5.2 E-government: Italy Going Against the Trend

The indicator regarding the use of public administration websites or apps reveals the most concerning trend in Italy. In 2022, 65.7% of individuals had used digital public administration services in the previous 12 months, which is in line with the European average (67.6%). Over the following three years, there has been a progressive and significant decline: 60.1% in 2023 and 55.1% in 2024, with a partial recovery to 57.7% in 2025. During the same period, the EU-27 average followed the opposite trend, increasing from 67.6% to 71.9%. Consequently, the gap between Italy and the European average, which was almost nonexistent in 2022, widened to approximately 15 percentage points in 2024–2025. Italy is the only major EU country to experience a clear and prolonged decrease in the use of e-government services over the observed period. The data are particularly critical when compared with leading countries: Denmark at 98.5% in 2024, Finland at 95.4%, the Netherlands at 96.0%, Sweden at 94.6%, and Ireland at 89.1%. Even countries that are traditionally less advanced in digitalisation are showing upward trends, such as Germany (66.5% in 2025), which leads to surpassing Italy. Only Romania (24.1%) and Bulgaria (36.0%) rank lower among the EU countries considered. This discrepancy between the growth of basic digital skills (+8.5 percentage points between 2023 and 2025) and the simultaneous decline in the use of e-government (-7.4 points between 2022 and 2024) is itself an anomaly that indicates the existence of specific barriers to the use of public administration services that cannot be attributed solely to a skills gap: quality and usability of portals, continuity of available digital services, user trust, and interoperability issues between systems.

Table 5. Use of public administration websites or apps (% of population aged 16–74 years, last 12 months).

Country	*2022*	*2023*	*2024*	*2025*
EU-27	67,6%	69,3%	70,0%	71,9%
Denmark	97,0%	97,7%	98,5%	98,0%
Finland	94,8%	95,5%	95,4%	96,1%
Netherlands	92,5%	94,8%	96,0%	96,2%
Ireland	80,8%	85,6%	89,1%	91,0%
France	82,6%	85,2%	87,2%	87,3%
Spain	79,8%	79,7%	79,7%	80,7%
Greece	67,6%	68,7%	66,3%	72,0%
Germany	51,2%	58,1%	60,3%	66,5%
Italy	**65,7%**	**60,1%**	**55,1%**	**57,7%**
Bulgaria	26,4%	29,7%	31,8%	36,0%
Romania	20,9%	22,6%	25,3%	24,1%

Source: Eurostat, isoc_ciegi_ac.

5.3 Territory and Differential Access to Digital Welfare

5.3.1 The Geography of Connection

In Italy, in 2024, the share of households without internet access at home is 13.8%, but this national average masks significant regional differences. In the North-East, the share drops to 11.2%, in the North-West to 13.0%, in the South to 17.4%, and in the Islands to 16.4%. The Centre is in an intermediate position (12.1%), closer to the northern divisions. However, the most significant insight is not the size of the gap, but the breakdown of the reasons given by households without a connection, which reveals profoundly different dynamics of exclusion across areas of the country. In the North, the main reason is "no one knows how to use the internet, " accounting for 63.9% of cases in the North-West and 60.8% in the North-East. Costs–both for devices and for the connection itself–are relatively minor factors (3% and 7%, respectively). The absence of internet in northern households is mainly seen as a skills deficit, not as a financial barrier. The most representative case is Lombardy: only 12.4% of households lack access, and costs are among the lowest in the country (3.5% for devices and 7.1% for the connection), while "no one knows how to use it" reaches 66.3%. In Lombardy, those without internet are not excluded for economic reasons but because they lack the skills to use it.

In the South, the proportion is reversed: "no one knows how to use it" drops to 53.6%, while costs rise–the cost of devices to 8.1% and the cost of the connection to 9.7%. The economic barrier becomes more significant than in the North, although it still remains secondary compared to the skill gap. The most extreme case is Calabria, with 21.5% of households without access (the highest rate in Italy), which also records the cost of devices at 11.1% and the cost of the connection at 12.8%, both the highest nationally. Here, "no one knows how to use it" drops to 48.9%: the main barrier is no longer skills but the actual cost of getting connected. This distinction has direct implications for digital inclusion policies: training initiatives may be effective in the North but are insufficient in the South, where the primary constraint is economic.

Table 6. Households without Internet access by geographical area and reason (%).

	No Internet	*Not useful*	*Cost of equipment*	*Cost of network*	*No one knows how to use*	*No broadband*
North-west	13,0%	20,2%	3,1%	7,3%	63,9%	2,9%
North-east	11,2%	26,9%	4,7%	6,8%	60,8%	5,3%
Central Italy	12,1%	23,9%	6,1%	8,9%	58,4%	3,8%
South	17,4%	23,9%	8,1%	9,7%	53,6%	2,2%
Islands	16,4%	27,2%	4,1%	9,6%	54,4%	1,4%
Italy	**13,8%**	**23,8%**	**5,4%**	**8,4%**	**58,4%**	**3,0%**

Source: ISTAT, Citizens and ICT Survey

In addition to this geographic divide between macroareas, there is an overlapping difference based on the size of the municipality, which affects the entire country regardless of its regional division. In municipalities with up to 2,000 inhabitants, the proportion of Internet users drops to 79.5%, compared to 83.5% in municipalities with over 50,000 inhabitants and 84.3% in metropolitan areas. The rural-urban gap is not limited to the South; it concerns inland areas in general, but in the South, these two dimensions of disadvantage tend to combine, creating the most deeply rooted conditions for digital exclusion in the country.

5.3.2 The Geography of Use: E-Government

If the territorial gap in access is significant, the gap in the use of digital public administration (PA) services is consistently wider, and this asymmetry is the most relevant analytical finding of Part Two. In the North-East, 84.8% of the population uses the Internet, and 35.4% uses PA informational services; in the South, 76.9% use the Internet, but only 20.5% use PA services. The difference in Internet use between the North-East and the South is approximately 8 percentage points; for e-government use, it is 15 percentage points. The gap does not remain the same as you move from access to use; it widens. This amplification can also be seen in the range of activities. Among those who have used the Internet in the past 12 months, only 29.1% have searched for information on PA services, benefits, and rights-less than one-third. The gap between searching and doing is even more revealing: informational activities are all around 23–29%, while as soon as you move into the area of concrete services, the numbers plummet-requests for social security benefits are at 9.0%, filling out tax returns at 9.4%. The digital PA system is mainly used as an information desk and not as a service delivery channel, and this is even more pronounced in southern regions.

At the regional level, the data are clear. Emilia-Romagna (35.2%), Lombardy (34.6%), and Trento (38.0%) lead in the use of public administration information services, while Calabria (16.8%), Sicily (16.9%), and Campania (18.6%) are at the bottom of the list. Regarding welfare services, the ratio is nearly three to one: Lazio (12.5%) and Lombardy (9.8%) versus Sicily (5.3%) and Calabria (6.6%). The correlation between the share of Internet users and the use of public administration information services at the regional level is extremely high ($r = 0.93$); however, the strength of the correlation does not imply proportionality: the digital government gap grows more rapidly than the access gap, indicating the existence of specific barriers that go beyond Internet availability-trust in institutions, familiarity with administrative procedures, availability of competent intermediaries, and perceived quality of online portals. Sardinia is emblematic in this regard: with a relatively low percentage of households without Internet access (12.9%, in line with the North), the region reports the use of public administration information services at 29.0%, closer to southern values than to northern ones. Access to the Internet alone is not a sufficient condition for benefiting from digital welfare.

Table 7. Use of public administration websites or applications by type of activity and geographical area (percentage of those who have used the Internet in the past 12 months)

	PA account info	*Databases*	*Forms*	*Appt.*	*Info service*	*Social Security*
North-west	-	-	27,3%	28,5%	33,3%	12,1%
North-east	30,7%	15,4%	31,8%	30,1%	35,4%	10,7%
Central Italy	32,1%	16,1%	26,3%	25,3%	31,8%	11,2%
South	26,8%	14,3%	14,8%	12,8%	20,5%	5,4%
Islands	16,1%	8,8%	13,9%	13,8%	20,0%	4,9%
Italy	**25,3%**	**13,1%**	**23,7%**	**23,0%**	**29,1%**	**9,4%**

Source: ISTAT, Citizens and ICT Survey

The size of the municipality echoes and reinforces this pattern even in e-government. In municipalities with up to 2,000 inhabitants, 25.3% of Internet users utilise public administration information services, compared to 35.4% in metropolitan areas, representing a ten-point gap for a function that, in theory, should be identical wherever there is an Internet connection. Small municipalities are already often disadvantaged by the closure of physical service counters and the gradual reduction of local services; the digital channel was supposed to compensate for this geographic marginality; instead, the data show that it replicates it. These findings are consistent with van Dijk's (2005, 2020) concept of the deepening divide: digital inequalities do not remain static but tend to intensify over time, as initial gaps in access are reproduced and amplified at the level of skills and actual use of services. The Italian case illustrates this dynamic with particular clarity, showing that the distance between those who access the internet and those who effectively use digital public services widens progressively as social disadvantage accumulates.

5.4 Age and education: multiplying factors

Aggregated data on Internet use show that 81.9% of the population aged 6 and over uses the Internet (Cfr. Table 5, 2024). This average masks a clear generational divide. Up to age 64, the picture is essentially homogeneous: all age groups range between 85.9% and 97.9%, with a peak in the 16–24 age group (97.9%). For those of working or school age, the Internet is practically universal. The decline begins with the 65–74 age group (68.1%) and becomes precipitous for those over 75, where only 31.4% use the Internet. Nearly seven out of ten older people are effectively excluded from the Web. This exclusion has special significance when analysing digital welfare: the over-75 age group has the greatest need for pension benefits, healthcare, and income support-exactly the services that the public administration is gradually digitising.

Table 8. People aged 6 years and over who have used the Internet in the last 3 months, categorised by sex and age group (%).

Age	*Males*	*Females*	*Total*
6-10	84,7%	85,2%	85,0%
11-15	95,6%	96,6%	96,1%
16-24	97,9%	98,0%	97,9%
25-34	94,1%	95,0%	94,5%
35-44	94,5%	95,4%	94,9%
45-54	93,6%	93,7%	93,7%
55-59	89,4%	90,4%	89,9%
60-64	88,1%	83,8%	85,9%
65-74	72,3%	64,4%	68,1%
75+	38,3%	26,5%	31,4%
Total	84,5%	79,5%	81,9%

Source: ISTAT, Citizens and ICT Survey

The level of education multiplies these effects in a nonlinear way. In younger age groups (6–24 years), educational attainment has little impact; university graduates, high school graduates, and those with only lower secondary school certificates all converge around 93–98%, because in that age bracket, the Internet is an almost universal tool. It is from age 45 onwards that education begins to make a difference, and in the 65 and over age group, the gap becomes enormous: 85.5% of older university graduates use the Internet, compared to 73.4% of high school graduates, while usage among those with only a lower secondary certificate drops to 34.7%. Nearly two out of three older people with low levels of education are offline.

Age and education do not operate as additive factors; instead, they multiply each other. An elderly person with low levels of education has two disadvantages that, together, become almost decisive. Regarding gender, the overall gap of five percentage points (men, 84.5%; women, 79.5%) is misleading when considered alone: up to age 59, the differences are minimal, and among 25–44-year-olds with lower secondary education, women even surpass men (90.5% vs. 87.5%). The gender gap appears entirely among the elderly with low levels of education: women over 65 years old with a lower secondary certificate stand at 30.9%, compared to 40.2% for men. Thus, the group most excluded from digital access in Italy can be identified with sociological precision: elderly women with low levels of education who also statistically have the highest welfare needs.

Note: The problem will not resolve itself automatically with generational turnover. Currently, individuals aged 45–64 years with only lower secondary education already show a 14-point gap compared to their university-educated peers (83.5% vs. 97.6%). When this cohort ages, it will carry with it a divide that age will only widen further.

Table 9. People aged 6 and over who have used the internet in the last 3 months, by age group and level of education (%)

Age	*Qualification*	*Males*	*Females*	*Total*
6-24	Graduate-Postgraduate	98,0%	97,3%	97,6%
	High School	98,6%	97,4%	98,0%
	Up to Middle School	92,5%	93,3%	92,9%
25-44	Graduate-Postgraduate	98,1%	97,7%	97,9%
	High School	95,9%	95,0%	95,5%
	Up to Middle School	87,5%	90,5%	88,7%
45-64	Graduate-Postgraduate	97,8%	97,5%	97,6%
	High School	94,8%	94,3%	94,6%

continued on following page

Table 9. Continued

Age	*Qualification*	*Males*	*Females*	*Total*
	Up to Middle School	84,9%	82,0%	83,5%
65+	Graduate-Postgraduate	87,2%	83,5%	85,5%
	High School	75,5%	71,2%	73,4%
	Up to Middle School	40,2%	30,9%	34,7%

Source: ISTAT, Citizens and ICT Survey

5.5 The Paradox of the Elderly

The most critical issue concerns the over-65 age group, and it is a structural paradox. Seniors are the main recipients of welfare pensions, healthcare services, attendance allowances, and social benefits; yet, they are precisely those who use digital channels the least to access these services. Among those aged 65–74 years, only 5.7% apply for welfare benefits online; for those over 75 years, the figure drops to 1.7%, which is essentially negligible. Meanwhile, the public administration is gradually reducing physical service counters and steering people toward digital solutions. The result is a system that, de facto, shifts the burden of access onto the most vulnerable groups: those unable to use digital channels must rely on a family member, a union representative, a tax assistance centre (when available), or else give up. The digitalisation of welfare, in the absence of support structures, risks not simplifying access to rights but merely shifting the bottleneck, making it less visible but no less selective.

Table 10. Use of public administration websites or applications by type of activity and age group (% of those who have used the Internet in the last 12 months)

Age	*PA account info*	*Databases*	*Forms*	*Appt.*	*Info service*	*Social Security*
14-17	2,2%	2,8%	7,6%	5,8%	13,8%	0,6%
18-19	8,3%	8,1%	17,5%	15,6%	24,7%	3,6%
20-24	18,0%	13,9%	22,7%	22,3%	33,5%	6,0%
25-34	30,2%	17,5%	29,8%	29,0%	37,9%	11,3%
35-44	34,0%	18,7%	31,8%	30,7%	39,2%	17,2%
45-54	33,9%	16,8%	30,8%	30,5%	38,1%	13,0%
55-59	32,2%	17,1%	28,7%	27,3%	33,6%	9,7%
60-64	31,0%	13,8%	25,8%	25,0%	29,6%	9,3%
65-74	24,6%	9,9%	19,8%	19,7%	22,6%	5,7%

continued on following page

Table 10. Continued

Age	*PA account info*	*Databases*	*Forms*	*Appt.*	*Info service*	*Social Security*
75+	7,7%	3,2%	7,6%	7,5%	7,4%	1,7%
Total	25,3%	13,1%	23,7%	23,0%	29,1%	9,0%

Source: ISTAT

This structural paradox directly instantiates Norris's (2001) concept of the democratic divide: the groups most dependent on public welfare provision are simultaneously those least able to access it through digital channels, producing a form of institutional exclusion that undermines the effective exercise of social rights and civic participation.

Taken together, the findings reveal a coherent pattern of cumulative disadvantage. Italy's lag in digital skills and declining e-government use at the European level are compounded, at the national level, by overlapping inequalities along territorial, generational, and educational lines. The groups most dependent on welfare provision — elderly individuals, women with low levels of education, residents of peripheral areas — are precisely those least able to access it through digital channels. This convergence of disadvantages challenges the universalistic principles on which welfare systems are founded.

6. CONCLUSIONS: DIGITAL COMPETENCE AS A CONDITION OF SOCIAL CITIZENSHIP

This chapter examines how the digitalisation of welfare systems intersects with the uneven distribution of digital competencies across the population, with particular focus on the Italian case. The central argument is that digital skills are not a secondary or optional attribute, but a genuine structural condition for accessing social rights in contemporary welfare states. The empirical analysis conducted in the preceding sections allows us to assess this claim with considerable precision, and the picture that emerges is both coherent and, in several respects, troubling. As Tomasello (2022) has argued, the transition from industrial to digital citizenship requires a fundamental rethinking of social rights: while Marshall's framework locates the guarantee of social rights within stable bureaucratic institutions, the digitalisation of welfare introduces a new layer of conditionality–one that is technically mediated, structurally unequal, and largely invisible in formal policy discourse.

At the European level, Italy exhibits a double lag that is directly relevant to the accessibility of digitalised welfare. First, the share of adults with at least basic digital skills (54.3% in 2025) remains below the EU-27 average (60.4%) and far from the 80% target set for 2030. This means that roughly one in two Italian adults lacks the competencies required to independently navigate the digital platforms through which an increasing number of welfare benefits and public services are now delivered. Second, and more critically, Italy registers a declining trend in the use of e-government services, at a time when most other major European countries are recording growth. The widening gap with the EU average (from approximately 2% to over 14% in just three years) signals that the problem is not merely one of skill deficit but reflects deeper structural barriers: institutional distrust, the inadequacy of intermediary support, and the opacity of digital administrative procedures. The decoupling between improvements in aggregate digital skills and declining use of public administration services suggests, as the literature on administrative burden has shown, that the barriers to digital welfare access cannot be reduced to a question of individual technical competence (Madsen, Lindgren, & Melin, 2021). Digital welfare systems risk transforming citizens into "accidental caseworkers"–individuals required to perform complex administrative tasks previously handled by professionals, without adequate support and with the full burden of error falling on themselves.

National data confirm and deepen this picture. The distribution of digital inequalities in Italy follows well-documented fault lines that the empirical analysis has been able to quantify with considerable precision. The North-South territorial divide is significant in terms of Internet access, but it becomes even more pronounced when the focus shifts to the actual use of e-government services, which is the dimension most relevant to welfare access. The generational structure of exclusion is particularly acute: among those aged 75 and over, barely one in fifty individuals uses digital channels to access social protection services, despite this being the age group with the greatest welfare needs. The compounding effect of low levels of education and advanced age produces the most extreme cases of exclusion, while the gender gap, rather than being evenly distributed across the population, is concentrated specifically among older women with low levels of educational attainment–a group that is both statistically large and highly dependent on public welfare provision. The Italian case is structurally shaped by the characteristics of its welfare regime: as research on the relationship between welfare state architectures and digital inclusion has shown, countries with family-based rather than universalistic provision tend to exhibit lower digital inclusion among older populations, precisely because the institutional infrastructure for supported access is less developed (Alexopoulou, Åström, & Karlsson, 2022). Italy exemplifies this pattern with particular clarity.

These findings have direct theoretical implications. The Marshallian conception of social citizenship rests on the principle that the state guarantees a set of rights to all its members, regardless of their individual capacities. The digitalisation of welfare does not formally revoke this principle, but it introduces a de facto condition of access that is unequally distributed across the population. Digital competence thus functions as what one might call a "gatekeeper resource": those who possess it can exercise their social rights autonomously; those who do not are forced into dependency on intermediaries when these are available, or face outright exclusion.

From a policy standpoint, the findings point to several concrete priorities. Investments in digital literacy, while necessary, are insufficient on their own; they primarily benefit those who are already partially digitally equipped, leaving the most excluded groups largely unaffected. In parallel, a deliberate policy of "digital mediation" is needed, which involves the institutionalisation of assisted access to welfare services through physical support points, trained intermediaries, and outreach services capable of reaching remote and peripheral areas. The evidence from comparative European research is instructive in this regard: welfare service centres–whether formalised as administrative desks, CAF offices[8], or patronage[9] networks–function as critical "analogue interfaces of the digital welfare state," spaces where citizens excluded from purely digital services can access support through human channels (Kaun & Liminga, 2023). Far from representing a residual or transitional arrangement, these intermediary structures constitute genuine welfare infrastructure, essential for translating formal entitlements into substantive access. The progressive reduction of in-person administrative counters, in the absence of adequate compensatory measures, risks functioning not as a modernisation of the welfare state but as a covert rationing of its benefits–selecting beneficiaries through technical barriers rather than through deliberate political choices, and producing what the literature has described as "digital by default" exclusion (Helsper, 2021).

Several limitations of the present study should be acknowledged. The analysis is based exclusively on secondary data from harmonised statistical surveys, which capture access and use patterns at an aggregate level but do not allow for an in-depth investigation of the mechanisms through which digital exclusion operates in specific welfare domains. Qualitative and ethnographic research would be necessary to document how individuals navigate–or fail to navigate–digital welfare platforms in practice and to assess the actual effectiveness of existing intermediary services. Furthermore, the analysis focuses on the demand side of digital welfare, mapping citizens' competences and behaviours, whereas the supply side–the design choices, usability standards, and accessibility provisions of digital welfare platforms–remains largely outside the scope of this work. This is due to the absence of suitable empirical data. Future research should address this dimension by examining how institutional design choices shape the accessibility of digital welfare, independent of users' skill levels, and by investigating whether and how intermediary support structures in Italy are effectively compensating for the digital exclusion documented here.

More broadly, this chapter contributes to a growing body of scholarship that interrogates the social consequences of administrative digitalisation and questions the dominant narrative of digital transformation as an inherently progressive and inclusive process. The evidence from the Italian case suggests that, without explicit and sustained attention to the conditions of equitable access, the digitalisation of welfare risks reproducing–and, in some respects, deepening–the very inequalities that welfare systems were designed to mitigate. The result is not a welfare state that has abandoned universalism in principle, but one that has allowed it to erode in practice through the accumulation of technical barriers that are individually small but collectively decisive. Whether this outcome is accepted as an unavoidable side effect of modernisation or addressed as a problem of social justice is ultimately a political question. The sociological task, as this chapter has attempted to demonstrate, is to make its contours visible.

REFERENCES

AgID. (2024). *Piano Triennale per l'Informatica nella Pubblica Amministrazione 2024–2026*. Agenzia per l'Italia Digitale.

Alexopoulou, S., Åström, J., & Karlsson, M. (2022). The grey digital divide and welfare state regimes: A comparative study of European countries. *Information Technology & People*, *35*(8), 273–291. DOI: 10.1108/ITP-11-2020-0803

Battisti, D. (2020). The digital transformation of Italy's public sector: government cannot be left Behind!. *JeDEM-eJournal of eDemocracy and Open Government, 12*(1), 25-39.

Civitarese Matteucci, S. (2016). Digitalisation and reforms of public administration in Italy. *Italian J. Pub. L.*, *8*, 127.

Eder, M., & Sjøvaag, H. (2024). Artificial intelligence and the dawn of an algorithmic divide. *Frontiers in Communication*, *9*, 1453251. DOI: 10.3389/fcomm.2024.1453251

Esping-Andersen, G. (1990). *The three words of welfare capitalism*. Princeton University Press.

European Commission. (2022). *EUROSHIP project: Closing gaps in social citizenship*. https://euroship-research.eu/

Goswami, M. R. (2025). The Algorithmic Citizen: How AI is Rewriting Rights, Representation and Responsibility. [ISRN]. *International Social Research Nexus*, *1*(3), 1–14. DOI: 10.63539/isrn.2025022

Gough, I. (1979). *The political economy of the welfare state*. Red Globe Press London. DOI: 10.1007/978-1-349-16122-5

Helsper, E. (2021). The digital disconnect: The social causes and consequences of digital inequalities.

Kaun, A., & Liminga, A. (2023). Welfare service centres: Maintenance, repair, and care at the analogue interfaces of the digital welfare state. *New Media & Society*, *27*(5), 3039–3054. DOI: 10.1177/14614448231220362

Marshall, T. H. (1950). *Citizenship and social class and other essays*. Cambridge University Press.

Norris, P. (2001). Digital divide: Civic engagement, information poverty, and the Internet worldwide.

Polanyi, K. (1944). *The Great Transformation*. Farrar and Rinehart.

Rebergen, M., Swart, J., & Broersma, M. (2025). Directing digital citizenship: How librarians mediate the Dutch digital welfare state. *Social Inclusion (Lisboa), 13,* 9949. DOI: 10.17645/si.9949

Snyder, I., Jones, A., & Lo Bianco, J. (2005). *Using information and communication technologies in adult literacy education: New practices, new challenges (Report).* National Centre for Vocational Education Research.

Tomasello, F. (2022). From industrial to digital citizenship: Rethinking social rights in cyberspace. *Theory and Society, 52*(3), 463–486. DOI: 10.1007/s11186-022-09480-6 PMID: 35676929

Van Dijk, J. (2020). The Digital Divide. Cambridge: Polity Press. *Communication, 2020.*

Van Dijk, J. A. G. M. (2005). *The deepening divide: Inequality in the information society*. SAGE Publications.

Vuorikari, R., Kluzer, S., & Punie, Y. (2022). DigComp 2.2: The Digital Competence Framework for Citizens – With new examples of knowledge, skills and attitudes. [EN. Publications Office of the European Union.]. *EUR, 31006,* •••.

ENDNOTES

1 SPID (Public Digital Identity System). A national digital identity system that allows users to securely access online public services using a single set of credentials.

2 CIE (Electronic Identity Card). A government-issued digital identity card that enables secure authentication and access to public administration services, both online and in person.

3 pagoPA. A national digital payment platform that standardises and facilitates payments to public administrations and public service providers.

4 ANPR (National Register of Resident Population). A centralised national database that integrates municipal population registers, enabling data sharing and interoperability across public administrations.

5 IO app A mobile application developed by the Italian government that provides a unified interface for accessing public services, receiving notifications, and managing interactions with public administrations.

6 INPS (National Institute for Social Security). The main public body responsible for managing pensions, social security benefits, and income support measures in Italy.

7 The National Recovery and Resilience Plan (PNRR) is Italy's national investment programme funded through the European Union's *Next Generation EU* recovery instrument, which aims to support post-pandemic economic recovery and accelerate digital transformation and public sector modernisation across Member States.

8 CAF (Tax Assistance Centres). Authorised private or semi-public organisations that provide administrative support to citizens, particularly for tax declarations and access to welfare benefits.

9 Patronato (Welfare assistance offices). Non-profit organisations that offer free assistance to citizens in accessing social security rights, including pensions, benefits, and administrative procedures.

Chapter 9

Rethinking the Family/Public Divide in Older Adults' Digital Facilitation:

Warming Up Digital Public Services

Giulia Melis
http://orcid.org/0000-0002-4699-021X
University of Milano-Bicocca, Italy

Mino Novello
http://orcid.org/0000-0002-4245-1809
Politecnico di Milano, Italy

ABSTRACT

As European welfare's digitisation advances, digital support strategies are increasingly relevant to assist the older segments of the population more at risk of digital and social exclusion. This chapter investigates digital support as social practices, both in familial environments and in formal public settings. Specifically, it adopts the concept of "warm expert" as an analytical lens to explore the nuances and tensions between intergenerational, family-based support practices and public institutional services of digital facilitation. It draws on two qualitative case studies conducted in Northern Italy: a longitudinal case study with older adults discussing their everyday life in digital societies and research with regional digital facilitation initiative workers. The findings from both case studies document the complex social

DOI: 10.4018/979-8-2600-3043-1.ch009

and power relations that underlie the different social contexts in which digital support is produced. Concluding remarks also contribute to the warm expert literature and discuss the findings' policy implications.

INTRODUCTION

In recent years, societies in the global North have undergone a profound digitisation process. In the European context, especially with the European Union funding from the NextGenerationEU programme, the post-pandemic reconstruction has encouraged member states to invest in more up-to-date institutional infrastructures to implement, among other goals, public targets concerning digital innovation. In Italy, the National Plan for Recovery and Resilience (PNRR) designated funds to digital transformation as one of the principal investment areas – together with ecological transition (Campedelli & Vesan, 2023; Italian Government, 2021; Signorelli et al., 2024).

As welfare institutions pivot toward digital citizenship, public services provision increasingly relies on digital technologies that reshape state-individuals' relationships. While digital policies claim greater efficiency and accessibility, they also shift the burden of navigating digital public services onto citizens themselves. Indeed, public services' digitisation generates profound challenges for older populations who risk facing greater rates of *(grey) digital divide* [GDD], namely the social exclusion due to the inability to engage with digital technologies that specifically impact older generations (Millward, 2003; Morris, 2007; Friemel, 2016). Survey data discusses GDD in Europe, documenting the small uptake of digital technologies within older age groups: in Italy, only 27.37% of adults aged 65-74 years old possess at least basic digital skills, compared to an EU mean of 33% (Eurostat, 2025). When focusing specifically on digital services and e-government, data shows that only a minority of older adults are able to successfully navigate digital services; although there is an enlarged adoption of e-government services, in Italy the gap between 55-64 and 65-74 years old increased from 12.8% in 2010 to 17.5% in 2023. Differences across states pertain not only to individual-level and sociodemographic characteristics (e.g., gender, education, and digital skills) but also to the quality of digital infrastructures and the overall welfare digitalisation process (Sala & Kochergina, 2025). Over the years, a comprehensive and multidimensional definition of the digital divide has generated a strand of research wherein this issue is not discussed merely in terms of access or competence but as an issue that also encompasses structural constraints and the socio-cultural contexts in which older individuals engage with digital technologies (Ragnedda & Ruiu, 2017). This phenomenon is particularly evident in Italy, where digitalisation initiatives under the PNRR collide with the rapid rate of population ageing.

Two distinct yet interconnected processes are currently unfolding: a crisis of the welfare state (Collington, 2022) and a crisis of the family institution (Naldini & Saraceno, 2022). On the one hand, public services' provision faces several challenges in terms of welfare system sustainability, an issue that policymakers seek to address through digitalisation as a means of cost reduction and efficiency boosting (e.g., Higgs & Gilleard, 2022). The Italian welfare system is grounded on the family as the main organisation responsible for the well-being of its members through intergenerational support and informal care. As a result, public policies tend to neglect the need for active welfare services that could help reduce individuals' reliance on family support but rather reinforce that same dependence. On the other hand, the family institution itself is changing, as declining birth rates and population ageing, along with heterogeneous family formation practices, reduce its capacity to provide informal support and care activities between generations that have long sustained social stability. With this regard, demographic ageing, and the changes in terms of population distribution affect both the organisation of the welfare system, particularly social security services, and family dynamics. While demography considers as older adults those reaching the threshold of 65 years old, we are aware that defining older age merely based on age criteria does not consider relevant aspects in older age. As underlined by Istat (2025), life expectancy has largely increased in the last decades, making room for other kinds of definitions, such as those assuming a dynamic threshold of residual life and entailing adults who today reach 65 years old still facing many years of good health conditions, activity and social participation. Moreover, new generations of older adults qualitatively differ from those of the middle of last century, for example, considering the increased education level (Istat, 2025).

As the rate of older adults grows, the demand for care and support services is expected to rise even though families are increasingly unable to meet those needs. From this perspective, welfare digitisation represents the point of convergence between these two different social processes: the crisis of the family institutions, which are finding it dramatically difficult to guarantee the provision of intergenerational care, and the digital transformation of public services, which is creating further support needs for people who are less technologically literate.

Considering how both the welfare system and the organisation of familial responsibilities are culturally embedded, in this contribution we propose adopting a framework that acknowledges how these dynamics vary significantly across different (i.e., familial and institutional) contexts. In this sense, we deem that the analytical lens offered by the grey digital divide, although providing a rich and sound body of empirical literature, does not fully grasp the complexity of older adults' digital practices. As we will argue, we propose to move beyond a deficit-oriented perspective and towards a theoretical lens that sees digital engagement as a socially situated practice. Within this framework, older adults' engagement with digital services is thus shaped by (and nested in) the social ties and cultural and contextual conditions in which it unfolds.

In this chapter we argue that digitisation of public services might represent a form of social exclusion for some groups of the population, such as older adults, for whom support in navigating digital ecosystems might be crucial. A similar role is often covered by family networks, especially in Italy, where the *digital-by-default* approach to public services becomes grafted onto a *familialism-by-default* welfare system. However, what happens when familialism is in crisis? Here we discuss the nuanced figure of warm experts *within* and *outside* the family, presenting cases of formal institutional digital support to older adults, such as *digital care work and technological support services for seniors* (TSSS). Specifically, through the analytical lens of the "warm expert", we intend to explore how familial and public support strategies facilitate older adults' engagement with digital services. Thus, we pursue two interrelated research questions to: (1.) examine how familial and close networks, alongside public formal settings, respond to older adults' needs for digital support within the context of welfare digitisation, and (2.) investigate the social dynamics that shape support practices across these two distinct settings.

To address these objectives, we draw on data derived from two qualitative case studies in the Lombardy region, in Northern Italy, that were both funded under the project Digital-by-Default[1]: the first one entails longitudinal narrative interviews with older adults in the rural Lodi area regarding their adaptation to a digitised society, while the second one explores the regional "Punti Digitale Facile" (Easy Digital Points) initiative from the perspective of facilitators and policymakers. By bridging these distinct studies, this contribution connects the experiences of older adults navigating digital public services and the organisational insights of those providing digital facilitation support.

The chapter opens with an introduction to the theoretical framework which guided our study by presenting the concept of "warm experts", used here as an analytical lens. As existing literature is divided among studies on family and close network members as assistants and research on institutional support, in this contribution we argue that the warm experts lens allows us to discuss and relate both environments for digital support. Then, we provide a background description on older adults' digital practices as subjective and social experiences, as well as on familial and close networks and public institutional settings where digital support strategies are enacted. Later, we present methods and data from the two case studies. In the "Findings" section we introduce an overview of older adults' needs in relation to welfare digitisation, and we depict familial digital support between care and dependence, and the public formal initiative explored in its *cold* and *warm* aspects. We finally discuss the nuances of "warm experts" in both familial and public settings, showing their promises and pitfalls and drawing concluding remarks.

THEORETICAL FRAMEWORK

As welfare provision and public services are undergoing digital transformations, support strategies for citizens who are potentially more vulnerable to social exclusion are increasingly needed. Especially in Italy, we need to consider how digital policy strategies may overlook the needs of older adults and of other populations more exposed to vulnerability and risks of social exclusion (Novello & Garavaglia, 2026). With this contribution we discuss the potential social exclusion generated by the advancing digital-by-default approach in welfare (Yates et al., 2015; Schou & Pors, 2019), focusing particularly on older adults (Olsson & Viscovi, 2023; Sourbati, 2015), and the fitting support strategies enacted to mitigate these issues. Such strategies emerge in a variety of contexts and modalities: usually, the informal social and familial networks are those who have been providing everyday assistance with digital tasks for older adults in recent years; however, formal public initiatives within institutional settings have gradually been implemented by disparate stakeholders.

To address these processes, we turn to the concept of the *warm expert* – a figure who blends technical guidance with emotional support, contextual adaptation, and interpersonal trust (Hänninen et al., 2021; Korpela et al., 2024). Originally ideated by Bakardjieva (2005), the concept particularly thrived in Finnish literature, in a hyperdigitalised society where, as it was observed, the knowledge gap hampered older individuals' request of assistance from IT professionals. The warm expert is neither exclusively a "trainer" nor a "technician" but someone who has a personal relationship with older users. Their importance lies in their key role as mediators between the (digitised) institutions and older individuals. Compared to the detachment of institutional procedures and digital infrastructures, warm experts are those who bridge the gaps between older adults and welfare institutions. From the perspective of older individuals, their role enables older users to navigate digital services not just by transferring skills but by building confidence, autonomy, and a sense of agency.

It is no surprise that empirical literature usually points out how this role is embodied by people belonging to older adults' close social networks – such as friends, acquaintances, and family members (Taipale, 2019; Martinez & Olson, 2022). To the best of our knowledge, in literature, with few exceptions (e.g., Guzzo, 2026) the term *'warm expert'* relates only to close social and familial networks; thus, with this contribution, we attempt to connect the warm expert concept with support roles performed outside the family and social networks in public formal settings. While several scholars (e.g., Korpela et al., 2023) tend to juxtapose the idea of a warm expert with the cold institutional support, we argue that this dichotomy is overly simplistic. The concept of warm experts might indeed be effectively applied to the practices of frontline workers supporting older adults in navigating digital environments. As we will outline in the following paragraphs, this suggested theoretical expansion is particularly urgent in the specific convergence of two structural conditions characterising the Italian context: a digital-by-default welfare model (Schou & Pors, 2019; Yates et al., 2015) and a persistent familialism-by-default (Saraceno & Keck, 2010). In this scenario, the state's withdrawal from direct service provision via digitisation implicitly delegates the burden of mediation to the family. As digital support is investigated in the two contexts of public institutional environments and family and close networks, regarding public support, we will present the example of *Technological Support Services for Seniors* (TSSS) (Tirado-Morueta et al., 2023) and the concept of *digital care work* (Kaun & Forsman, 2024). Although promising, *digital care work* results specific to public support figures, being less suitable than the *warm expert* to relate with familial and close network environments. To address this phenomenon, we considered various theoretical and empirical strands. To begin with, such frontline workers can be conceived as street-level bureaucrats, drawing on the concept from Lipsky (2010) and the vast following literature in policy research, considering the aspects of working via face-to-face encounters and representing a public organisation. This specific research stream is mostly concerned with elements of discretion, which might interact with policy design and discretionary practices are at the centre of reflections in the stream even when it comes to digitisation processes (see, for instance: Alshallaqi, 2024; Busch et al., 2018; Busch & Henriksen, 2018; Johansson, 2025). However, the intent of the present study is not to contribute to the debate on how digitalisation might curtail or enable street-level discretion, but rather to focus on the social practices of digital support.

We have also examined the seminal work on emotional labour (Hochschild, 1979, 1983) which describes the management of emotions that characterises workers (women, in particular) in the service sector (see also Wharton, 2009). Research stemming from this broad debate focuses primarily on specific categories of service-sector professionals that involve interaction with customers, patients or other people (e.g., social workers, health professionals, teachers, etc.), also including workers in public services (Guy et al., 2014). Empirical research in this field focuses primarily on the organisational dimension and how this shapes the way in which service professionals comply with specific guidelines that shape their interactions in the workplace (Erickson & Grove, 2008; Leidner, 1999; Virkki, 2007). Moreover, to the best of our knowledge, literature addressing interaction with digital technologies covered the switch from in-person service to online interactions among others (Nyanjom & Naylor, 2021). Some scholars have proposed investigating the interaction between warm experts and emotional labour (see Li, 2025; Wu & Chen, 2026). However promising, these studies nevertheless focus on informal digital support as a means of promoting active participation among older adults, but are difficult to apply to the phenomenon of digital support provided both in the informal and familial social context and by frontline service workers. In this sense, as we will discuss, the warm expert literature seems more appropriate to critically examine the social dimension of digital support and to compare the strengths and limitations of the different social contexts in which digital facilitation takes place. This concept accounts for the complexity of digital support relationships whilst allowing us to explore those aspects that are often overlooked by policy designs: specifically, the 'expert' dimension, which is typically associated with family relationships, and the 'warm' dimension, which is not usually considered in frontline digital support relationships.

Engagement with digital technologies as a social practice

To address the phenomenon of older adults' engagement with digital services, we refer to digital practices as subjective and social experiences. Drawing on studies on media and technology domestication into the household (Haddon, 2011; Silverstone & Hirsch, 1992) and on Miller's appropriation framework (1987), this body of work describes the adoption and familiarisation of digital technologies as a process through which users gradually incorporate these objects into their own everyday routines. Scholars in this field take into special consideration the role of culture and social context: social actors and potential digital users attribute meaning to digital technologies, negotiating their role in a culturally mediated system of values. In particular, this literature highlights that patterns of digital adoption are not merely an issue of access or competence – they also encompass elements related to the social sphere. *Digital cultures* may vary across gender, age categories, life course paths, and social roles. With this in mind, it is important to consider the heterogeneity of older individuals, avoiding the risk of overgeneralisation (Loos, 2012; Hargittai & Dobransky, 2017). Diverse cultural contexts may thus shape specific media ideologies (Gershon, 2010), which shape beliefs, constraints, and affordances. In this respect, several scholars documented specific generational identities that influence older individuals' digital patterns (Aroldi et al., 2011; Haddon & Mante-Meijer, 2016; Loos et al., 2012; Loos & Ivan, 2024; Taipale et al., 2017). Far from being a monolithic age group, some embrace technology; others may resist it or subvert it, and many navigate it selectively, based on their life experiences, social networks, and perceived benefits (Hänninen et al., 2021). Empirical studies highlight generation-based digital practices (Colombo et al., 2018), wherein younger generations, e.g., from the family and the extended family networks, are often the social drivers for older adults' gradual engagement with digital technologies (Taipale, 2019). Studies also document socially situated experiences that blur traditional dichotomies between use and non-use (Carlo & Diodati, 2026; Fernández-Ardèvol, 2016; Gallistl et al., 2021) and challenge both the interventionist logics (Peine & Neven, 2019) and techno-enthusiastic ideas about the expectations for older adults to reach autonomy in the use of digital technologies (Carlo & Sourbati, 2020; Ragnedda, 2018). Following these critical debates, we discuss older individuals' agency in mediating technology use within the family and institutional contexts (Gallistl et al., 2021; Loe, 2010).

Regarding digital services, several scholars support the need to adopt a user-centred perspective that pays attention to older adults' preferences and meanings (Sourbati, 2009; Laukka et al., 2024). Moreover, empirical literature has highlighted shared practices of use (Hänninen et al., 2021) that challenge individualistic assumptions about digital literacy and participation. This is also supported by recent studies that document how digital literacy does not predict digital services use among older adults, although those who reported seeking digital assistance (both from family and public formal settings) also reported higher usage intentions (Jokisch et al., 2022).

Digital support between familialism-by-default and digital care work

The digital transformation of public services – typically framed in a logic of enhancing efficiency, accessibility and bureaucratic simplification (Layne & Lee, 2001) – has increasingly shifted the burden of access onto citizens, thereby compounding the effect of ongoing welfare retrenchment (Collington, 2022). However, for those lacking digital access or literacy – as could be the case for many older adults – this burden could be mitigated by various forms of support coming from public employees, volunteers, or family members. Yet familial support can be understood as ambivalent. Although often represented as *warm* and affectionate in literature on warm experts and on cultural narratives, it can also reflect inequalities and gendered care expectations. Ultimately, this dynamic may create frustrating relationships both for the person providing care and the receiver. Empirical studies in this field document these nuances: although scholars often document older adults' preference for technical support within the family (among others, Haase et al., 2025), they have also shown how older adults' engagement with digital technologies is hampered by stereotypes among family and close networks (Birkland, 2024) and how media practices might produce intergenerational conflicts (Ivan & Nimrod, 2021). Family support, thus, plays a multifaceted and often contradictory role in digital support for older adults, acting as a primary gateway for technology adoption while potentially creating barriers to independent learning and technology use (Hunsaker et al., 2019; Korpela et al., 2024; Schreurs et al., 2017). As family members – particularly those from younger generations – serve as essential supporters, motivators, and occasionally, sources of frustration for older adults navigating the digital world.

Especially in Italy, more than in other European contexts, the family has historically served as the primary provider of care – including, increasingly, digital support. Family members often act as *warm experts*, as they offer personalised support. This process, however, reflects the dominant model of *familialism-by-default*, where welfare responsibilities are delegated to the family (Saraceno & Keck, 2010). However, this model is under strain from multiple interconnected perspectives. First, at the macro-level the nuclear family as a caring institution is transformed by emergent demographic changes: declining birth rates, population ageing, and changing family structures indeed reduce the family's capacity to provide informal care (Albertini & Pavolini, 2017) – including digital support. Then, at the micro-level, family relations are influenced by an idea of "care as a burden" (Cahill et al., 2009; Foster & Walker, 2021; Warnes, 1993) that older adults might not want to impose on younger family members. As this process is largely studied in literature regarding care work (e.g., Pope et al., 2016; Barrett et al., 2026), a similar trend might emerge considering familial digital support (e.g., Schreurs et al., 2017). Thus, formal digital assistance and literacy initiatives outside of the familial environments, often implemented through public policy, offer a crucial support strategy. They serve older adults who lack or choose not to rely on kinship ties, as well as those who prefer navigating digital ecosystems with the aid of formal channels, rather than relying on the availability of family or social networks (Hunsaker et al., 2019).

Regarding public support strategies, contributions in the field of cultural and media studies, analysing the new forms of work related to the digitalisation processes, advanced the concept of *digital care work* – a form of emotional and practical labour performed by street-level bureaucrats who, beyond their formal duties, provide personalised assistance to bridge the digital divide (Kaun & Forsman, 2024). This work is rarely recognised as such: it is rather invisible, unpaid, or under-resourced, yet it represents an essential means to promote digitally – and socially – inclusive services. Within this context, the idea of emotional labour, largely associated in literature with service and care work, is extended to professionals performing digital support tasks – such as librarians, in the case study by Kaun and Forsman (2024). Thus, the social and emotional dimension of care lies at the centre of the concept of *digital care work*.

Other examples of digital support emerging from public institutional environments are described in the literature as *Technological Support Services for Seniors* (TSSS), namely «community-based services promoted by public institutions to facilitate material access to the internet and literacy support for older people» (Tirado-Morueta et al., 2023: 1413). Thus, we can understand public institutional digital support as digital access points, helpdesks, or training programmes designed to assist older adults in acquiring the necessary skills and confidence to effectively utilise digital tools for everyday bureaucratic and service tasks. However, institutional support often struggles to tackle down the social and intersubjective dimension of care. As the dominant perspective on welfare remains efficiency-driven, the design of support services hardly values and takes into consideration the need to promote situated relationships of care between service professionals and older users, encouraging sustained support and universal access.

METHODS

Starting from the premises discussed in the theoretical framework, the overall aim of this contribution is to investigate the role of familial and public initiatives in supporting older adults' engagement with digital services, adopting the concept of "warm expert" as an analytical perspective. Specifically, we address the following, and interrelated, research questions:

1. Within the context of welfare digitisation, how do familial and close networks, as well as public formal settings, respond to older adults' needs for digital support?
2. What social dynamics shape the support practices in the two different settings?

The data for this analysis derive from two qualitative case studies conducted in different areas of the Lombardy region, in northern Italy. The first one relates to the changes of everyday life and social and digital resources of older adults living in a cluster of villages in the southern province of Lodi, drawing on longitudinal narrative interviews that address participants' experiences and representations about the gradual shaping of a digitised society. The second study focuses on the regional implementation of the PNRR initiative "Punti Digitale Facile" (Easy digital access points), from the perspective of facilitators and policymakers. Bridging results from two different studies on the context represents an added value of this contribution, allowing us to discuss the experiences of older adults engaging with digital public services in relation to the ones of those working for digital facilitation services and organising them.

The "Older Adults' Everyday Life" longitudinal case study ILQA

The ILQA longitudinal case study investigates older adults' well-being and everyday life in a post-pandemic and increasingly digitised society. It first started in 2020 during the pandemic as exploratory research. The area covered by the case study covers a cluster of ten villages located in the southern part of the Lombardy region that ILQA. The aim of the research was to analyse the relationship between the use of digital technologies to maintain social relationships and the impact on older adults' well-being. The study was prompted by the digital acceleration that followed the pandemic (Gallistl et al., 2021), a phenomenon which has also led to an increase in social and digital inequalities (Litchfield et al., 2021). The study is conducted on a purposive sample of 40 older men and women over 65 years old. Participants are a heterogeneous group in terms of family composition, gender, and socioeconomic status. With regard to digital competencies, overall, participants possess basic literacy skills but experience some difficulty in carrying out various tasks related to everyday life; some of them had low to zero digital skills, while others showed high digital skills. However, everyone had basic access to digital technologies in order to take part in the interview (namely, they owned at least a smartphone with WhatsApp). Overall, participants are an active group of individuals: although some of them present health or social conditions, none of them reported serious elements of vulnerability, economic issues or signs of cognitive decline. All the research design phase, first-wave participants' recruitment processes, and data collection have been conducted fully remotely. Data is collected through yearly narrative video interviews, adopting inclusive and non-ageistic procedures aimed at maximising participation (Melis et al., 2021; Garavaglia et al., 2023), along with participants' engagement strategies such as annual in-person meetings and video messages with research updates and festivity greetings (Melis et al., 2022) that have been enacted in the effort to sustain research relationships in-between waves (Neale, 2020). In that respect, the preliminary research encounters with participants have been crucial to build participants' trust and negotiate the consent throughout the different waves. After the emergency pandemic had ended, the panel participants were interviewed about the changes in everyday life and the ageing process in an increasingly digitised society, with a particular focus on the digitisation of public services. Data for this analysis are based mainly on wave 5 interviews, which took place in the years 2024-2025 and focused on the digitisation of welfare services, digital-by-default innovation processes, and the related risks of social exclusion. 32 participants took part in the 2025 interview: 12 men and 20 women, with a mean age of 75 years old; most of them possess a secondary education, with only 3 participants with primary education and 1 with tertiary education.

The "Helpdesk Digital Support" case study design [HDS]

The HDS case study investigates the "Rete dei servizi di facilitazione digitale" (Network of Services for Digital Facilitation) in Lombardy, with the aim of better understanding the implementation of a policy for supporting citizens in the so-called digital transition of welfare and public administration. Funded by Italy's PNRR, the initiative operates through a network of local helpdesks and digital facilitators. According to the Region's website, As of November 18, 2024, there were a total of 322 points across the entire region. Data were collected via semi-structured interviews with key informants as well as local coordinators and frontline facilitators. To account for heterogeneity of municipalities within the Region, the research design ensured representation from all provinces, with the exception of Varese, where no interviews could be secured. Furthermore, to capture the diversity of urban, peri-urban, and rural contexts, municipalities were sampled based on the ISTAT "aree interne" classification, with the intentional oversampling of rural areas, where such services are typically less prevalent. Semi-structured interviews were conducted mostly online, through the web-conference software Webex (except for one interview in the organisation's space), between January and October 2025. The HDS study comprises 8 single interviews and 5 group interviews, with a total of 19 interviewees: 5 key informants, 5 local coordinators, and 9 facilitators. Specifically, the key informants are members of the regional administration and a provincial (Pavia) administration, of one labour services association and one professional training institution with a strategic role in the policy implementation. The local coordinators and facilitators are members of professional training organisations in the Sondrio and Bergamo provinces (rural areas), one ageing association in the Cremona province (peri-urban area), a labour services association in the Como province (urban area), a social services association in the Milano province (urban area), a local association in the Lodi context (peri-urban area) and one municipality in the Milano province (urban area). While 9 interviewees are women, 10 are men, providing a certain gender balance in responses. The majority of interviewees (10) are middle-aged adults, while 3 of them are young adults (2 key informants and 1 facilitator), and 4 interviewees are older adults (1 local coordinator and 3 facilitators).

Data Analysis

All the data collected within the two case studies has been transcribed verbatim, ILQA and archived following the procedures adopted in each research team (AUTHORS' WORK). The two datasets have undergone a qualitative thematic analysis (Boyatzis, 1998; Braun & Clarke, 2006) using NVivo 15, adopting a two-step procedure: first, data analysis was conducted separately for each case study; then, the results were compared and integrated across a selected set of common analytical dimensions. The separate data analysis allowed the peculiarities of each empirical context to emerge. Specifically, in the ILQA case study, the analysis focused on the experiences and representations of older people in relation to the digitalisation of welfare and public services. Particular attention was paid to the digital support practices within family and local networks, the potential and limitations of digital literacy courses, as well as the digital support services provided in the area. In the HDS case, the analysis focused on the working practices of frontline service workers. Data analysis explored in depth the interaction between digital facilitators and older adults who have accessed the service, focusing on the tensions between the institutional design of the service and the care strategies implemented at an individual level.

After this first step, we compared the preliminary findings to identify points of convergence and tension between the two. Starting from the preliminary coding frame, we developed a codebook using as a sensitising concept (Blumer 1954; Charmaz, 2003) the literature on ageing and warm experts. We proposed a set of criteria that allowed us to identify the defining features of each context: specifically, tailored, sustained, trustworthy interactions were elements that identified *warmness*, whereas universal, once-only, top-down interactions identified the *coldness* in digital support practices. Moreover, we also coded *expertise* to take into consideration the competence that emerges both with respect to the digital technologies and in relation to the support provided. Finally, we coded *representations of ageing* to cover older adults' subjective accounts of digital support in relation to the ageing process – e.g., personal attitudes regarding digital technologies, issues of autonomy and agency, as well as their representations of dependence and burden when needing digital support. To highlight the complexity of the two domains in which digital support takes place, the findings presented in the next section will be discussed separately to present support in the family context and in public contexts.

FINDINGS

As mentioned in the methods section, the analysis is focused on comparing the practices of digital support and digital care work (Kaun & Forsman, 2024) that have been enacted in the different contexts taken into consideration, namely the family dimension and the institutional support, drawing from the literature on *warm experts* (Bakardjieva, 2005; Hänninen et al., 2021; Korpela et al., 2024; Martinez & Olson, 2022; Taipale 2019). In that respect, the preliminary exploration of the data from the ILQA case study has provided an overview of older individuals' needs in relation to digital welfare services. According to the scholars that highlight the lack of homogeneity among the older population (Hargittai & Dobransky, 2017), the data portrays a variety of profiles differing not only in terms of socioeconomic background and life trajectories but also in relation to digital experiences and attitudes. Overall, ILQA participants do not appear overly "technophobic". They recognise the usefulness of welfare digitisation processes, but despite the challenges they experience, they often produce contrasting attitudes toward these policies. Specifically, older individuals seem to find themselves caught between the expectations of being able to keep up with welfare innovations and the difficulties of pursuing these updates. In this regard, they try to navigate digital services by exploring welfare platforms through self-education, asking people from their close social networks for assistance or, when available, attending digital literacy training courses or other initiatives. However, the interviews sometimes reveal a certain level of discomfort with the methods employed to overcome these challenges. For example, they seem unsatisfied with the digital literacy courses they have attended over the years, which, according to them, do not seem to be able to consolidate their skills, especially when it comes to tasks they have never encountered before.

To begin with, we present the experience of Sandra: she is a widow, lives alone and has no children but she keeps in touch with her extended family on a daily basis. Her weeks are full of volunteering activities, which also give her the opportunity to attend many training courses, such as those designed to familiarise her with the use of digital technologies. She supports the need for older adults to remain active and independent as long as possible, and for that she recognises the importance of possessing at least basic digital literacy. However, as documented in this excerpt, Sandra shows dissatisfaction with the course methods. Despite her commitment, she says, the course is unable to convey skills that last:

> *Well, they teach you, and you can see, learn, etc., but you still need someone to be there with you for a while, right? It's not like if they show you [once], then you learn. [...] At the time you thought you would have remembered, but in the end, you went back where you were before, didn't you? I mean, if you tried at home, maybe you missed a few steps... unless you wrote everything down, but in the meantime [that you take notes], the teacher goes on! And so, I really think that in order to learn, you need to have someone close by who guides you while you're doing it, at least for a while, until you have internalised the mechanisms... [ILQA, INT12, W5, F, 75-79]*

As a first example, Sandra's interview is particularly relevant because it highlights the issue faced by someone who, despite presenting a significant amount of social and cultural capital, nevertheless complains about her inability to transfer it into digital capital (Ragnedda 2018), proving the complex interaction between the different sources of privilege, social and digital inequalities.

This preliminary overview can now be expanded by considering Tina's experience. Widowed with two children, with a son that lives with her while her daughter lives nearby, on her own, Tina is engaged in volunteering as well but she presents some peculiarities: in the first place, she had a more difficult life path than Sandra, resulting in a different social background; in the second place, she only partially shares Sandra's opinions on the relationship with public institutions and welfare services. While admitting to having little familiarity with navigating digital services autonomously, she argues that independence in the use of digital services should not be an obligation, and, instead, she is eager to ask for assistance from offices and services provided by the institutions:

I don't even touch it! I wouldn't be able to do it myself, for goodness' sake! However, I don't think that we should do everything by ourselves [...], staying at home all the time. There are services that provide us with what we need; they're almost free... [...] I like to go there and ask, get information, have a quick chat... I get things explained to me... I still go to the offices, to all of them. [ILQA, INT37, W5, F, 70-74]

What appears most useful in Tina's interviews, apart from the existence of institutional services that undertake such delicate tasks on her behalf, is the opportunity to interact with the people who work in these various offices. Their presence seems to bring a sense of humanity to these tasks, and their reliability helps reduce the sense of defeat that sometimes arises when one is unable to successfully navigate digital services. Here we see another excerpt from Tina, who describes the relationship she pursues when going to the municipal offices to ask for help after trying unsuccessfully to obtain information by browsing their website:

Well, I [go] even to get information about the offices' opening hours, for example, which is not updated, and a lot of other things. [...] Now there's a new employee in the municipal office, but the site is not very updated and not easy to use either... even the employees have admitted it! They say they're trying to improve it; it's an old site... I don't understand it technically. I trust what they tell me, but yes, there is this difficulty here. [ILQA, INT37, W5, F, 70-74]

It is interesting to mention how the employees of public offices realise and share the difficulties that can be encountered when trying to access digital services. From what we are able to observe, they often anticipate such challenges and offer to assist with certain tasks that are necessary to access digital welfare services.

Preliminary analysis from the ILQA case study, such as Tina's account, anticipates the complexities of the warm expert figure that we will discuss in the following sections. As we will argue, data indeed shows, on one hand, the nuances of family-based practices of digital support; on the other hand, it suggests that relationships of trust and digital support are not limited to the familial sphere but might extend to institutional environments and professionals with whom older adults engage in digital support relationships.

Digital support in familial contexts

Preliminary data explorations document how older adults' experiences in navigating digital services' ecosystems are grounded in pre-existing relationships and situated trust: a dynamic that within the empirical literature finds its most thorough expression in the *warm expert* figure, who offers digital support within the intimate sphere of familial networks. The excerpts presented so far showed how the relational intersubjective dimension of trust resulted in being poignant in support relationships. We here deepen our investigation into the nuances of the warm expert role, understanding the dynamics unfolding *within* the context of familial networks – and later we will discuss them *outside* the family, in formal support environments. Indeed, interviews with frontline workers at helpdesks (HDS) confirm that trust is one of the foundational elements underpinning the digital support older adults receive in the domestic context. The following passage underlines how children are often the ones entrusted with *private* issues, such as digital identity:

Older adults struggle, as I was saying... Also because of the mistrust, I mean, SPID for them is something extremely private, so private they already don't trust it. If they have it, the child is managing it. And the child can't be bothered... [HDS, INT05_1, Facilitator, Lodi, middle-aged adult, W]

Following the opinion of helpdesk workers, younger family members act as a trusted intermediary who legitimise the digital service ecosystem itself. Crucially, the older adults' hesitation to engage directly with SPID often reflects a perceived deficit in digital agency, rather than a lack of technical capability; the digital realm may be regarded as unsafe, as well as hostile and emotionally inaccessible. In this context, the role of younger family members – especially sons and daughters – outstrips technical assistance, shifting toward an emotional safeguard that makes technology usable, bridging the gap between fear and action. However, this reliance may introduce a new vulnerability as older adults' access to welfare services becomes contingent on family members' availability, highlighting a fragility in this informal support model. Similarly, the following quote from a helpdesk coordinator underlines the double-edged nature of familial support:

It's not easy, also because the aim is to promote the service [...] On the other hand, we need to understand if the citizen really has the need for it, because maybe the older adult sometimes says "I'll never make it" or "well, I have my nephew, my son...". For example, [...] my father lives in Campania and I use my father's SPID. So, my father doesn't even know what SPID is, while I know it's there and I use it. Thus, if among your networks you have the nephew, or the child, or the daughter-in-law or a younger family member supporting you... It's clear you will make it. Let's say who comes here - a man of between 90 and 94 years old came once - I mean, to get engaged is not, is not easy, so it was a nice feeling for me too. So, it's also a bit subjective. [HDS, GRINT04_2, Coordinator, Como, middle-aged adult, W]

Thus, while the presence of a younger family member could guarantee access to digital service in some situations, it may simultaneously reinforce the older adult's self-perception of inadequacy. The coordinator's observation that engagement is "not easy" and "subjective" underscores a critical tension: the goal of "promoting the service" clashes with the reality that informal networks often act as a substitute for, rather than a bridge to, digital agency.

The interviews with older digital users show in more depth the ambivalences that emerge from family practices of digital support. In the following excerpt, Mariano relates with frustration the reversal of social roles between him and his children and the power imbalances that this entails: although his adult children seem to be willing to help him when he has difficulty accessing welfare services, apparently they do not seem inclined to take the time to teach him how to perform these tasks independently, justifying this choice on the basis of their father's alleged inability to learn.

R: Is there anything you would like to learn that you find particularly difficult?
I: What makes me angry is when I say to my children, "Explain it to me!" "Yes, but afterwards you don't remember; it's useless! When you need something, you ask me!"... They ignore me like this and that's that! I argue, "I've taught you some things; maybe I know a little more than you think," but nothing, "if you need anything, just ask." We'll see… it's just that when I ask… they're always busy, never have time, you know… That's life; I have to be patient, even though I've never been patient! [ILQA, INT21, W5, M, 75-79]

This example shows the contradictions that arise in family caregiving. When support is not paired with efforts to encourage autonomy in navigating digital services, the practical role of support that their children assume leads to a loss of agency and invalidates the older adults' sense of self.

Furthermore, data from the interviews with the helpdesk workers (HDS) confirm that digital support within families is not always the preferred modality of help for older adults. Among the elements reported at the helpdesks in the decision to seek institutional support is the older adult's perception of the unavailability of the younger family members, frequently compounded by the distress caused by their children's perceived lack of time and attentiveness. As shown by the following excerpt, individuals with existing family networks might nevertheless refer to the helpdesks when younger family members are not available for support:

Older adults, not exclusively alone, [are coming for support] because they often tell us, "I come here because my son never has time to listen to me", some came for this reason, so not exclusively people living alone. I mean people with a familiar network [HDS, GRINT02_1, Coordinator, Cremona, older adult, W].

As a complex social arena, the enactment of digital support within the family is grounded in complex mutual care practices, power relationship imbalances and other social roles that complicate the picture. In the example, pressuring younger family members with the expectation to obtain digital support might be met with the refusal of assuming undesirable care roles.

Furthermore, even when they are willing to provide support, younger family members may often lack both the technical expertise and the soft/teaching skills required to deliver adequate and comprehensive digital support, as we can read in some excerpts here reported.

She was a relatively young lady, married with daughters, [...] and as a matter of fact at home she couldn't make it, because they [daughters] were telling her "No, mum, don't do this task because you blow it." The husband as well. So, she was like "what do I do now?" So, I need to turn to someone, let's say, neutral, who may understand me." She indeed was thanking us later, she came twice, and I have to say without our help she wouldn't improve as she was desperately hoping to. [....] The husband was mocking her and the daughters even worse. "Do not touch absolutely anything, otherwise nothing works." [...] It is a point of pride for the person going back home and saying "now I feel confident, I can operate autonomously, I don't need anyone" [HDS, GRINT02_1, Coordinator, Cremona, older adult, W].

In this quote we understand once again how digital support should not be discussed in dichotomous terms, wherein the warmth of the family dynamics is opposed to the detachment of institutional practices. In this regard, data from both case studies documents several occasions wherein familial support is not perceived as *warm*. In situations of scarcity of resources, such as time or teaching skills, younger family members may opt to entirely perform tasks for an insecure older adult, thus neglecting the procedures that older individuals need to perform or even raising issues for their autonomy.

Here we present another testimony from Tina's interview, from the ILQA case study. Tina draws a parallel between the digitisation of welfare services, as opposed to traditional practices involving physical offices and face-to-face interactions, and the issue of autonomy in old age. Indeed, given her difficulty in accessing adequate digital support, Tina feels that having to rely on her daughter to manage sensitive data that is only available online poses a risk not only to her privacy but also to her autonomy.

[I sense] A little agitation, a little worry... They take away my independence; I always have to ask someone to help me do my things. I might not even tell my daughter about my bank account, for example, or my health status, so that she doesn't worry or else... So, I wonder, why am I forced to have my medical records sent to me via computer? So that I have to ask my daughter to deliver me my medical records and have a chance to have a look at them before giving them to me? Instead, I could very easily go out, to the hospital or the designated office, ask for my medical records, even pay my 20 euros – I don't know whether

you're supposed to pay or not – but still go home with my paper... Why should I always ask other people to do it? [ILQA, INT37, W5, F, 70-74]

On the one hand, we are unaware of Tina's daughter's attitude towards digital assistance, as her role as a warm expert is not necessarily a free choice but rather another implicit demand in the ongoing process of welfare digitisation. On the other hand, Tina's experience addresses the multiple levels of autonomy simultaneously at stake, wherein the use of digital services – and therefore the inability to access and navigate on her own – seems to be the least important. What appears to worry her the most are, in fact, the risk of losing control of her personal data and the lack of autonomy in managing a relationship with her daughter, which, due to the need for digital support, inevitably changes the nature of intergenerational relationships.

In light of this issue, in Tina's experience, the material affordances of institutional support services emerge as a symbol of resistance, counteracting the erosion of independence. Indeed, such erosion could be conceived as a direct consequence of the coercive compliance required by digital services' environments. This dynamic also highlights that lack of access and competence to successfully navigate digital services should not be confused with lack of older adults' agency, which may manifest, for example, in the choice to seek institutional digital support. It is with this perspective in mind that we will analyse the experiences that take place when older adults turn to service and helpdesk professionals, presented in the next section.

Warming up the support within public institutions

The critical issues that emerged while discussing the role of warm experts in the family context show that close family ties are not necessarily the best choice for older adults when it comes to assistance with digital welfare services. In this section, we will address public digital support through the warm expert perspective. As we will argue, data often documents how the dichotomous perspective which contrasts the qualities of digital support within familial environments with the coldness of relationships with workers in public institutions may return a naive and simplistic picture. Frontline workers at helpdesks, generally assumed to be operating within the *cold* policy initiative framework, indeed shape *warm* interactions with older users as well in order to assist them with digital public services tasks.

The analysis of ILQA data also revealed that the role of the warm expert was more blurred than the traditional boundaries between family and institutional contexts. For example, Sandro's interview provides us with a clear example of this phenomenon. Overall, he seems to conduct an active life within and outside the family. He helps look after his grandchildren and his older brothers and sisters while relying on his daughter's help with the most difficult administrative tasks. Meanwhile, he is also an active member of his small community. The sense of belonging and the mutual support that comes from the close connections with the various members of his small community, as he says, is what appears to help him overcome some of the difficulties he faces in using digital services. In this excerpt, he documents how he managed to activate the digital public identity (SPID, *Public System of Digital Identity*), which is necessary to access all kinds of welfare services, such as Italy's national security agency (INPS, *National Institute of Social Security*) and navigate all his health records:

I got it at the post office. I went to pay a bill and the employee – this is typical of small towns – said, "INTERVIEWEE, let's do the SPID!" "Look, I would do it, but I don't have [my documents] with me," I replied. "Look, you don't need anything. Come here, I'll do it for you right away!". I gave him my personal details, and within a few seconds I received the text message. [...] I had wanted to do it for a while because I really needed for the INPS and for my health records... [ILQA, INT09, W3, M, 65-69]

These experiences are mirrored in the HDS case study, wherein data shows how helpdesk professionals strategically appropriate warm practices to bridge the gap between rigid institutional processes of policy implementation and the lived realities of older users. This tension is particularly evident in the training phase: facilitators frequently describe the official training programme as impersonal and technically focused, failing to equip them with the intersubjective and relational tools necessary for the daily interaction. As one coordinator and frontline worker noted:

In my opinion, training is, besides sad, anonymous, because [...] it's you and your PC, this voice speaking, slides moving. They are beautiful, really, [...] they did interesting things. [...] However, it is a little bit cold and people, especially older people, don't need it to be so cold. It's already so cold, the social world, you know? So, I find it, and we find it, wrong to also have a relationship with technology that is so cold. We indeed created this nice synergy [emphasised by the interviewee], this friendly connection, you know? So it's not a mathematical operation to make, but a more humanistic operation. One that brings to basic problems resolution, related to technology, which remains the focus of my presence to their side when we meet. [HDS, INT02_1, Coordinator, Sondrio, middle-aged adult, M]

Other structural deficits are identified by various interviewees, such as the "once only" design of the initiative, which allows only one access to helpdesks by a single citizen. Frontline workers face efficiency-oriented design that overlooks support continuity and intersubjective *warm* elements. To compensate, they rely heavily on resources such as their own personal dispositions, specifically their availability, patience, and in some cases, expansive personalities, to humanise the service provided. In doing so, the professional boundary often blurs, as facilitators may find themselves transcending their formal role to act as friends, surrogate children, or even guardians of safety for the older adults they assist. This shift is vividly captured by the aforequoted interviewee, who explained:

I have an open and outgoing personality, so I immediately can create a father-son/ mother-son kind of relationship every time. And being very welcoming, people are more trusting. [HDS, INT02_1, Coordinator, Sondrio, middle-aged adult, M]

This care work extends well beyond the expected roles of skills transmission and the physical boundaries of the helpdesk. In some instances, the trust established is so profound that it leads to interventions in the private sphere of the older adult's lives, addressing vulnerabilities that are entirely non-digital. As another facilitator described regarding winter evenings:

During winter, it was night and someone even entrusted me to give them a ride back home. Now, a random unknown Mr. X says "I can give you a ride, if you want". But they are older folks you know? [I've felt bad] to see them go home by foot, "if you want, I'll give you a lift". And they were saying yes to me. So, even unasked, they'd tell me where they lived. I mean... it takes trust for an older folk to be given a ride home. [HDS, INT05_1, Facilitator, Lodi, middle-aged adult, W]

Furthermore, to overcome the limitation of the "once-only" access rule, front-line workers often reinterpret the policy to provide recurrent support. Facilitators strategically organise small, recurring groups that return to the helpdesk, working iteratively on individual issues within a collective setting. By fostering recurrence and peer-to-peer social interaction, these workers effectively bridge technical learning needs with crucial social dimensions in their support practices. Thus, the effectiveness of helpdesks is reported to depend less on the Region's structural framework given for the policy measure and more on the individual worker's ability to capture the full spectrum of older adults' support needs – needs that transcend mere technical assistance to encompass crucial intersubjective and social dimensions.

DISCUSSION AND CONCLUDING REMARKS

The social transformations produced by the digitisation of welfare, as part of a broader process of digital innovation in contemporary societies, have led to a re-configuration of social relationships and given rise to new risks of social exclusion. Older adults, who present on average less digital competence than younger age groups, might encounter more difficulties in complying with the request to switch their interactions with the public sphere to online-only environments, thus resulting in potential sources of marginalisation. For these reasons, it is necessary to take into account the practices of digital support that have been enacted within familial and close networks to mitigate the difficulties faced by older generations, along with the experiences of public support recently implemented to overcome these issues.

To address this phenomenon, the overall aim of this contribution has focused on the role of familial and public strategies in supporting older adults' engagement with digital services, adopting the concept of "warm expert" as an analytical perspective.

In doing so, in this contribution we have presented the integration of two case studies, both conducted in the Lombardy region in Italy: longitudinal research on older adults' everyday practices in digitised societies (ILQA) and an investigation on helpdesk digital support services and frontline workers' practices of support (HDS). The combined analysis of the two case studies allowed us to grasp the challenges related to the digitisation of welfare services from different perspectives: on the one hand, the interviews with older participants, as digital services' users, focused on the social issues in relation to the use of digital services, looking at the relationships of support in the familial and close networks and with public service professionals; on the other hand, the interviews with frontline workers in digital assistance services showed how their role was performed in the support encounter, highlighting the differences between the top-down institutional design of public support services and the bottom-up social and subjective strategies put into practice. In this sense, the "warm expert" concept proved to be a promising analytical perspective, as it makes it possible to identify the nuances in both domains wherein digital support takes place. Specifically, findings show that digital support provided within familial contexts is embedded in a complex network of relationships of mutual care where attitudes towards digital support collide with attitudes towards ageing: for this reason, requests for support directed at family members, although on average more likely to be available, carry with them the risk of further reducing older people's independence. At the same time, the caregiving responsibilities that already exist within family dynamics can lead to digital support being perceived as a double burden: on the one hand, older people may avoid asking their family members for digital support so as not to feel like a burden. On the other hand, it is important to recognise that, in a familistic culture, family members simultaneously feel the burden of providing constant support, without necessarily having the skills or resources to do so. Moreover, findings show that the interactions within public support services can also foster the sense of trust and familiarity needed to empower older adults when it comes to everyday digital tasks. However, it is important to emphasise that this opportunity is left entirely to the initiative of frontline service professionals.

With our research questions, we attempted to investigate the social dimension of support strategies enacted by familial and close networks, as well as by formal public initiatives, to assist older adults in navigating digital service ecosystems. This analysis originates from a complex context in which a top-down, centralised process of digitisation appears characterised by a digital-by-default approach (Schou & Pors,

2019; Yates et al., 2015) that places the responsibility to continually adapt to new digital platforms onto individuals, with insufficient public support. Considering this void, the main burden falls on family and informal networks. This dynamic reflects Italy's longstanding tradition of familialism-by-default (Saraceno & Keck, 2010). Within these structural patterns, this tendency is also increasingly showing the pressures caused by demographic changes that are eroding its foundations. Data in this respect confirms that familial and close social ties remain the main resources that older adults rely on when they need help accessing digital welfare services.

At the same time, however, our findings reveal the issues associated with these practices of support: the digital care work (Kaun & Forsman, 2024) within the family is often documented as demanding and carried out without specific preparation nor the intent to transfer digital competences onto older family members. A crucial distinction thus emerges between the delegation of digital tasks and the act of enabling older individuals to access and manage their engagement with welfare services on their own. This mechanism, although carried out unintentionally by younger family members, appears to be producing a reversal of intergenerational power relations wherein the autonomy and agency of older adults, rather than being supported, risk being inevitably undermined.

Our research question intended also to investigate practices of support within the public institutional sphere enacted by the helpdesk digital support service, especially taking into consideration frontline service workers. Findings in this domain show that the "coldness" metaphor used to represent public institutions' structural detachment from citizens and digital users, often fuelled by the lack of formal support due to inaccessible design and the very same digital-by-default approach, does not fully capture the social practices of digital support that are performed within interactions between older users and support service professionals. Contrary to this picture, frontline workers often emerge as capable of adapting universal procedures to situated support encounters. These workers are shown to be negotiating the coldness of digital welfare designs by performing caring support practices that largely surpass their professional mandate, offering reassurance and translating digital and bureaucratic complexity into accessible, enduring processes. If we discuss these findings through the warm expert lens, we could add a new perspective to digital support literature: if usually the warm familial practices are juxtaposed to the cold public formal initiatives, we here argue that a micro-level approach to institutional practices reveals how often rigid policy protocols are reinterpreted based on everyday support needs. This process, however, entails a fundamental care work in providing digital support, a dimension at the core of the warm expert concept which tends to remain unacknowledged. If a caregiving burden and emotional availability is often taken for granted within familial networks, with the downside of placing care expectations onto younger family members, the care aspects of digital facilitation performed by workers risk being under-recognised and underpaid (Kaun & Forsman, 2024).

Thus, based on these remarks, we identify two considerable policy implications of this work. The first one relates to the need to design adequate, *warmer* public digital support, tailored for older adults' specific experiences and needs and considering the heterogeneity of digital practices among this target population. Specifically, building on our findings, *warmer* support could be obtained by envisioning recurrent access, relational continuity, and adequate staffing. A tailored design of digital public support service could also provide guidelines on how to adapt these interactions to older adults' specific needs while recognising that support services that are implicitly expected to go the extra mile in order to provide a more efficient intervention might also overlook the risk of emotional labour. With that in mind, the suggestion is to fully recognise the care work performed by frontline workers. This requires integrating communication and care models into professional training programmes and ensuring adequate remuneration for the job, rather than taking emotional labour for granted.

By all means, while promising, the results here presented show various limitations. First, our study is situated in a specific regional geographical context. Thus, an expansion on a larger, national scale would be beneficial in order to advance knowledge on the topic. Secondly, despite our attempt to combine similar case studies, it is worth mentioning that our results partially referred to different contexts: specifically, the ILQA study was conducted in the southern province of Lodi, while the HDS study refers to different areas within the larger Lombardy region, with only one interview conducted with a frontline worker in the same area of the ILQA case. Moreover, the present study does not analyse data coming directly from family members and close networks: interviews with these kinds of informants would have deepened findings on the role of the family in digital support. Therefore, we invite future research addressing this phenomenon to also investigate these processes in the situated contexts in which support strategies are implemented, paying attention to the different social groups at stake – older digital users, family members and close networks, and frontline digital support service workers – in order to disentangle the complex interplay of each of these actors in this phenomenon.

REFERENCES

Albertini, M., & Pavolini, E. (2017). Unequal Inequalities: The Stratification of the Use of Formal Care Among Older Europeans. *The Journals of Gerontology. Series B, Psychological Sciences and Social Sciences*, *72*(3), 510–521. DOI: 10.1093/geronb/gbv038 PMID: 26224754

Alshallaqi, M. (2024). The complexities of digitization and street-level discretion: A socio-materiality perspective. *Public Management Review*, *26*(1), 25–47. DOI: 10.1080/14719037.2022.2042726

Aroldi, P., Fortunati, L., Gebhardt, J., & Vincent, J. (2011). Generational Belonging Between Media Audiences and ICT Users. *Broadband Society and Generational Changes*, *5*(3), 51–67.

Bakardjieva, M. (2005). *Internet Society: The Internet in Everyday Life*. Sage Academic Books.

Barrett, A., Consolandi, M., Fattorini, E., & Vecchione, K. (2026). Altruistic Ageing: How Age Inequality Contributes to Care Work's Construction as a Burden. *Ageing and Society*, *46*, e4. DOI: 10.1017/S0144686X25100342

Birkland, J. L. (2024). How Older Adult Information and Communication Technology Users Are Impacted by Aging Stereotypes: A Multigenerational Perspective. *New Media & Society*, *26*(7), 3967–3988. DOI: 10.1177/14614448221108959

Blumer, H. (1954). What is wrong with social theory? *American Sociological Review*, *19*(1), 3–10. DOI: 10.2307/2088165

Boyatzis, R. E. (1998). *Transforming Qualitative Information*. Sage.

Braun, V., & Clarke, V. (2006). Using thematic analysis in psychology. *Qualitative Research in Psychology*, *3*(2), 77–101. DOI: 10.1191/1478088706qp063oa

Busch, P. A., & Henriksen, H. Z. (2018). Digital discretion: A systematic literature review of ICT and street-level discretion. *Information Polity*, *23*(1), 3–28. DOI: 10.3233/IP-170050

Busch, P. A., Henriksen, H. Z., & Sæbø, Ø. (2018). Opportunities and challenges of digitized discretionary practices: A public service worker perspective. *Government Information Quarterly*, *35*(4), 547–556. DOI: 10.1016/j.giq.2018.09.003

Cahill, E., Lewis, L. M., Barg, F. K., & Bogner, H. R. (2009). "You Don't Want to Burden Them": Older Adults' Views on Family Involvement in Care. *Journal of Family Nursing*, *15*(3), 295–317. DOI: 10.1177/1074840709337247 PMID: 19474397

Campedelli, M., & Vesan, P. (2023). Welfare Digitalizzato, Welfare Digitale e i Nuovi Rischi Sociali Digitali: un'Introduzione. *Politiche Sociali, 2*. Advance online publication. DOI: 10.7389/108019

Carlo, S., & Diodati, F. (2026). Ageing and Mobile Phones: Tactical Uses/Nonuses in Postpandemic Italy. *Mobile Media & Communication, 14*(1), 89–107. DOI: 10.1177/20501579251359072

Carlo, S., & Sourbati, M. (2020). Age and Technology in Digital Inclusion Policy: A Study of Italy and the UK. *ESSACHESS–Journal for Communication Studies*, 13.2 (26), 107-127.

Charmaz, K. (2003). Grounded theory: Objectivist and constructivist methods. In Denzin, N. K., & Lincoln, Y. S. (Eds.), *Strategies for Qualitative Inquiry* (pp. 249–291). Sage.

Collington, R. (2022). Disrupting the Welfare State? Digitalisation and the Retrenchment of Public Sector Capacity. *New Political Economy, 27*(2), 312–328. DOI: 10.1080/13563467.2021.1952559

Colombo, F., Aroldi, P., & Carlo, S. (2018). 'I Use it Correctly!': The Use of ICTs among Italian Grandmothers in a Generational Perspective. *Human Technology, 14*(3), 343–365. DOI: 10.17011/ht/urn.201811224837

Erickson, R. J., & Grove, W. J. (2008). Emotional labor and health care. *Sociology Compass, 2*(2), 704–733. DOI: 10.1111/j.1751-9020.2007.00084.x

Eurostat (2025). *Individuals' Level of Digital Skills by Sex and Age* https://ec.europa.eu/eurostat/databrowser/view/eq_dskl07/default/table?lang=en

Fernández-Ardèvol, M. (2016). An Exploration of Mobile Telephony Non-Use among Older People. In E., Domínguez-Rué, & L.E., Nierling. (Eds.). *Ageing and Technology: Perspectives from the Social Sciences* (pp. 47-66). Transcript Verlag. DOI: 10.14361/9783839429570-003

Foster, L., & Walker, A. (2021). Active Ageing across the Life Course: Towards a Comprehensive Approach to Prevention. *BioMed Research International, 2021*(1), 6650414. DOI: 10.1155/2021/6650414 PMID: 33623785

Friemel, T. N. (2016). The Digital Divide Has Grown Old: Determinants of a Digital Divide Among Seniors. *New Media & Society, 18*(2), 313–331. DOI: 10.1177/1461444814538648

Gallistl, V., Rohner, R., Hengl, L., & Kolland, F. (2021). Doing Digital Exclusion – Technology Practices of Older Internet Non-Users. *Journal of Aging Studies, 59*, 100973. DOI: 10.1016/j.jaging.2021.100973 PMID: 34794717

Gallistl, V., Seifert, A., & Kolland, F. (2021). COVID-19 as a "digital push?" Research experiences from long-term care and recommendations for the post-pandemic era. *Frontiers in Public Health, 9*, 660064. DOI: 10.3389/fpubh.2021.660064 PMID: 34041216

Garavaglia, E., Caliandro, A., Melis, G., Sala, E., & Zaccaria, D. (2023). Contrasting ageism in research on older adults and digital technologies: A methodological reflection. In Rosales, A., Fernández-Ardèvol, M., & Svensson, J. (Eds.). *Digital ageism: How it operates and approaches to tackling it.* (pp. 248-265). Routledge.

Gershon, I. (2010). Media Ideologies: An Introduction. *Journal of Linguistic Anthropology, 20*(2), 283–293. DOI: 10.1111/j.1548-1395.2010.01070.x

Guy, M. E., Newman, M. A., & Mastracci, S. H. (2014). *Emotional labor: Putting the service in public service*. Routledge. DOI: 10.4324/9781315704852

Guzzo, M. del R. (2026). The Multiple Faces of Warm Experts. In V. G., Duffy, Q., Gao, & J. Zhou. (Eds.). *HCI International 2025* – Late Breaking Papers (pp. 52–68). Springer Nature Switzerland. DOI: 10.1007/978-3-032-13022-8_5

Haase, M., Bosse, M., Sackmann, S., & Meyer, G. (2025). IT Skills of Young and Older People: A Qualitative Study. *International Journal of Human-Computer Interaction, 41*(4), 2301–2311. DOI: 10.1080/10447318.2024.2319916

Haddon, L. (2011). Domestication Analysis, Objects of Study, and the Centrality of Technologies in Everyday Life. *Canadian Journal of Communication, 36*(2), 311–324. DOI: 10.22230/cjc.2011v36n2a2322

Haddon, L., & Mante-Meijer, E. (2016). *Generational Use of New Media*. Routledge. DOI: 10.4324/9781315584270

Hänninen, R., Taipale, S., & Luostari, R. (2021). Exploring Heterogeneous ICT Use among Older Adults: The Warm Experts' Perspective. *New Media & Society, 23*(6), 1584–1601. DOI: 10.1177/1461444820917353

Hargittai, E., & Dobransky, K. (2017). Old Dogs, New Clicks: Digital Inequality in Skills and Uses Among Older Adults. *Canadian Journal of Communication, 42*(2), 195–212. DOI: 10.22230/cjc.2017v42n2a3176

Higgs, P., & Gilleard, C. (2022). Techno-Fixes for an Ageing Society. *Aging & Mental Health, 26*(7), 1303–1305. DOI: 10.1080/13607863.2021.2008308 PMID: 34823393

Hochschild, A. R. (1979). Emotion work, feeling rules, and social structure. *American Journal of Sociology*, *85*(3), 551–575. DOI: 10.1086/227049

Hochschild, A. R. (1983). *The Managed Heart: Commercialization Of Human Feeling*. University of California Press.

Hunsaker, A., Nguyen, M. H., Fuchs, J., Djukaric, T., Hugentobler, L., & Hargittai, E. (2019). "He Explained It to Me and I Also Did It Myself": How Older Adults Get Support with Their Technology Uses. *Socius: Sociological Research for a Dynamic World*, *5*, 2378023119887866. DOI: 10.1177/2378023119887866

Istat (2025). *Rapporto annuale 2025*. Roma

Italian Government. (2021) «*PNRR - Piano Nazionale di Ripresa e Resilienza. Presidency of the Council of Ministers.*» https://www.governo.it/sites/governo.it/files/PNRR.pdf

Ivan, L., & Nimrod, G. (2021). Family Conflicts and Technology Use: The Voices of Grandmothers. *Family Relations*, *70*(1), 104–119. DOI: 10.1111/fare.12530

Johansson, J. (2025). Research on digital discretion—The subjectification of street-level work in public administration. *The Review of Policy Research*, *42*(1), 122–148. DOI: 10.1111/ropr.12637

Jokisch, M. R., Schmidt, L. I., & Doh, M. (2022). Acceptance Of Digital Health Services Among Older Adults: Findings on Perceived Usefulness, Self-Efficacy, Privacy Concerns, ICT Knowledge, and Support Seeking. *Frontiers in Public Health*, *10*, 1073756. DOI: 10.3389/fpubh.2022.1073756 PMID: 36582385

Kaun, A., & Forsman, M. (2024). Digital Care Work at Public Libraries: Making Digital First Possible. *New Media & Society*, *26*(7), 3751–3766. DOI: 10.1177/14614448221104234

Korpela, V., Pajula, L., & Hänninen, R. (2023). Older Adults Learning Digital Skills Together: Peer Tutors' Perspectives on Non-Formal Digital Support. *Media and Communication*, *11*(3), 53–62. DOI: 10.17645/mac.v11i3.6742

Korpela, V., Pajula, L., & Hänninen, R. (2024). Investigating the multifaceted role of warm experts in enhancing and hindering older adults' digital skills in Finland. *International Journal of Lifelong Education*, *43*(5), 509–522. DOI: 10.1080/02601370.2024.2353176

Laukka, E., Lakoma, S., Harjumaa, M., Hiltunen, S., Härkönen, H., Jansson, M., Leskelä, R., Martikainen, S., Pennanen, P., Verho, A., & Torkki, P. (2024). Older Adults' Preferences in the Utilisation of Digital Health and Social Services: A Qualitative Analysis of Responses to Open-Ended Questions. *BMC Health Services Research*, *24*(1), 1184. DOI: 10.1186/s12913-024-11564-1 PMID: 39367429

Layne, K., & Lee, J. (2001). Developing Fully Functional E-Government: A Four Stage Model. *Government Information Quarterly*, *18*(2), 122–136. DOI: 10.1016/S0740-624X(01)00066-1

Leidner, R. (1999). Emotional labor in service work. *The Annals of the American Academy of Political and Social Science*, *561*(1), 81–95. DOI: 10.1177/000271629956100106

Li, Y. (2025). Vlogging as mediated mobility: Warm Experts 3.0 engaging in peer production and digital labor in the era of short videos. *International Journal of Cultural Studies*, *28*(3), 562–579. DOI: 10.1177/13678779241298707

Lipsky, M. (2010). *Street-Level Bureaucracy, 30th Anniversary Edition: Dilemmas of the Individual in Public Service*. Russell Sage Foundation.

Litchfield, I., Shukla, D., & Greenfield, S. (2021). Impact of COVID-19 on the digital divide: A rapid review. *BMJ Open*, *11*(10), e053440. DOI: 10.1136/bmjopen-2021-053440 PMID: 34642200

Loe, M. (2010). Doing It My Way: Old Women, Technology and Wellbeing. *Sociology of Health & Illness*, *32*(2), 319–334. DOI: 10.1111/j.1467-9566.2009.01220.x PMID: 20149150

Loos, E., Haddon, L., & Mante-Meijer, E. A. (Eds.). (2012). *Generational Use of New Media*. Ashgate.

Loos, E., & Ivan, L. (2024). Not Only People Are Getting Old, the New Media Are Too: Technology Generations and the Changes in New Media Use. *New Media & Society*, *26*(6), 3588–3613. DOI: 10.1177/14614448221101783

Loos, E. F. (2012). Senior Citizens: Digital Immigrants in their Own Country? *Observatorio (OBS*). Journal*, *6*, 1–23.

Martinez, C., & Olsson, T. (2022). The Warm Expert – A Warm Teacher? Learning about Digital Media in Intergenerational Interaction. *Convergence (London)*, *28*(6), 1861–1877. DOI: 10.1177/13548565211070409

Melis, G., Sala, E., & Zaccaria, D. (2021). Remote recruiting and video-interviewing older people: a research note on a qualitative case study carried out in the first Covid-19 Red Zone in Europe. *International Journal of Social Research Methodology, 25*(4), 477-482.

Melis, G., Sala, E., & Zaccaria, D. (2022). The Role of Information and Communication Technologies in Researching Older People During the Covid-19 Pandemic: The Case of the Italian Longitudinal Study on Older People's Quality of Life During the Covid-19 Pandemic (ILQA-19). In *International Conference on Human-Computer Interaction* (pp. 53-68). Cham: Springer International Publishing.

Miller, D. (1987). *Material Culture and Mass Consumption*. Blackwell.

Millward, P. (2003). The 'Grey Digital Divide': Perception, Exclusion and Barriers of Access to the Internet for Older People. *First Monday, 8*(7). Advance online publication. DOI: 10.5210/fm.v8i7.1066

Morris, A., & Brading, H. (2007). E-Literacy and the Grey Digital Divide: A Review with Recommendations. *Journal of Information Literacy, 1*(3), 1–13. DOI: 10.11645/1.3.14

Naldini, M., & Saraceno, C. (2022). Changes in the Italian Work-Family System and the Role of Social Policies in the Last Forty Years. *Stato e Mercato, 42*(1), 87–115.

Neale, B. (2020). *Qualitative Longitudinal Research: Research Methods*. Bloomsbury Publishing.

Nyanjom, J., & Naylor, D. (2021). Performing emotional labour while teaching online. *Educational Research, 63*(2), 147–163. DOI: 10.1080/00131881.2020.1836989

Novello, M., & Garavaglia, E. (2026). Ageing and technology in the policy discourse on public services digitalisation: a missed opportunity?. *Ageing & Society, 46*, e6.

Olsson, T., & Viscovi, D. (2023). Digitalised Welfare: Access, Usage, and Outcomes Among Older Adults. *Media and Communication, 11*(3), 18–28. DOI: 10.17645/mac.v11i3.6694

Peine, A., & Neven, L. (2019). From Intervention to Co-constitution: New Directions in Theorizing about Aging and Technology. *The Gerontologist, 59*(1), 15–21. DOI: 10.1093/geront/gny050 PMID: 29850812

Pope, N. D., Riley, J. E., Haberkorn, J., & Ely, G. E. (2016). Being "Easy": Women's Desire to Accept Help in Later Life. *Journal of Women & Aging, 28*(5), 352–362. DOI: 10.1080/08952841.2014.962863 PMID: 26933929

Ragnedda, M. (2018). Conceptualizing Digital Capital. *Telematics and Informatics, 35*(8), 2366–2375. DOI: 10.1016/j.tele.2018.10.006

Ragnedda, M., & Ruiu, M. L. (2017). Social Capital and the Three Levels of Digital Divide. In G., Muschert & M., Ragnedda (Eds.). *Theorizing Digital Divides* (pp. 21-34). Routledge. DOI: 10.4324/9781315455334-3

Sala, E., & Kochergina, E. (2025). Is E-Government an Opportunity for All? Identifying Barriers and Enablers of E-Government Use Among Older Adults in Europe. *Social Sciences & Humanities Open, 12*, 102158. DOI: 10.1016/j.ssaho.2025.102158

Saraceno, C., & Keck, W. (2010). Can we Identify Intergenerational Policy Regimes in Europe? *European Societies, 12*(5), 675–696. DOI: 10.1080/14616696.2010.483006

Schou, J., & Pors, A. S. (2019). Digital by Default? A Qualitative Study of Exclusion in Digitalised Welfare. *Social Policy and Administration, 53*(3), 464–477. DOI: 10.1111/spol.12470

Schreurs, K., Quan-Haase, A., & Martin, K. (2017). Problematizing the Digital Literacy Paradox in the Context of Older Adults' ICT Use: Aging, Media Discourse, and Self-Determination. *Canadian Journal of Communication, 42*(2), 359–377. DOI: 10.22230/cjc.2017v42n2a3130

Signorelli, S., Torrecillas Jodar, J., Papazoglou, M., & López Cobo, M. (2024). *Mapping EU Level Funding Instruments 2021-2027 to Digital Decade Targets.* European Commission, Joint Research Centre. Publication Office of the European Union. https://data.europa.eu/doi/10.2760/45054

Silverstone, R., & Hirsch, E. (Eds.). (1992). *Consuming Technologies: Media and Information in Domestic Spaces*. Routledge.

Sourbati, M. (2009). 'It Could be Useful, but not for me at the Moment': Older People, Internet Access and E-Public Service Provision. *New Media & Society, 11*(7), 1083–1100. DOI: 10.1177/1461444809340786

Sourbati, M. (2015). Age(ism) in Digital Information Provision: The Case of Online Public Services for Older Adults. In Zhou, J., & Salvendy, G. (Eds.), *Human Aspects of IT for the Aged Population. Design for Aging* (pp. 376–386). Springer International Publishing., DOI: 10.1007/978-3-319-20892-3_37

Taipale, S. (2019). *Intergenerational Connections in Digital Families*. Springer International Publishing. DOI: 10.1007/978-3-030-11947-8

Taipale, S., Wilska, T. A., & Gilleard, C. J. (Eds.). (2017). *Digital Technologies and Generational Identity*. Routledge. DOI: 10.4324/9781315398624

Tirado-Morueta, R., Rodríguez-Martín, A., Álvarez-Arregui, E., Ortíz-Sobrino, M. Á., & Aguaded-Gómez, J. I. (2023). The Digital Inclusion of Older People in Spain: Technological Support Services for Seniors as Predictor. *Ageing and Society*, *43*(6), 1409–1435. DOI: 10.1017/S0144686X21001173

Virkki, T. (2007). Emotional capital in caring work. In Charmine E.J. Härtel, Neal M. Ashkanasy, & Wilfred J. Zerbe (editors), *Research on Emotionin Organizations. Volume 3: Functionality, intentionality and morality*. Emerald Group Publishing Limited. Pp. 265-285. https://doi.org/DOI: 10.1016/S1746-9791(2007)3

Warnes, A. M. (1993). Being Old, Old People and the Burdens of Burden. *Ageing and Society*, *13*(3), 297–338. DOI: 10.1017/S0144686X00001069

Wharton, A. S. (2009). The sociology of emotional labor. *Annual Review of Sociology*, *35*(1), 147–165. DOI: 10.1146/annurev-soc-070308-115944

Wu, X., & Chen, S. (2026). From "Warm Expert" to "Warm Steward": Digital Backfeeding as Everyday Intergenerational GenAI Learning in Chinese Families. *International Journal of Human-Computer Interaction*, •••, 1–28. DOI: 10.1080/10447318.2026.2668041

Yates, S. J., Kirby, J., & Lockley, E. (2015). 'Digital-by-Default': Reinforcing Exclusion Through Technology. *Defence of welfare, 2*, 158-161.

KEY TERMS AND DEFINITIONS

Digital Care Workers: a figure of street-level bureaucrat performing a form of emotional and practical labour, beyond their formal duties, providing personalised digital assistance (Kaun & Forsman, 2024)

Digital-by-Default: a social system wherein public services are provided through digital means, without an on-site alternative (Schou & Pors, 2019; Yates et al., 2015)

Familism-by-Default: a social system that is heavily dependent on the support provided by family members (Saraceno & Keck, 2010)

Generational Media Practices: a theoretical approach that explores the shared practices of media use and how these meanings are socially constructed as part of a generational identity (Haddon & Mante-Meijer, 2016; Loos et al., 2012; Loos & Ivan, 2024; Taipale et al., 2017)

Grey Digital Divide: drawing from the broader concept of 'digital divide', which addresses the social exclusion due to the inability to engage with digital technologies due to lack of access, attitudes, support, etc. (see, among others, van Dijk, 2005; Hargittai, 2003; Ragnedda & Muschert, 2013), the 'grey digital divide' is focused on the digital divide that specifically impacts older generations (Millward, 2003; Morris, 2007; Friemel, 2016)

TSSS: Technological Support Services for Seniors, community-based initiatives driven by public institutions aimed at ensuring older adults' material access to the internet and providing digital literacy support (Tirado-Morueta et al., 2023)

Warm Experts: a figure who blends technical guidance with emotional support, contextual adaptation, and interpersonal trust in providing digital support (Bakardjieva, 2005; Hänninen et al., 2021; Korpela et al., 2024)

Chapter 10
The Challenges of Digital Transformation in Rethinking Welfare:
Innovative Strategies for Preventing and Combating Gender-Based Violence

Daniele Battista
http://orcid.org/0009-0005-8418-8374
University of Salerno, Italy

Emiliana Mangone
http://orcid.org/0000-0002-9958-4346
University of Salerno, Italy

Giuseppe Masullo
http://orcid.org/0000-0003-0818-6981
University of Salerno, Italy

ABSTRACT

The prevention and fight against gender-based violence represents a privileged area for questioning the welfare system and identifying innovative strategies capable of responding to emerging needs, also considering the digitalization of society, which has shifted some of these forms of violence from physical (offline) environments to digital (online) environments, primarily involving women and members of the LGBTQIA+ community as victims. This chapter therefore aims, on the one hand, to frame the issue of preventing and combating gender-based violence to rethink – from an integrated digital perspective – the contemporary welfare system, while

DOI: 10.4018/979-8-2600-3043-1.ch010

also addressing the ambivalent nature of technologies, which can strengthen the protection of victims but also create new risks if not adequately designed and contextualized. On the other hand, it also emphasizes the need for an integrated approach that combines technological innovation, social justice, and the protection of fundamental rights.

INTRODUCTION

The series of crises of recent decades has demonstrated that vulnerability is increasing due to multiple sociocultural and natural transformations, the latest example being the pandemic caused by the spread of the SARS-CoV-2 virus, which has been experienced globally. This changing context has created the need for a new welfare governance framework that can provide social responses to citizens' real needs and, above all, combine resources and quality. This is especially true given that the expansion of rights is accompanied by a declining capacity for public funding, shifting the focus from ensuring well-being to the problem of cost containment. The future challenge lies in the qualification of spending, which must address the tripolar structure of choice (need, preferences, goods), thus transcending the rational choice model (preferences, goods). However, it is essential to reconcile the scarcity of resources with the interests of improving citizens' living conditions. This leads—as a basic prerequisite for revitalizing welfare policy planning—to the attempt to build strong partnerships that serve as a point of intersection between formal structures (institutions) and illegitimate informal ones (all other organized social actors). This allows for the implementation of integrated interventions and services that don't only act when harmful or undesirable events have already occurred or spread, but that have a preventative function (Demurtas & Mangone, 2025; Mangone, 2016). This approach typically follows two paths: on the one hand, it coincides with the attempt to avoid moments of difficulty without the slightest concern for transforming situations (the state of well-being, once achieved, must remain unchanged), but such a situation is poorly reconciled with the mutability of human existence; on the other hand, it considers the possibility of recovering elements that moments of difficulty bring with them, attempting to redirect them in a positive direction. Choosing between these two dimensions (avoiding the crisis and redirecting it) is certainly not a simple or automatic task. Rather, this ambiguity represents the crux of the matter, where integrated interventions, including promotion and education, can be introduced to mobilize positive resources and prevent the difficult moment from becoming chronic.

The prevention and fight against gender-based violence represents a privileged framework for questioning the welfare system and identifying innovative strategies capable of responding to emerging needs (Strid et al., 2021), also considering the digitalization of society. Starting from this premise, we intend to emphasize the need to "refocus" the discussion on the network perspective within interventions to prevent and combat various forms of "sexist and sexual" violence. Moreover, top-down intervention measures prove ineffective without grassroots citizen engagement. This engagement is not only linked to the ability of community networks to support victims of violence and discrimination originating in local communities, but also to contribute to the spread of a broader and more shared culture of equal opportunities and the fight against violence and discrimination. Furthermore, it is necessary to consider the changes in communication systems that have caused some of these forms of violence to migrate from physical (offline) environments to digital (online) environments, primarily involving women and members of the LGBTQIA+ community as victims, but without reducing the negative effects (Donato, Eslen-Ziya & Mangone, 2022). Although gender-based violence refers to multiple categories of victims, data shows that it is predominantly women (see Demurtas & Mangone, 2025) who are most exposed.

Recent literature highlights how online gender-based violence is not a homogeneous phenomenon, but rather a set of differentiated practices that vary based on social contexts and levels of public exposure. Data from the European Union Agency for Fundamental Rights (2026), for example, show how women active in public spaces are subjected to more intense and systematic forms of abuse, especially during times of heightened media visibility. At the same time, the multifaceted nature of cyber violence is highlighted here, combining threats, harassment, and non-consensual dissemination of content, making it a cumulative rather than episodic process.

This applies even to those women who, by common sense, are not perceived as vulnerable. It also affects all female figures engaged in the public sphere, regardless of their level of experience and notoriety. A case in point is the one involving several British female MPs who were frequently exposed to a complex set of digital harassment, ranging from microaggressions and sexist comments to intimidating or threatening messages, with significant psychological, professional, and social impacts. This emerges as a structural issue, in which online violence intersects with gender, ethnicity, and public visibility, representing not only a dispute over individual protection but also a central issue for the quality of democracy, political representation, and equal access to public life. Specifically, Southern and Harmer (2021), analysing messages addressed to Members of Parliament on X (Twitter at the time), found that women are more likely to receive uncivilized tweets, containing stereotypes, or questioning their political legitimacy, as well as being the target of attacks that describe them as "unqualified" or unwanted in the public sphere. This hostile climate is particularly salient as the use of social media has now become an integral part of political work, exposing representatives to stigmatizing communications with a high frequency. Further empirical evidence confirms that online violence against women engaged in politics is not an episodic phenomenon, but rather a clear and recurrent structural dynamic that tends to target selectively specific categories of individuals, particularly those situated at the intersection of gender, ethnic background, and public visibility. From this perspective, the report by Amnesty International (2022) highlights that women parliamentarians receive a significantly disproportionate amount of abusive content compared with their male counterparts, and that such exposure increases further in the case of representatives belonging to ethnic minorities. In particular, the analysis of approximately one million tweets directed at 177 British women MPs between January and June 2017 showed that 20 Black, Asian, and minority ethnic parliamentarians accounted for 41% of all abusive messages recorded, despite representing a numerically much smaller share than their white colleagues[1].

More generally, exposure to intimidation and threats more frequent online than during campaigning contributes to structural barriers to women's participation. While these studies do not always demonstrate a direct causal link between individual incidents of abuse and abandonment of office, the body of evidence suggests that cyberviolence represents a democratic problem, as it can limit women's freedom of expression, personal safety, and full participation in political life.

This scenario highlights the inherent complexity of violent phenomena, which therefore prompts us to consider and analyze the determinants that lead to the necessary implementation of a coordinated system of interventions that integrates different policies and local services, as well as digital technologies. This is aimed at preventing and combating violence, protecting and supporting victims on their journey to empowerment, and holding perpetrators accountable.

In light of the above, this chapter aims to frame the issue of preventing and combating gender-based violence as a strategic framework for rethinking—from an integrated digital perspective—the contemporary welfare system. Digital technologies are not intended as stand-alone solutions, but rather as enabling infrastructures capable of expanding access to services, strengthening local networks, and facilitating safe and timely contact between victims and support systems. From this perspective, digital welfare plays a central role in enhancing interventions, provided that technological tools are integrated into a multilevel governance system based on collaboration between public institutions, local services, the third sector, and local communities. The effectiveness of digital solutions depends on their integration with local social services, continuity of support, and attention to crucial elements such as usability, security, and privacy protection. Prevention is therefore understood as a dynamic process, in which digital welfare can contribute to the early identification of situations of vulnerability and support empowerment, preventing violence from becoming structural. At the same time, the chapter highlights the ambivalent nature of technologies, which can strengthen victim protection but also create new risks if not adequately designed and contextualized.

In conclusion, the chapter offers a critical reflection on digital welfare as a lever for more inclusive and effective policies in the fight against gender-based violence, emphasizing the need for an integrated approach that combines technological innovation, social justice, and the protection of fundamental rights. To achieve this goal, the chapter's structure begins with a first section that frames the issue of preventing and combating gender-based violence, aiming to rethink the contemporary welfare system from an integrated digital perspective. It then addresses the ambivalent nature of technologies, which can strengthen victim protection but also create new risks. Finally, it reflects on the need for an integrated approach that combines technological innovation, social justice, and the protection of fundamental rights.

GENDER-BASED VIOLENCE ONLIFE: AN INTRODUCTORY FRAMEWORK

Gender-based violence is one of the most complex and persistent challenges for contemporary welfare systems, representing both a serious violation of human rights and a significant public health problem that must be addressed.

The term Gender-Based Violence (GBV) – used as a sort of "umbrella" term – includes all forms of gender-based violence, both online and offline (physical, sexual, psychological, economic, sexual harassment, gender-based harassment, and environmental harassment). Therefore, this concept describes a continuum of violence, violations, behaviours, and abuses based on sex and gender (Hearn et al., 2022; Strid et al. 2021). This approach stems from the 1995 United Nations Beijing Conference and highlights the need to examine gender violence as a phenomenon not limited to women alone, but involving all categories of people (including transgender and/or non-binary people, etc.) who are oppressed and excluded because of their gender identity and expression, and because of a non-heteronormative sexual orientation. The GBV approach, on the one hand, highlights the devastating effects of oppressive patriarchal practices; on the other, it opposes the theory of the naturalness of normative heterosexuality and the male-female binary that underlies violence against women. These dichotomous logics, which homogenize differences within the male/female binary and, therefore, victim/perpetrator, are challenged precisely because they fail to recognize the heterogeneity of practices, models, and representations of gender violence and the variety of meanings in historically constructed contexts of domination. Broadening our focus to include categories considered "outside the norm" more forcefully underscores the socially constructed nature of gender, the outcome of processes that can be traced back minimally to nature and mostly to processes of sociality. These processes, while reproducing the gender order, simultaneously engage with novel processes of subjectivation that challenge it.

Factors such as age, disability, migration background (Mangone et al., 2018), sexual orientation, and socioeconomic status give rise to different forms of violence and generate specific conditions of vulnerability, which require targeted and diversified interventions. From this awareness emerges the need to adopt an intersectional perspective, capable of grasping how experiences of violence develop at the convergence of multiple systems of oppression and consequently require policies capable of interpreting and addressing this complexity (Demurtas & Mangone, 2025). As Jennifer C. Nash writes, intersectionality is "analytic that asks how we might reconceptualize discrimination, harm, violence, and power around the experiences of the multiply rather than the singly marginalized" (Nash, 2021, p. 129).

Gender-based violence is a frequent and global phenomenon. According to the World Health Organization (WHO, 2025), an estimated 840 million women globally (of whom 682 million have experienced it from an intimate partner) – approximately 30% of women aged 15 and over – have experienced physical and/or sexual violence from an intimate partner, sexual violence from a person other than their partner, or both at least once in their lifetime. Rates of depression, anxiety, unwanted pregnancies, sexually transmitted infections, HIV, and other long-term health problems are higher among women who have experienced violence than among women who have not. Most violence against women is committed by husbands or current or former partners.

In recent decades, sociology has devoted considerable attention to the topic of violence, which for many years was relegated to the exclusive realms of law and criminology. The Enlightenment illusion of a modern society dominated by reason has led to a delay in sociologists' exploration of this concept and, consequently, of many of its fields of research, which for years have focused specifically on acts of physical harm – a "limited" concept of violence, neglecting the "broader" concept that refers to conceptual analogies such as structural violence or symbolic violence, not to mention concepts of non-physical forms of violence such as discrimination and racism, exploitation, or social exclusion (Fornari & Masullo, 2023). Broadening the spectrum of phenomena covered by the term violence through a micro and macro definition, including situations of self-directed, interpersonal, and finally institutional violence, has allowed sociology to highlight, even for gender-based violence, that it is not simply a tool for resolving conflicts of an identity, political, or ideological nature, but can be conceived as a social force in itself, whose counteraction requires the use of complex, diversified approaches that call for multidimensional prevention analysis strategies.

Violence against women is, in fact, one of the issues in which government institutions are currently investing significant resources, both in terms of research and prevention services and policies. This interest in the phenomenon is further strengthened by the exponential increase in cases of male violence against women, of which femicide is just the tip of a complex iceberg, which includes crimes such as domestic violence, psychological violence, economic violence, and, finally, new categories that include crimes such as stalking.

Since the 1970s, feminist and gay liberation movements have played a decisive role in exposing the structural nature of patriarchal violence, highlighting its roots in systemic inequalities and pervasive power dynamics. These movements have challenged the social and cultural institutions that legitimize male domination, while also denouncing the shortcomings of public policies in effectively recognizing and combating these forms of oppression. In a historical period characterized by limited capacity for intervention by state institutions, feminist movements have provided concrete responses to women survivors of male violence through the creation of safe spaces and specialized services. These services, in some national contexts, have been distinguished by the primacy of the political dimension over a professionalizing approach and by the centrality attributed to female desire, self-determination, and planning (Corradi & Stöckl, 2016). These experiences have highlighted the urgent need for a welfare system capable of addressing the structural roots of gender-based violence, promoting a broader reflection on the role of public policies in transforming the social conditions that enable it. Given this framework, it is necessary to question the concrete ways in which anti-violence policies and interventions are embedded within welfare systems. It is at the meso and micro levels that the real effects of integrated strategies for preventing and combating violence are observed, measuring the system's effective capacity to ensure the safety of survivors and their pathways to escape violence (Demurtas & Mangone, 2025).

From this perspective, preventing and combating gender-based violence is a complex social process that cannot be limited to strengthening individual skills and abilities, but must include interventions aimed at modifying the social, environmental, and economic conditions that impact the well-being and health of individuals and communities. Consistent with this approach, the WHO has recognized gender-based violence as a serious public health problem, developing a framework for the prevention of violence against women based on the United Nations Framework for Action (UN Women, 2015) and subsequently updated considering new empirical evidence (UN Women, 2020; WHO, 2019). This model identifies seven key strategies – including strengthening interpersonal skills, empowering women, ensuring accessible services, and transforming attitudes, beliefs, and social norms – emphasizing the need for multilevel and integrated interventions.

The recognition of gender-based violence as a structural phenomenon and a violation of fundamental rights was further strengthened in Europe by the ratification of the 2011 Istanbul Convention, which represented a turning point for regulatory development and policy planning aimed at preventing violence, protecting victims, and holding perpetrators accountable. However, despite regulatory progress, significant challenges remain in implementing anti-violence policies, as evidenced by difficulties in funding anti-violence centers and shelters, differences in the operational practices of specialized and generalist services, and the weak integration between anti-violence measures and sectoral policies aimed at supporting the economic, employment, and housing independence of women survivors of violence (Masullo & Picarella, 2025). These challenges have emerged particularly clearly during the COVID-19 pandemic, which has exacerbated women's vulnerability and, at the same time, prompted the introduction of innovative practices, including programs dedicated to the rehabilitation and accountability of perpetrators.

At the same time, the increasing digitalization of society has transformed the ways in which gender-based violence manifests itself, making the continuity between offline and online environments increasingly evident. In recent years, the implosion of new communication technologies in our lives has created new representations of violence, new typologies or allowing older forms of violence to gain greater visibility.

Forms of "*Technology-Facilitated Gender-based violence*" (Chalovska Dimovska, 2024) such as cyberstalking and the non-consensual dissemination of sexually explicit images become embedded within pre-existing violent relationships, amplifying their effects and prolonging their impact over time (Donato, Eslen-Ziya & Mangone, 2022). These phenomena disproportionately affect young women and members of the LGBTQIA+ community, intensifying existing vulnerabilities and generating new challenges for welfare systems (EIGE, 2018; FRA, 2020). This scenario has favoured the emergence of an "onlife" perspective (Floridi, 2015) on gender-based violence, which has also been progressively recognized at the European regulatory level, as demonstrated by Directive (EU) 2024/1385 on combating violence against women and domestic violence.

From the first half of the 20th century to the present, society has experienced a significant acceleration of transformation processes, closely linked to technological development. Technical progress has fostered the transition from a traditional industrial society to a post-industrial one, profoundly redefining social, economic, and cultural structures. The most recent innovations, attributable to computerization, the spread of the internet, robotics, and artificial intelligence, mark the advent of the fourth and fifth industrial revolutions (Addeo & Masullo, 2021). Technological change, however, is not considered a neutral factor, but rather a process capable of impacting social relations and forms of power organization. Post-industrial society is generally described as being founded on the centrality of knowledge, the use of intelligent technologies, and the valorisation of creativity. These transformations produce ambivalent effects: alongside new opportunities for participation and communication, practices of exclusion, control, and violence emerge, disproportionately affecting socially marginalized groups, including women, minors, and LGBTQIA+ people.

Within the framework of gender studies, the relationship between digital technologies and gender-based violence (GBV) can be analyzed on two interconnected levels: the "interpersonal level" concerns the dynamics of violence that manifest within intimate and everyday relationships – with partners, family, friends, peers, and colleagues. The "structural level", on the other hand, concerns relationships with social institutions and state infrastructures, highlighting how violence is rooted in social structures themselves. From this perspective, power asymmetries translate into systemic inequalities that limit access to resources and life opportunities (Jurėnienė, 2026). GBV perpetrated at the individual level cannot therefore be interpreted as an isolated phenomenon, as it reflects and reinforces broader structural patterns, such as sexism and racism. Since the beginning of the 21st century, these dynamics have spurred the development of policies and regulatory instruments at the international and national levels, promoted by organizations such as UNESCO, the European Commission, and the European Parliament, with the aim of preventing gender-based violence, particularly against children.

In recent years, institutional and academic attention has further expanded to include, alongside traditional forms of physical, psychological, emotional, and economic violence, manifestations of technological violence. Legislative and social responses today largely focus on digital environments, recognized as spaces where existing power relations are reproduced and amplified. Social networking platforms, instant messaging services, online discussion sites, forums, dating apps, and digital gaming environments represent, in this sense, central contexts for the sociological and gender analysis of abuse and violence.

From a sociological and gender perspective, technology is therefore an intrinsically ambivalent field. While on the one hand, it has expanded and reorganized the ways in which gender-based violence can manifest and spread, on the other, it offers potentially effective tools to combat it. The same digital infrastructures that can reproduce power asymmetries can be reoriented in an emancipatory manner, assuming an active role in prevention, protection, and support processes (Battista & Coppola, 2025). It is within this tension that the use of digital technologies as a resource for welfare and anti-violence policies is located. Moreover, precisely within this context of sociocultural transformation, the use of a virtual framework fits as an innovative strategic resource. Digital tools, in fact, allow for expanded access to support services, promoting more timely, flexible, and personalized forms of assistance, in line with the digitalization processes of contemporary social protection systems (Mazzucato, 2021). On the other hand, technological systems contribute to the development of prevention and awareness-raising practices through online campaigns, information platforms, and anonymous reporting systems that reduce barriers to access for victims, often linked to social isolation or fear of retaliation. However, this process is not without its ambivalence, as while it can strengthen the empowerment of those involved, it also risks reproducing structural inequalities linked to the digital divide, technological surveillance, and potential exposure to new forms of online control and abuse (van Dijk, 2020). In this sense, integrating technologies into anti-violence policies requires a critical and multidimensional approach, capable of combining technological innovation, protection of rights, and the centrality of the relational and territorial dimensions of social intervention. In this diverse landscape, therefore, digital technologies assume a strategic role as enabling welfare infrastructures, capable of expanding access to services, strengthening local support networks, and promoting the early emergence of situations of vulnerability. Dedicated applications, digital platforms, and secure communication tools can help lower the barrier to accessing help by offering rapid, discreet, and potentially anonymous ways to contact anti-violence centers and social services (Epiphanio & Oms, 2025). These tools are particularly relevant from a preventative perspective, as they can support and empowerment programs and strengthen the welfare system's ability to intervene before violence becomes chronic.

Integrating digital technologies into strategies to prevent and combat gender-based violence, however, requires a critical approach that is aware of the ambivalences associated with their use. The digital divide, understood both as inequality in access to technology and differences in digital skills, can exclude the most vulnerable women and limit the effectiveness of digital tools (Amato, 2025). Women's lower investment in STEM education, and their consequent lower familiarity with new technologies, are among the factors explaining why women use the internet and digital applications less than men. Globally, according to the International Telecommunication Union (ITC), "The digital gender gap continues expanding in many developing countries, creating a specific need to support digital gender equality. Globally, in 2022, 62% of men are using the Internet, compared with 57% of women. Only 19% of women in Least Developed Countries (LDCs) used the Internet in 2020, compared to 86 percent in developed world (in 2019)" (ITC, 2023), despite the pandemic having forced women to engage more with new communication technologies.

Likewise, issues related to personal data protection, communications security, and the ethical design of technological tools take on central importance to prevent processes of re-victimization or new forms of control by perpetrators of violence.

This necessitates multilevel governance based on collaboration between public institutions, local services, the third sector, and local communities. Preventing and combating gender-based violence therefore represents a strategic area for rethinking welfare from an integrated digital perspective, consistent with the principles established by the Istanbul Convention (2011) and the most recent European policies. Digital welfare, if embedded in solid local networks and geared toward the protection of fundamental rights, can contribute to strengthening the system's preventive capacity and promoting more inclusive and effective interventions, addressing gender-based violence as a structural phenomenon that continually affects the physical and digital spaces of social experience.

DIGITAL VIOLENCE AND GENDER INEQUALITIES IN SOCIO-TECHNICAL ECOSYSTEMS

The massive proliferation of digital infrastructures has significantly revamped modes of social interaction, giving rise to unusual relational configurations that combine the technological and cultural dimensions. Following this perspective, the analysis of *affordances* – understood as the set of action possibilities offered by digital environments – has emerged as a central theoretical direction for grasping the dynamics of online hostility. These various affordances cannot be labelled neutral but should be conceived as sociotechnical systems that mediate relationships between individuals and can, sometimes unintentionally, facilitate harmful behaviours such as threats and verbal aggression. Moreover, the increase in exchanges via *social apps* is accompanied by a rise in digital violence, underscoring the need to perceive these environments as segments capable of triggering certain social behaviours. This connotation highlights the "double-faced" nature of technology in combating this emergency. While, in some ways, helping apps provide a direct channel between victims and potential law enforcement and support agencies, at the same time, these same apps could provide perpetrators with additional tools to perpetrate forms of violence and social oppression, exacerbating the digital and social control of victims (Cardoso et al. 2019). Apps dedicated to victim assistance perform a liberating function, facilitating access to support services, reporting of risk situations, and initial contact with social safety nets. However, there are emerging patterns of re-articulation of the forms of control exercised by perpetrators within digital ecosystems. But this issue cannot be the exclusive prerogative of individual deviations; rather, it must be viewed as the outcome of a complex interface between technological architecture, social norms, and power relations. Platforms formally aspire to guarantee safe and equitable participatory experiences, a landscape that fits within a broader and more robust socio-technical framework involving the joint analysis of technological infrastructures (algorithms, platforms, moderation systems) and social dynamics (cultural norms, structural inequalities, social capital). This makes it possible to understand how vulnerabilities are not evenly distributed, but rather stratified. Indeed, global research shows that women continue to experience a wide range of online harassment, including insults, cyberstalking, threats, defamatory campaigns, and the non-consensual dissemination of intimate images. Far from constituting a neutral space of participation, the digital ecosystem reproduces many of the gender inequalities already present in the offline sphere, often amplifying them through anonymity, the rapid circulation of content, and the limited accountability of perpetrators. International estimates confirm the structural dimension of the phenomenon. According to UN Women, between 16% and 58% of women worldwide report having experienced forms of online violence or harassment, depending on national contexts, research methodologies, and the specific forms of abuse considered. A global survey cited by the United Nations further found that 38% of women had directly experienced episodes of digital violence, while 85% stated that they had witnessed such abuse or knew other women who had been victims of it. Among the most recurrent forms of abuse are sexist insults, threats of physical and sexual violence, coercive surveillance through digital tools, and the unauthorized dissemination of intimate material. The latter practice, increasingly facilitated by generative artificial intelligence, represents one of the most invasive manifestations of online gender-based violence. According to recent data, between 90% and 95% of deepfakes currently circulating online contain non-consensual pornographic content, and approximately 90% of those depicted are women. The consequences do not remain confined to the virtual sphere. Numerous studies show that online violence produces concrete effects on women's psychological well-being, freedom of expression, and public participation. Anxiety, fear, hypervigilance, stress, withdrawal from social media, and self-censorship are among the most frequently documented outcomes. In a recent study conducted in the United Kingdom, only 24% of women interviewed reported feeling comfortable expressing political opinions online, compared with around 40% of men, suggesting that perceptions of digital risk may translate into a reduction of women's public voice. The phenomenon becomes even more critical when it targets women journalists, activists, academics, or political figures. UN Women reports that one in four women journalists has received online threats of physical violence, including death threats, while many professionals state that they have reduced their public exposure or altered their working routines for safety reasons. Overall, these findings suggest that digital violence against women should not be interpreted merely as a form of communicative deviance, but rather as a mechanism of symbolic and material exclusion that restricts full and equal access to online public spaces. In this sense, digital harassment today represents one of the most significant ways through which relations of power and gender hierarchies are being reconfigured within technological environments.

This discrepancy between the ideal of inclusiveness and the reality of lived experiences suggests that online constructions can reproduce – and sometimes increase – inequalities already entrenched offline (Sauerborn et al. 2022). Among the potential for action most frequently associated with this manifestation, anonymity certainly plays a central role, since the possibility of concealing or manipulating one's, identity reduces the perception of personal responsibility, attenuates mechanisms of social control, and even creates conditions favourable to behavioural disinhibition (Woodlock, 2016). This logic contributes to the normalization of aggressive language and persecutory practices, making the digital environment a highly fertile ground for the expression of hostility that would otherwise be difficult to emerge in face-to-face contexts. At the same time, the scalability of platforms – i.e., the ability to simultaneously reach very large audiences – amplifies the scope of attacks, transforming isolated incidents into collective experiences of symbolic violence (Recuero, 2024). Undoubtedly, the impact of these dynamics is particularly evident when adopting a gender perspective. Empirical evidence indicates that, although men and women may be exposed to harmful content to a similar extent, women are more frequently targeted by misogyny, cyberstalking, and other forms of abuse, as well as reporting a more significant psychological impact (Duncombe, 2020). An international study (Amnesty International, 2017) based on an online survey of approximately 4,000 women (aged 18-55) in eight countries (Denmark, Italy, New Zealand, Poland, Spain, Sweden, the United Kingdom, and the United States) found that 23% of respondents reported having experienced online harassment or threats at least once. Percentages vary significantly at the national level, ranging from 16% in Italy to 33% in the United States, and among those who have experienced these episodes, almost half perceived them as motivated by misogyny or sexism, while over a quarter reported threats of physical or sexual aggression. More than half of the harassment was attributed to strangers, confirming how social distance and the anonymity of digital spaces can encourage this type of behaviour. Wider data collected by international agencies undeniably attest to the global diffusion of the phenomenon; in fact, according to the UN Women knowledge portal on tech-facilitated violence (2025), between 16% and 58% of women and girls have experienced some form of cyber violence based on the geographic region considered; for example, in European Member States and OECD countries, approximately 23% of adult women reported incidents of online abuse or harassment at least once.

At the European level, the most recent report by *Women Against Violence Europe* notes that cyberstalking, digital surveillance, and the use of spyware are among the forms of cyberviolence most reported by women and girls, and that several countries have observed an increase in image-based abuse and the non-consensual sharing of intimate content (Trindade Pereira & Zaba, 2026). In Greece, for example, women represent over 69% of victims in cyberstalking cases. In the US context, however, an analysis by the *Pew Research Center* (2021) reveals that approximately 41% of adults online have experienced at least one form of online harassment, with a significant share of cases classified as more severe (physical threats, stalking, or sexual harassment). Furthermore, women, and especially young women, are more likely than other demographic groups to report sexual harassment or stalking than men. These diverse sources converge in highlighting not only the pervasiveness of digital harassment globally, but also the methodological and terminological difficulties in measuring it. They also confirm a strong gender component in experiences of online abuse, with women tending to experience both more diverse behaviours and more negative psychological impacts than men. However, the consequences of these experiences extend far beyond the virtual sphere, appearing as events capable of structurally impacting the biographical trajectories of victims. The scientific literature within the field of gender-based online violence studies highlight how repeated exposure to online harassment and threats is associated with symptoms of anxiety, depression, hypervigilance, and post-traumatic stress, as well as forms of social isolation and progressive self-exclusion from digital public spaces. This line of research is more broadly situated within studies on cybervictimization and the psychosocial effects of hostile communication mediated by online platforms, which have shown that the continuity and pervasiveness of online aggression amplify its emotional impact compared to traditional forms of offline harassment (Hinduja & Patchin, 2010). Notably, it has also been demonstrated that prolonged exposure to cyberharassment behaviours is strongly correlated with increased levels of psychological distress and a reduction in perceived well-being, particularly among individuals who are highly publicly exposed (Abarna et al., 2022). A sort of cumulative effect of negative online interactions comes into play, capable of generating avoidance strategies toward digital platforms and a decline in social and political participation, thereby contributing to forms of self-exclusion from the digital public sphere.

These flows produce a "silencing" effect, that is, a reduction in discursive and political participation, with direct implications for the quality of the public sphere and gender representation. Furthermore, as we will see, the persistence and replicability of digital content exacerbates reputational damage and the perception of vulnerability, making the experience of abuse potentially ongoing over time. From this perspective, online violence emerges as a continuum between online and offline, as its psychological, social, and economic repercussions materialize in the daily lives of those affected (Henry & Powell, 2018). Digital violence, therefore, is increasingly recognized as real violence, capable of producing tangible psychological, social, and economic effects. Cyberstalking, revenge porn, pornographic deepfakes, and sextortion represent just some of the manifestations of a situation that is not confined but can reverberate in the daily lives of victims, inducing fear, isolation, and reputational damage (Bjelajac & Filipović, 2021). The current scenario therefore allows us to move beyond reductive interpretations of online violence as simply the result of deviant behaviour. The structural characteristics of platforms—including content persistence, visibility, and ease of aggregation—can transform a single hostile act into a coordinated campaign, multiplying the potential for harm. Along this path, digital hostility appears closely intertwined with the logic of the attention economy, which rewards polarizing and conflictual content, contributing to the normalization of incivility (Ross et al., 2021). As reiterated, at present, it must be considered that online violence lies on a continuum with offline violence. Digital aggression not only reflects pre-existing social hierarchies, but can also reinforce them, consolidating forms of symbolic exclusion that limit the presence of women in public spaces—be they physical or virtual. If much of contemporary political and cultural debate now takes place on platforms, self-exclusion driven by the fear of attack risks translating into a new form of democratic inequality.

In light of these considerations, it is clear that understanding cyber violence requires a multidimensional approach, capable of integrating diverse perspectives. Addressing individual behaviours alone is not enough; it is necessary to rethink platform architectures, strengthen moderation policies, and promote gender-sensitive design models. Only through a sociotechnical understanding of the phenomenon will it be possible to envision truly inclusive digital environments, where participation is not hindered by the fear of hostility. Ultimately, online attacks against women represent not only a problem of individual safety, but also a question of social justice and the quality of the digital public sphere. Ensuring respectful spaces for interaction means protecting the right to freedom of expression, visibility, and citizenship – essential elements for an increasingly interconnected society.

Digital Platforms: Risks and New Support Strategies

The rapid emergence of digital platforms in public debate has made it essential to analyse their structural characteristics to understand the propagation of hostile conduct in online space. As already explained, one of the most frequently analysed elements in relation to the phenomenon under examination is undoubtedly anonymity. It represents a key factor both in shaping the dynamics of digital hostility and in the dynamics of requests for support and reporting, since the possibility of concealing or manipulating one's identity, while attenuating the mechanisms of individual accountability, also reduces the pressure of social control for victims. Anonymity, however, should not be interpreted as one of the predominant affordances that, interacting with social norms, platform cultures, and group dynamics, contributes to creating favourable conditions for the expression of hostility and, at the same time, for reporting. Moreover, the possibility of registering anonymous or pseudonymous accounts, particularly popular on X (formerly Twitter), is frequently used. Anonymity reduces social accountability mechanisms, alleviates the fear of reputational sanctions, and can foster processes of disinhibition, through which users feel legitimized to express content that they would be unlikely to share in offline contexts or in digital environments characterized by greater identifiability (Santana, 2014). It is no coincidence that Rowe (2015) has long revealed how the open and public nature of the platform favours the visibility of aggressive comments, while Kornikoff (2021) has emphasized how moderation policies and terms of service can sometimes prove insufficient in preventing the spread of hate content. From what can be gathered, it seems reasonable to conclude that X has the highest incidence of incivility and abuse compared to other social media platforms. On the other hand, Facebook and Instagram have different communication architectures that shape interaction mechanisms. Facebook generally requires the use of real identities, increasing users' identifiability and encouraging more rational and less hostile discussions (Jaidka, 2022), given the lack of a rigid character limit. Furthermore, its network structure, based primarily on friendships or relatively defined communities, tends to confine discussions within more homogeneous social groups. Instagram, while sharing a certain emphasis on personal identity with Facebook, stands out for the centrality of visual communication and the possibility of using temporary tools such as Stories. Recent studies indicate that some female figures have exploited Instagram to construct alternative narratives, circumventing gender stereotypes and strengthening their public image (Bast et al. 2022). Nonetheless, it is not immune to this issue, as targeted harassment targeting women has also been documented. Integrating a gender perspective is essential to fully understand the complex landscape of online communication dynamics. Participatory cultures present on various digital platforms can contribute to the dissemination and normalization of misogynistic content (Massanari, 2017). At the same time, the role of algorithms becomes central in determining the visibility of content, contributing to amplifying controversial messages and reinforcing certain narratives within digital environments (Marwick & Caplan, 2018). At this point, the interaction between user practices and algorithmic logic represents a crucial element in analysing the construction and circulation of gender discourses on social media platforms. All this, however, starts from a basic assumption: that topics related to gender, women's rights, or equality policies tend to generate higher levels of hostility (Oz et al. 2018). Overall, this analysis of different channels highlights how this is not a uniform phenomenon, but the result of a complex interaction between technological architecture, social norms, and power dynamics.

Digital platforms can be understood as sociotechnical spaces in which interaction structures shape communicative practices and relationships between users (boyd, 2010). The affordances of each platform, such as anonymity, visibility, content persistence, and the possibility of performative sharing, contribute to structuring communicative spaces with varying degrees of hostility and with different modes of moderation and regulation of public discourse (Papacharissi, 2015). Including the gender dimension also allows us to understand how these environments can be particularly ambivalent for women, impacting the quality of debate, forms of democratic participation, and public expression (Jane, 2017), but also all possibilities for publicly or anonymously reporting violence (regardless of its nature). Therefore, online gender inequalities are intertwined with other forms of social exclusion, contributing to the reproduction of symbolic and relational hierarchies even in contemporary digital environments.

Although digital technologies are often analysed in relation to their critical aspects, it is important to adopt a more complex and non-deterministic perspective, recognizing the dual nature of digital environments. In this sense, digital technologies should not be considered exclusively as tools for reproducing violence or exclusion, but also as potential resources for building support networks, empowerment, and social resilience. They can also constitute new communication channels that allow victims to interact more directly, anonymously, and securely with support services (Meyer, 2016). In recent years, in fact, there has been a significant expansion in the offering of digital applications and solutions that offer women – and non-normative gender identities – new ways of assistance or initial contact. These devices, thanks to their unique characteristics such as free access, immediacy, and anonymity, allow people to seek support and report abuse and violence to others within a digital "listening space", perceived as protective and immune (Westmarland & Kelly, 2013). In Italy, for example, several apps exist (for example, *YouPol* and *App1522-Anti-violence and Stalking Helpline*, the former operated by the State Police and the latter originally launched as a telephone hotline—promoted by the Department for Equal Opportunities at the Presidency of the Council of Ministers—and later transformed into an app). Both provide a direct, immediate, and relatively discreet channel between citizens, those in need (women in particular), and law enforcement, contributing to the need to increase the vulnerable population's perception of safety and ease of access to help. One aspect that deserves specific attention regarding these two apps is their affordances, which go beyond simply providing communication tools, but profoundly shape the relationship between those seeking help and those offering it. The ability to save content, create archives of evidence, and customize reporting methods helps empower victims, who can develop a more comprehensive and informed plan to escape the violence. The very ability to maintain a partially anonymous identity and adjust the level of public exposure constitutes a crucial opportunity to reduce social stigma and mitigate the fear of retaliation. Other apps are versatile tools, capable of meeting a variety of needs (see, for example, *Viola Walkhome* or *Where Are U*, the official app for the European Emergency Number 112), but many other examples are found in other countries. This latter app, downloadable for free, allows women in need, as well as other citizens, to quickly connect to Operations Centers and communicate an ongoing emergency by voice or with just a few clicks. This allows emergency operators to immediately determine the caller's exact location using the smartphone's GPS.

In light of what has been described so far, it clearly emerges that in the fight against gender-based violence, technology can prove to be a "double-edged sword" (Boethius et al., 2022): if on the one hand, apps can represent a direct link between victims and potential agencies for combating and supporting them (perhaps law enforcement agencies or support associations), on the other hand they - precisely because they are specific - can provide the potential aggressor with further elements to tighten the digital and social control of victims and still perpetrate forms of violence. In fact, the possibility of maintaining anonymity and discretion represents a crucial element of protection, while the lack of continuity between digital intervention and local support risks producing an action devoid of concrete effectiveness (Woodlock, 2016). Considering this, technology is not a solution or a tool, much less neutral. It must be integrated into forms of digitalized welfare, taking into account the diverse needs of various segments of the population (Díaz Gorfinkiel et al., 2021) – in this specific case, victims of gender-based violence – without overlooking the fact that the quality of support depends on the usability of the tools and their ability to address the specificities of individual experiences in complete anonymity and security. This is to more effectively address victims' needs and strengthen the support and protection network against gender-based violence.

In this context, the quality of support depends on the usability of the tools and their ability to address the specificities of gender-based violence experiences. The design of accessible interfaces, the presence of multilingual resources, and the protection of privacy are essential conditions to ensure that the provision of assistance is not confined to a horizon of merely symbolic solidarity.

Furthermore, access to digital affordances is itself stratified and unequal. Not all victims have the necessary technological skills or sufficient communication skills to navigate cyber-helping tools. The consequence is that platforms risk generating unequal solidarity, where the effectiveness of intervention depends on the individual's ability to activate available resources. In this sense, the affordance of cyber-helping becomes not only an opportunity, but also a field of collective responsibility, requiring us to reflect on the need to accompany technological innovations with educational interventions and the strengthening of local community networks.

CONCLUSION

When considering the design of innovative digital strategies and tools to prevent and combat gender-based violence, however, it must be clarified that not all victims of violence have the necessary technological skills or sufficient communication skills to navigate cyber-helping or cyber-supporting tools. The quality of support, therefore, depends on the usability of the tools and their ability to address the specificities of experiences of gender-based violence (as we have seen, technology carries significant risks both in its use and in the perpetuation of online violence). Designing accessible and integrated interfaces, providing multilingual resources, and protecting privacy are essential to ensuring that the provision of assistance is not confined to merely symbolic solidarity, but is implemented through concrete support and assistance. What must be avoided to consider digital resources as a genuine support and assistance for victims of gender-based violence is that platforms, rather than being a tool for assistance, become yet another instrument for generating unequal solidarity, where the effectiveness of the intervention depends on the individual's ability to activate available resources rather than the ability to integrate various welfare services. In this sense, the affordance of cyber-helping and/or cyber-supporting becomes not only an opportunity if it integrates the information function (a set of procedures, methods, and tools needed to manage information; here, by management, we mean all the operations of collecting, classifying, associating, and retrieving it) with the communication function, but also a field of collective responsibility, which requires reflecting on the need to accompany technological innovations with educational interventions and the consolidation of local community networks. A redefinition of the communication/information system is necessary and must move toward a circular system (formal and informal) between victims of gender-based violence and the services, and between the services themselves. Only a conscious integration of technology (the entire digital world) and community support can generate pathways out of violence based on continuity, protection, and full recognition of the dignity of those involved.

Building on the ambivalent nature of digital technologies outlined in this chapter, future research should more systematically investigate how this "double-edged" condition shapes both risks and opportunities within anti-violence strategies. In particular, several research questions emerge: how do different platform affordances simultaneously enable support and facilitate control or abuse? Under what conditions do digital tools enhance victims' empowerment rather than reproduce forms of unequal access and "unequal solidarity"? How do local welfare systems mediate the integration of digital solutions, and to what extent can they mitigate the risks associated with technological exclusion? Moreover, the intersections between gender, visibility, and social position profoundly influence both exposure to digital violence and access to protection and support resources. This trajectory makes it possible to grasp in depth how vulnerabilities are not evenly distributed, but rather stratified. Such an approach enables the design of more targeted, inclusive, and context-sensitive interventions. In this way, empirical research and public policies can be more effectively integrated and made more impactful. These trends in contemporary society require a rethinking of how welfare policies are planned and implemented, aiming to combine available resources with improvements in the living conditions of survivors of violence, while simultaneously ensuring the enforceability of rights. Innovative strategies must, therefore, be based on an "integrated logic" that coherently captures the objectives underlying the protection and guarantee of the well-being of victims of gender-based violence. From this perspective, the integration of social, territorial, and technological networks is therefore essential, leading to the construction of a sort of hub that gathers available resources under a single platform, as well as the active participation of all stakeholders, not only as recipients but as partners in policy design.

Only then will the resources provided (including digital reporting tools) not be perceived as isolated tools of a single institution, but rather as part of a broader, coordinated network of actors united to achieve a common goal.

Welfare thus becomes digital and integrated if all actions undertaken to combat gender-based violence are coordinated among different actors in the local network and, above all, if they are made visible, in digital spaces, to women who wish to access them.

REFERENCES

Abarna, S., Sheeba, J. I., Jayasrilakshmi, S., & Devaneyan, S. P. (2022). Identification of cyber harassment and intention of target users on social media platforms. *Engineering Applications of Artificial Intelligence, 115*, 105283. DOI: 10.1016/j.engappai.2022.105283 PMID: 35968532

Addeo, F., & Masullo, G. (2021). Research Methods in the Digital Society: Challenges and opportunities. *Italian Sociological Review*, 11(4S), 153- 369. https://doi.org/DOI: 10.13136/isr.v11i4S.428

Amato, R. (2025). *Collecting Data on Technology-Facilitated Violence Against Women: Challenges and Ways Forward.* Council of Europe.

Amnesty International. (2017, 20 November). *Amnesty reveals alarming impact of online abuse against women.* https://www.amnesty.org/en/latest/press-release/2017/11/amnesty-reveals-alarming-impact-of-online-abuse-against-women/

Amnesty International. (2022, 20 April). *Black and Asian women MPs abused more online.* https://www.amnesty.org.uk/knowledge-hub/all-resources/online-violence-women-mps/

Bast, J., Oschatz, C., & Renner, A. M. (2022). Successfully overcoming the "double bind"? A mixed-method analysis of the self-presentation of female right-wing populists on Instagram and the impact on voter attitudes. *Political Communication, 39*(3), 358–382. DOI: 10.1080/10584609.2021.2007190

Battista, D., & Coppola, M. (2025). Gender-Based Violence and Cyber-Helping: The Affordance of Dedicated Apps Between Opportunities and Obstacles. *Welfare e Ergonomia, 2*, 169–180.

Bjelajac, Ž., & Filipović, A. (2021). Specific characteristics of digital violence and digital crime. *Pravo-teorija i praksa, 38*(4), 16-32.

Boethius, S., Åkerström, M., & Hydén, M. (2022). The double-edged sword – abused women's experiences of digital technology. *European Journal of Social Work, 26*(3), 506–518. DOI: 10.1080/13691457.2022.2040437

Boyd, D. (2010). Social network sites as networked publics: Affordances, dynamics, and implications. In *A networked self* (pp. 47–66). Routledge.

Cardoso, L. F., Sorenson, S. B., Webb, O., & Landers, S. (2019). Recent and emerging technologies: Implications for women's safety. *Technology in Society, 58*, 101108. DOI: 10.1016/j.techsoc.2019.01.001

Chalovska Dimovska, N. (2024). *Analysis of Technology facilitated Gender-Based Violence*. United Nations Development Programme.

Corradi, C., & Stöckl, H. (2016). The lessons of history: The role of the nation-states and the EU in fighting violence against women in 10 European countries. *Current Sociology, 64*(4), 671–688. DOI: 10.1177/0011392116640457

Demurtas, P., & Mangone, E. (2025). Ripensare il welfare per prevenire e contrastare la violenza di genere: Sfide e opportunità per un sistema integrato. *Welfare e Ergonomia, 2*, 7–26.

Díaz Gorfinkiel, M., Díaz Gandasegui, V., & Gómez García, M. V. (2021). New technology proposals for tackling intimate partner violence: Challenges and opportunities. *Technology in Society, 67*, 101714. DOI: 10.1016/j.techsoc.2021.101714

Donato, S., Eslen-Ziya, H., & Mangone, E. (2022). From offline to online violence: New challenges for the contemporary society. *International Review of Sociology, 32*(3), 400–412. DOI: 10.1080/03906701.2022.2133405

Duncombe, C. (2020). Social media and the visibility of horrific violence. *International Affairs, 96*(3), 609–629. DOI: 10.1093/ia/iiaa055

EIGE. (2018). *Gender equality and youth: opportunities and risks of digitalisation*. Publications Office of the European Union., DOI: 10.2839/148393

Epiphanio, F., & Oms, C. (2025). The use of digital technology to prevent violence against women: A scoping review of recent literature. *International Journal of Technological Learning. Innovation and Development, 16*(2), 134–152. DOI: 10.1504/IJTLID.2025.146723

Floridi, L. (2015). *The Onlife Manifesto. Being Human in a Hyperconnected Era*. Sprnger.

Fornari, S., & Masullo, G. (2023). Ripensare il fenomeno della violenza nella digital society. In S. Fornari, & G. Masullo (Eds.), *Forme di violenza e rischi per le persone* (monographic issue). *Sicurezza e scienze sociali*, 3, 7-10. DOI: 10.3280/SISS2023-003001

FRA. (2020). *A long way to go for LGBTI equality*. Publications Office of the European Union., DOI: 10.2811/7746

Hearn, J., Strid, S., Humbert, A. L., Balkmar, D., & Delaunay, M. (2022). From Gender Regimes to Violence Regimes: Re-thinking the Position of Violence. *Social Politics, 29*(2), 682–705. DOI: 10.1093/sp/jxaa022

Henry, N., & Powell, A. (2018). Technology-facilitated sexual violence: A literature review of empirical research. *Trauma, Violence & Abuse, 19*(2), 195–208. DOI: 10.1177/1524838016650189 PMID: 27311818

Hinduja, S., & Patchin, J. W. (2010). Bullying, cyberbullying, and suicide. *Archives of Suicide Research, 14*(3), 206–221. DOI: 10.1080/13811118.2010.494133 PMID: 20658375

ITC. (2023). *Bridging the gender divide* (last Update November). https://www.itu.int/en/mediacentre/backgrounders/Pages/bridging-the-gender-divide.aspx

Jane, E. A. (2017). 'Dude… stop the spread': Antagonism, agonism, and# manspreading on social media. *International Journal of Cultural Studies, 20*(5), 459–475. DOI: 10.1177/1367877916637151

Jurėnienė, V. (2026). Technology-Driven Gender Violence. In Shaw, S. M., Santos, X. M., Mayilsamy, J., Veni, K., Pallarés Ameneiro, L., Rosaline, Z., & Lockhart, J. (Eds.), *Resisting Gender Violence* (pp. 159–179). Oregon State University.

Mangone, E. (2016). Implicazioni normative e istituzionali nello sviluppo integrato del welfare. In Del Forno, M. (Ed.), *Nel complesso mondo del welfare. Idee, metodi e pratiche* (pp. 93–104). FrancoAngeli.

Mangone, E., Masullo, G., & Gallego, M. (Eds.). (2018). *Gender and Sexuality in the Migration Trajectories. Studies between the Northern and Southern Mediterranean Shores*. Information Age Publishing.

Marwick, A. E., & Caplan, R. (2018). Drinking male tears: Language, the manosphere, and networked harassment. *Feminist Media Studies, 18*(4), 543–559. DOI: 10.1080/14680777.2018.1450568

Massanari, A. (2017). # Gamergate and The Fappening: How Reddit's algorithm, governance, and culture support toxic technocultures. *New Media & Society, 19*(3), 329–346. DOI: 10.1177/1461444815608807

Masullo, G., & Picarella, L. (2025). Men's involvement in preventing gender violence: Socio-educational and cultural strategies for an integrated welfare. *Welfare e Ergonomia, 2*, 39–50.

Mazzucato, M. (2021). *Mission economy: A moonshot guide to changing capitalism*. Penguin.

Meyer, S. (2016). Examining women's agency in managing intimate partner violence and the related risk of homelessness: The role of harm minimisation. *Global Public Health: An International Journal for Research, Policy and Practice, 11*(1-2), 198–210. DOI: 10.1080/17441692.2015.1047390 PMID: 26110781

Nash, J. C. (2021). Intersectionality. In The Keywords Feminist Editorial Collective (Ed.), *Keywords for gender and sexuality* (pp. 128-133). New York University Press.

Oz, M., Zheng, P., & Chen, G. M. (2018). Twitter versus Facebook: Comparing incivility, impoliteness, and deliberative attributes. *New Media & Society, 20*(9), 3400–3419. DOI: 10.1177/1461444817749516

Papacharissi, Z. (2015). We have always been social. *Social Media + Society, 1*(1), 2056305115581185. DOI: 10.1177/2056305115581185

Pew Research Center. (2021). *The State of Online Harassment.* https://www.pewresearch.org/internet/2021/01/13/the-state-of-online-harassment/

Recuero, R. (2024). The platformization of violence: Toward a concept of discursive toxicity on social media. *Social Media + Society, 10*(1), 20563051231224264. DOI: 10.1177/20563051231224264

Ross, A. R., Chadwick, A., & Vaccari, C. (2021). Digital media and the proliferation of public opinion cues online: Biases and vulnerabilities in the new attention economy. In *The Routledge companion to political journalism* (pp. 241–251). Routledge. DOI: 10.4324/9780429284571-22

Rowe, I. (2015). Civility 2.0: A comparative analysis of incivility in online political discussion. *Information Communication and Society, 18*(2), 121–138. DOI: 10.1080/1369118X.2014.940365

Santana, A. D. (2014). Virtuous or vitriolic: The effect of anonymity on civility in online newspaper reader comment boards. *Journalism Practice, 8*(1), 18–33. DOI: 10.1080/17512786.2013.813194

Sauerborn, E., Eisenhut, K., Ganguli-Mitra, A., & Wild, V. (2022). Digitally supported public health interventions through the lens of structural injustice: The case of mobile apps responding to violence against women and girls. *Bioethics, 36*(1), 71–76. DOI: 10.1111/bioe.12965 PMID: 34668600

Southern, R., & Harmer, E. (2021). Twitter, incivility and "everyday" gendered othering: An analysis of tweets sent to UK members of parliament. *Social Science Computer Review, 39*(2), 259–275. DOI: 10.1177/0894439319865519

Strid, S., Humbert, A. L., Hearn, J., & Balkmar, D. (2021). States of violence: Exploring welfare state regimes as violence regimes by developing a violence regimes index. *Journal of European Social Policy, 31*(3), 321–336. DOI: 10.1177/09589287211002370

Trindade Pereira, I., & Zaba, M. (2026, 19 January). *How is cyberviolence against women and girls spreading across Europe?* https://www.euronews.com/my-europe/2026/01/19/how-is-cyberviolence-against-women-and-girls-spreading-across-europe

Van Dijk, J. (2020). *The Digital Divide*. Polity Press.

Westmarland, N., & Kelly, L. (2013). Why extending measurements of "success" in domestic violence perpetrator programmes matters for social work. *British Journal of Social Work, 43*(6), 1092–1110. DOI: 10.1093/bjsw/bcs049

WHO. (2019). *RESPECT women: Preventing violence against women* (WHO/RHR/18.19). https://iris.who.int/bitstream/handle/10665/312261/WHO-RHR-18.19-eng.pdf?sequence=1

WHO. (2025). *Violence against women prevalence estimates, 2023: global, regional and national prevalence estimates for intimate partner violence against women and non-partner sexual violence against women*. World Health Organization. https://iris.who.int/handle/10665/383559

Women, U. N. (2015). *A Framework to Underpin Action to Prevent Violence Against Women*. https://www.unwomen.org/sites/default/files/Headquarters/Attachments/Sections/Library/Publications/2015/Prevention_Framework_unwomen_nov2015.pdf

Women, U. N. (2020). *Overview: How to Use the RESPECT Framework Implementation Guide*. https://www.unwomen.org/sites/default/files/Headquarters/Attachments/Sections/Library/Publications/2020/RESPECT-implementation-guide-Overview-en.pdf

Women, U. N. (2025, 13 November). *Digital abuse, trolling, stalking, and other forms of technology-facilitated violence against women and girls.* https://www.unwomen.org/en/articles/faqs/digital-abuse-trolling-stalking-and-other-forms-of-technology-facilitated-violence-against-women

Women, U. N. (2025, 18 November). *Online safety 101: What every woman and girl should know*. https://www.unwomen.org/en/articles/explainer/online-safety-101-what-every-woman-and-girl-should-know

Woodlock, D. (2016). The Abuse of Technology in Domestic Violence and Stalking. *Violence Against Women*, *23*(5), 584–602. DOI: 10.1177/1077801216646277 PMID: 27178564

ENDNOTES

1 A further relevant element concerns the strong concentration of abuse on single, symbolically exposed figures. In the same study, Diane Abbott alone was the target of 31.6% of all abusive tweets analysed; during the six weeks preceding the 2017 general election, this proportion rose to 45.14%, equivalent to an average of 51 abusive messages per day. This finding suggests that digital violence often operates through intensive targeting campaigns against highly visible women, especially when they belong to minority groups. The structural nature of the phenomenon also emerges from broader comparative analyses. In an international study promoted by Amnesty International involving women journalists and politicians in the United Kingdom and the United States, it was found that in 2017 one problematic tweet directed at a woman was posted every 30 seconds. Although the sample included different professions, the finding confirms the pervasiveness of hostile communicative environments toward women occupying public and opinion-shaping roles. Recent studies further confirm that online hate directed at women in politics frequently contains a strong misogynistic component. The Ofcom (2025) study, based on surveys and qualitative interviews with 23 women who were current or former members of the British Parliament, found that participants described online abuse as constant and pervasive, often characterised by rape threats, death threats, and sexist language. Many interviewees also believed that such a climate discourages some women from entering politics and, in several cases, has contributed to the withdrawal of female representatives from public life.

Chapter 11
Welfare and AI:
Female Representation and Social Inequalities

Mirella Ferrari
http://orcid.org/0009-0005-3710-5767
University of Milano Bicocca, Italy

ABSTRACT

This research paper aims to analyse the risk of social exclusion – and in particular gender-based exclusion – fuelled by artificial intelligence, highlighting, amongst other current trends, those relating to processes of masculinisation present in AI platforms, with a particular focus on welfare. The literature review on the impact of Artificial Intelligence reveals an under-representation of women in scientific fields and STEM disciplines. It also highlights the presence of bias. The research further highlights the presence of inequalities in AI, not only in terms of gender. An approach to process transformation that integrates reflexivity, pluralism and participation can minimise inequalities in AI and, consequently, in welfare services.

INTRODUCTION: THEORETICAL FRAMEWORK: EMERGING TRENDS AND APPROACHES

When addressing the topic of "*artificial intelligence*", we cannot refrain from dwelling on the terms that, to some extent, we perceive as juxtaposed.

Intelligence is perceived as innate and, therefore, "natural"; whereas the term "artificial" refers to the intentionality of human action capable of objectifying its own cognitive faculties in technological devices, categorizing constructive practices that aim at the synthetic and artificial replication of natural processes.

DOI: 10.4018/979-8-2600-3043-1.ch011

Insofar as it is natural and finite, human action is irreversible and, as such, stimulates the search for "ends" (Hans, 2009), that is, those forms of conduct directed toward the exploration of the meaning of action. Such finitude constitutes the driving force of behaviours and expressions of natural intelligence, which articulates multiple productions and manifestations.

Artificial intelligence, by contrast, is configured as an algorithmic simulation devoid of ontological intentionality. It is not oriented toward the exploration of "ends", but toward the optimization of means, operating within a system of pure calculability in which action is, by its nature, indifferent to meaning.

Some scholars maintain that AI represents the human attempt to emancipate cognitive function from bodily limits (Miano, 2013; De Simone, 2020; Esposito, 2022), pursuing the ambitious objective of creating an unlimited ontological productivity, freed from the spatio-temporal limitations that afflict the body.

From healthcare to work and education; from the economy to industry; from information to communication and even to individual behaviours, our existences and our relationships, today, can no longer be conceived without the contribution of technology (Floridi, 2015).

The adoption of artificial intelligence in welfare systems is becoming increasingly central in the global scientific debate, involving not only academic institutions but also governments, public and private organizations, as well as technology companies.

The introduction of artificial intelligence into the processes of distributing social benefits pursues the ambitious goal of transforming the *welfare state,* by providing greater efficiency and personalization of services, as well as a more equitable management of resources (Airoldi, 2021; Burrell & Fourcade, 2021), reducing waste and optimizing distribution at the territorial level. The integration of AI into welfare systems, although representing an extraordinary opportunity to improve equity and efficiency, is not without challenges.

Numerous countries have attempted to regulate the use of generative artificial intelligence (Santosuosso, 2020; Vantin, 2018) in different ways: by introducing legislation that integrates aspects of traditional law with concepts such as "ethics, dignity, non-discrimination, social well-being, and sustainable development," as in Europe; by promoting a market-oriented approach aimed at encouraging investment, as in the United States; or by experimenting with a regulatory framework that combines state control with the standardization of ethical principles, as in China.

The revolution connected to the use and diffusion of AI implies the artificial global categorization of behavioral and social patterns through the application of categories that necessarily tend toward the simplification of human action within the narrow algorithmic boundaries (Murru & Selva, 2025): ethnicities, genders, emotional states, human geographies are thus classified through a superficial ontological knowledge, without taking into account human complexity and contexts. Barret (et al. 2019) warns us about this, insisting on the superficiality and simplification of social ontologies.

In order to account in this contribution for the evolution of the welfare state mediated by artificial intelligence, it has been necessary to consider three different areas of research: the traditional one concerning welfare and its developments over the last decades; that of the female condition explored by feminist literature and technoscience; as well as that of the revolution we are experiencing produced by the introduction of AI into our everyday life.

Looking at the literature, several trends emerge: those who believe that the introduction of AI in the public welfare service constitutes a unique opportunity for development and social progress; and those who believe that AI conceals considerable risks, which may even lead to an exacerbation of already existing disparities, creating a veritable "society of bias" (Suresh & Guttag, 2020).

We note that, beyond support for or the most stringent criticism of AI, the debate often moves within deterministic logics, anchored to the discursive characterization of inevitability (Vicseck, 2020). The dominant issue, when exploring the theoretical framework, is directed at the recurring problem of "bias", understood as the core of algorithmic fragility.

In the algorithmic universe, automated systems govern or are directed and programmed to manage many aspects of contemporaneity, including among others social inequalities, unemployment, justice, subsidies and much more (Benjamin, 2019).

"Machine learning"(ML) is built on the reflection of human judgment and priorities, according to classes of ideas or thoughts, generated through processes of simplification and categorization inherent in individual reflections (Crawford, 2024). ML crystallizes and simplifies reality, in order to allow categorization, transforming, complex thoughts into algorithms.

This way of proceeding in its conception encounters the pernicious obstacle of stereotypes. The solution for several analysts and scholars of the field consists in removing or minimizing distortions, known as "bias" (Silberg & Manyica, 2019).

In this regard the approaches identified in the literature are different. Media and cultural studies, which have long documented inequalities between social groups; phenomena of social exclusion, and privileges dictated by belonging to dominant groups, even simply for the long-standing issue of access to the technologies themselves (Pascale, 2013; Silberg & Mayika, 2019) with respect to the modeling of AI.

A first approach focuses on the territorial dimension and maintains that inequities and inequalities cannot be absent from AI (Airoldi, 2021). Let us consider even only the possibility of access to AI, which the "Global North" enjoys in comparison with the "Least Developed Countries" (Sadowski, 2020; Couldry, & Mejias, 2019; Gray & Suri, 2019), a phenomenon already highlighted.

Bourdieu several years ago spoke in advance in this regard of "digital exclusion" (Bourdieu, 1983). Particularly interesting appear the reflections concerning global neo-colonization mediated by technologies (Bhambra, 2014), which refer to the considerations on the "new forms of virtual colonialism" by Foucault (1996, p.135), which identify in the Global North a tendency to perpetuate forms of exploitation and impoverishment of the Global South. North America, Europe and East Asia are the main competitors in this "new conquest of virtual frontiers" (Couldry, & Mejias,2019) mediated by AI.

A second approach highlights the presence of stereotypes and prejudices in software design, because they are intrinsically present in the collectivity. Such stereotypes would have been introduced into the system by the developers themselves, unintentionally, because they are intrinsically present in their *common sense* (Grieve et al., 2025; Pronzato, 2024; Bell et al., 2016). As if to say that technology, which is the product of contemporary society, which shows deep fractures, inequalities and injustices, can only be the imprint of the different models of inequity present at the global level; and the algorithm can only reproduce them accurately. Some sociologists of language confine "bias" within the natural process of computer programming, rendering "deviations and errors" a spontaneous and impartial fact, because they are the product of an inequitable society. According to this approach the "bias" themselves would prove to be truthful, precisely because they adhere to reality (Grieve et al., 2025). Artificial intelligence is becoming established as an epistemic technology (Alvarado, 2023) capable of exercising the process of gatekeeping (Miragoli, 2025) within public discourse. *LLMs* (Large Language Models) draw upon the infinite repertoire of cultural language, feeding a variety of inventories that are themselves potentially infinite.

The linguistic practices, on which AI draws, are so extensive that they align with widespread "common sense" (Bender et al., 2021), which naturally incorporates prejudices and stereotypes. According to Bender, AI is nothing more than a "stochastic parrot" (ibidem) that reproduces stereotypes, generating probable forms of thought that contain factual correctness at the expense of purely creative forms. In the processes of design and training, criteria of alignment with social desirability intervene, rather than creatively controversial forms or positions contrary to common sense. The risk is that of a tendency toward cultural homogenization (Sorice, 2021) and of the generation of forms of thought, that do not contradict genericity, but rather articulate it in its infinite forms, constructing an "artificial common sense" (McCarthy, 2022).

Others, on the contrary, believe that "bias" represent a dangerous deviation to be isolated and corrected, in order to build a more equitable world, in which the consolidation of the already existing social exclusion is not witnessed (Gehl Sampath, 2021; Park & Humphry, 2019; Van DijK, 2006; Joyce & Cruz, 2024).

Work and organizational sociologists have highlighted the emergence of new organizational models, reconfigured by algorithmic systems to the detriment of workers (Bailey et al., 2020; Kellog et al. 2020). Utopian and dystopian predictions of robots with human-like features have often been the main object of study of this branch of sociology.

Educational sociologists have identified the risk of a weakening of human relationships, correlable to an increase in "virtual human relationships" (Boyd & Holton, 2018). Wajcman (2017) has contextualized AI within the perennial human anxiety in the face of progress and its disorientation when confronted with novelty.

There are those who, like Burrell and Fourcade (2021), foresee in the current technological revolution the risk of a concentration of power in areas such as: health; security; justice; and education in the hands of an "elite of technologists".

The role of sociology may prove valuable, as it boasts a long history of arguments concerning the human condition (Arendt, 1958), its action (Bourdieu, 1980); the contexts within which the individual acts (Parsons, 2021); behavioural phenomena and trends, as well as the fields in which AI is increasingly used, namely justice; education; health; and welfare.

TECHNOLOGY, GENDER AND STEM DISCIPLINES

Having analysed the scientific literature, we shall continue our exploration, taking into account other aspects relevant to our investigation. First and foremost, as we wish to examine the correlation between women and technology, we believe it is useful to consider, in quantitative terms, the representation of women in the STEM sector; we shall then analyse the types of bias present in IT platforms that contribute to the exclusion of women from the STEM sector. Finally, we shall continue our analysis by examining the social construct underlying the female gender, in order to identify the possible causes of the lower representation of women in the IT sector.

Nowadays, technology has assumed relevance not only in the constructive models of common thought but also an identity value in the processes of socialization, education and critical capacity of reading events and interpreting information at all levels and degrees of education. We estimate that, in this context, it is important to attempt to understand what the constraint is that still links technology to the processes of socialization, which contribute not only to the co-construction of individual identities but also to the creation of stereotypes and prejudices.

We know that technology, similarly to other means, values and abilities conforms to normative expectations, correlated with gender differences (Ruble et al. 2006). The internalization of social normative expectations on the one hand and self-expressive values on the other root in boys and girls essentialist gender beliefs, which rest on stereotyped cultural schemas. Value systems encourage the transmission of masculine and feminine attributes functional to the construction of social identity. The genders would behave in the same way toward technology.

Scholars in the field (De las Cuevas et al., 2022; England, 2010; Correll, 2004) maintain that gender stereotypes evoke preferences with respect to the universe of STEM disciplines both at the level of study and at the occupational level, and that such stereotypes would contribute to the greater male presence in the field of AI. The way in which we are socialized to technologies influences gender and use. On the one hand the types of technologies, their design and meanings are created within social relationships, and on the other technologies are the reflection of these same relationships, beliefs, and pre-existing values.

A rich scientific literature increasingly helps us to outline the general framework within which AI operates and develops, revealing advantages and disadvantages of generative intelligence (Wang & Degol, 2017).

Gender biases have received attention with respect to the tracking and datafication of the body (Kristensen & Prigge, 2017). Numerous studies highlight the exclusion of the female gender in the design of digital technologies and the lack of testing on women (Eubanks, 2018; Noble, 2018), which would contribute to the reduced trust of the latter toward AI.

Gender differences in normative expectations; in access; in the perception of technology as well as in different economic possibilities tend to exclude women from technological developments, confining them to other fields of knowledge, although in history there have been several female contributions to scientific progress. By way of example we recall Ada Lovelace Byron considered the inventor of *software*, that is the first computer program; or Hedy Lamarr, to whom is owed the invention of a *modulation system* to encode information to be transmitted over *radio waves*, which aroused the interest of the secret services and laid the foundations of modern cryptography; or again Katherine Johnson who was hired by NASA for her qualities and competences in the area of mathematics and physics. Despite these early and brilliant presences, the sector of technologies and even more of AI is dominated mostly by men. The technological field is pervaded by a rather rooted and deep gender gap, which has shaped the expectations and destinies of entire generations up to our days.

To these historical stereotypes another problem is added that risks further marginalizing women, namely their underrepresentation in probability calculation models. Already in 2010 the need was felt at the planetary level to counter female exclusion, so much so that the United Nations Entity for Gender Equality and Empowerment of Women began to promote gender equality and female empowerment in an attempt to counter gender inequalities with the aim of building a more equitable and inclusive society.

Historically women in STEM sectors (Science, Technology, Engineering and Mathematics) have been underrepresented and from a 2021 survey (Hansen et al., 2024) this trend continues to perpetuate itself even today: in fact the female workforce presence covers only 28% according to the WEF Report 2024.

Although the gender gap evolves differently from country to country; a cross-national pattern of disproportions between female and male presence emerges, which in turn influences women's participation and the technological transition.

Italy in 2024 was in 87th place in the "index gender gap" out of 146 countries; and in 111th for the "female presence in the economic sector". Iceland, Finland and Norway were the States that ensured greater gender equality, occupying the top positions at the global level; although Europe, as a whole, ensured a good performance in the areas of education; health; and politics reaching 75% of women employed in the mentioned sectors. Europe also shows a constant growth over the last twenty years, aimed at gender equality, which although slow appears appreciable. The female situation reveals, also, a low presence in managerial positions and in decision-making roles in all the sectors explored by the WEF survey. Only in the educational sector has our country obtained a better position placing itself at the 56th level out of 146.

The STEM sector, among those investigated, shows greater difficulties. For decades women have been marginalized from access to education and to scientific and technological professions, and their abilities often ignored.

The disparity, however, is not only the result of decades of voluntary marginalization but also of cultural factors, which relegated women to subordinate roles, and directed them to fields of knowledge and to professions considered for them more "appropriate". This mechanism of social marginalization, perpetrated for centuries, has reinforced the phenomenon of female underrepresentation in many areas of knowledge and of scientific production, as well as industrial.

One need only consider the absence of clinical studies in the medical field on cardiovascular risk, which for many years were conducted primarily on male samples. Such a process has developed pathological prediction algorithms of the cardiac system on typically male symptoms. Such predictive mappings have had the consequence of not being precisely replicable on the female gender, which reported different symptoms; thus diagnoses revealed errors or delays in treatments (Vogel et al., 2021). AI was wrong, because it was trained on computational models that rested on stereotypes, which classified the female gender in the same way as the male one.

Another study shows, instead, the positive use of AI for in vitro fertilization, significantly increasing implantation rates and optimizing the fertilization process (Vermilyea, 2020).

Beyond gaps in the design of AI there also exists the variable of the perception of privacy, which discourages women from the use of generative intelligence (Armantier et al., 2024).

The gender gap in connectivity and in digital skills could lead to a marginalization of women's role in society in the coming decades on the economic; commercial; political; health; educational level and in many other fields in which AI has already massively penetrated. To avoid this scenario it will be necessary to invest in knowledge and skills.

The *Alliance for Affordable Internet* (A4AI) has estimated that by closing the female digital gap an economic value equal to 524 billion dollars could be generated at the global level.

It appears that a cultural challenge of planetary scale awaits us. Italy in the global framework is situated in an intermediate position compared to other countries in the level of education: 69% of women possess a diploma compared to men, who reach 64%. At the level of tertiary education women graduates in Italy are 25% and men 18%. The report "Education Levels and Employment Returns" by Istat (2025) depicts a complex picture of the Italian labour market, highlighting imbalances between levels of education and employment opportunities. There emerges, in fact, a significant gender disparity: although women are on average more educated than men, their employment rate remains considerably lower. This gap stands at 59% for women against 79% for men, highlighting a persistent gender employment difference in the country. To this is added the drastic underrepresentation of women in the STEM sector with 9 percentage points less. The Italian labour context moreover also shows a transversal fragility, which relegates the latter to the phenomenon of "involuntary part-time" carried out by 49% of women, reaching the share of 73% in southern Italy. Although this tendency decreases with the increase in the level of education, even among female graduates it stands around 42% (Report ISTAT 2025).

25% of young people (aged 25–34) hold a STEM degree: among them, 37% are men and 16% are women. This gap is reflected in the employment outcomes of women themselves. We observe that, across all the economic sectors explored, the phenomenon of "trasversal segregation" occurs (Clark, 1982; Hakim, 1992).

A review of the OECD Report (2022) and EUROSTAT (2026), which investigates women's presence in the AI sector, also reveals trends that corroborate what has been highlighted so far. The global impact of AI shows different risks across different latitudes, further marking the clear distinction between the Global North and the Global South. If we consider Latin America, where the majority of firms are small and medium-sized and women's presence is predominant in manufacturing and services, the critical issue is not only that of under-dimensioning compared with large American companies; but also that of labour exclusion, caused by layoffs resulting from the introduction of AI in both manufacturing and services (Young et al., 2021). The gender gap and some potential forms of exclusion also persist in these regions of the world, to which women may be exposed to a greater extent.

An analysis of the data highlights the urgency of improving women's participation; increasing awareness of women's potential; and strengthening their skills in the STEM sector. In this exploration as well scientific evidence emerges showing women relegated to involuntary part-time work; underrepresented in the STEM field; forced into lower wages, or worse, exposed to a greater risk of dismissal compared to men. Young's study also anticipates the profound trend toward automation that will affect many productive sectors, which for thousands of women will translate into concrete segregation (Huang et al., 2021) with the loss of employment; whereas men will be less exposed because they occupy intermediate and managerial roles that are not easily replaceable by AI (Gmyrek et al., 2023).

RISK OF EXCLUSION IN DIGITAL WELFARE SERVICES: TYPES OF BIAS

Artificial intelligence currently stands as one of the most disruptive technological innovations, exerting a pervasive influence across all fields of knowledge and at every social level. Although its consolidation is relatively recent, the historical roots of AI are much deeper and date back to the 1940s, when the simulation of human thought through neural networks was first experimented; the Turing test (1956) conventionally marks its birth. Numerous milestones have marked the advancement of this technology up to the present day.

What should be emphasized here is the "historical-cultural" factor, which has influenced AI since its origins. It is the result of a documented evolution that has shaped both its architecture and its objectives. Initially, AI was strongly influenced by "symbolic rationalism", namely the idea that a symbolic system possessed the necessary and sufficient means for intelligent action, and that intelligence was grounded in the manipulation of abstract symbols according to logical rules (Wajcman & Young, 2023; Newell & Simon 1976; Weizenbaum, 1976).

AI is also conditioned by at least one additional factor, namely the "social factor", as it is not a neutral technology but rather the product of the values; economic needs and power structures of the society that created it (Noble, 2018; Green & Viljoen, 2020; Crawford, 2021).

Society, as a historical and cultural expression, is traversed by prejudices and permeated by stereotypes which, as social constructs, perform specific functions within the social system (Longworth, 2021; Tipaldo, 2019; Lamont, 2000).

According to the most recent approaches in the sociology of science prejudice constitutes a powerful mechanism within the digital community, whose objective is to discredit experts and scholars in the field, in order to protect one's own worldview: a tendency described by Tipaldo as "epistemological narcissism" (2019).

Prejudices and stereotypes, therefore, are to some extent functional to the construction of an epistemological framework of thought, which AI designers whether intentionally or unintentionally introduce into algorithmic implementation. Such conditioning factors as cultural devices are capable of contributing to the reproduction of social hierarchies and gender inequalities.

The considerable quantity and diversity of "cognitive biases" (Tversky & Kahneman, 1974; Garrido-Muñoz et al., 2021; Fahse et al., 2021; Shelby et al. 2023) has prompted numerous scholars to develop classifications, which we briefly present here.

There are at least five *cognitive biases*:

- anchoring, also known as the "truth trap", occurs when the social actor anchors to a single value or element that becomes decisive for evaluating one's own actions and those of others, effectively limiting the critical analysis of the context (Tversky & Kahneman, 1974);
- cost biases that induce the overestimation of the value of the costs or losses of an action, influencing future choices and leading to irrational behaviour;
- desire biases which refer to desirability and affect the mind with illusory thoughts;
- finally there is *framing* which occurs when a specific interpretative framework limits our judgement.

Among the other distortions we include the *representativeness heuristic*, which is represented by a cognitive mechanism through which we violate the rules of probability. The mind tends to evaluate an event, relying on stereotypes rather than on objective statistical data (ibidem).

Among the other biases, however, those which most concern our scientific exploration are gender biases. Gender bias is defined as the entire system of prejudices and stereotypes, which rests on the systematic discrimination of one gender in relation to another (Basta, Costa-Jussà et al., 2019). These biases have their roots in cultural and social preconceptions, which are already embedded in linguistic structures and in data and, consequently, are reflected in learning systems.

In the recruiting sector, the Amazon case (Craciun et al., 2020) exemplifies the phenomenon of algorithmic bias applied to gender stratification. The machine learning system, fed by historical datasets characterized by a male overrepresentation, had internalized and encoded a preference for male profiles, interpreting gender identity as an indicator of competence. This process over time generated systemic discrimination, in which the algorithm operated an automatic devaluation of female social and cultural capital, methodically penalizing candidates coming from markedly female institutions or associations.

The impact of gender biases is very profound both at the individual and collective level, since it limits the opportunity for social action; subordinates aspirations (Spencer et al., 1999); conditions individual perception and thought and can convey common sense.

There are also system biases. These biases reflect the characteristics of the training data. Historical data incorporate already existing prejudices and social imbalances and reproduce the same imbalances in the predictive capacities of AI systems.

Such a phenomenon proves particularly problematic in those contexts where AI supports relevant decisions in crucial sectors such as justice; public health; welfare; finance; as well as personnel selection. An emblematic case is represented by predictive policing systems in the United States (Gebru, 2020), which demonstrates how automation can institutionalize asymmetries and social inequalities. AI, by analysing historical data relating to searches and arrests, has triggered a negative feedback mechanism, intensifying monitoring activities in areas already historically subject to surveillance. This practice has not produced an objective mapping of illegality, but rather has replicated systemic discrimination to the detriment of African American communities. Artificial intelligence has therefore operated a technological validation of "system biases", transforming the partiality of historical data into a disproportionate strategy of territorial control.

The same situation has occurred in the credit sector, labelling certain social categories, such as women or ethnic minorities, as "bad debtors"; whereas it is precisely these same categories that would need to reconcile low income with flexible repayment times (Crawford, 2017).

In the Public Administration (PA), where the use of AI tools to evaluate candidates in public competitions is increasing, the risk of systemic biases becomes even more critical, because it involves equitable access to public services and career opportunities. Studies on facial recognition systems have revealed error rates of 35% on the faces of African American women compared to just 1% on the faces of Caucasian men. Well known are the studies (Buolamwini & Gebru, 2018) which highlight rather significant errors in the facial recognition of three popular companies in the high-tech sector: Microsoft, IBM and FacePlusPlus, the three systems show difficulty in recognizing African American women.

The application of AI in public competitions or in welfare services of the PA could prove problematic, because it could use biometric systems such as those listed above, and a response provided by an African woman would not be recognized and, therefore, invalidated, marginalizing the latter from the selection or from the service. Moreover the use of these systems in access to public offices could produce discriminatory gender practices.

In welfare services, the adoption of AI algorithms without adequate controls can turn into an instrument of systematic exclusion, making vulnerable groups and women less visible or penalized in the access to fundamental rights.

CONSTRUCTION OF GENDER: DOES AI REWRITE THE FEMALE GENDER OR CRYSTALLIZE MILLENARY STEREOTYPES?

Sociological research over the decades has revealed how the processes and social structures, which create and sustain gender differences, are often summarized with the expression "social construction of gender" (Rubin, 1975; Piccone & Saraceno, 1996; Saguy, 2025).

In recent years one of the most debated issues, in gender studies in particular and in sociology in general, examines the impact of AI on the construction of masculinity.

AI positions itself not as a neutral agent but as an agent that constructs social structures, as well as a "socialization agent" thanks to the continuous creation of new algorithms (Noble, 2018) capable of reinforcing or challenging traditional gender models. Noble demonstrates that AI, in fact, does not merely find, associate or store information, but creates meaning. In her study she analyses how search engines, based on machine learning algorithms, systematically associate certain words with stereotyped images or concepts. For example when Google associates the term "girls" with predominantly hypersexualized results, it performs an act of social construction. The user, not perceiving that it is a social construction, internalizes the gender stereotype as real and truthful (Gillespie, 2024). Technology validates the process as neutral, since the human - machine relationship guarantees impartiality in common sense. Noble goes further to argue that technological socialization is more powerful than that of the family or traditional social agencies, because AI presenting itself, precisely, as "neutral" offers users a truthful exploration of the world. Very young people do not perceive the risk of indoctrination and the possible influence exercised by the platforms.

The theoretical framework addressing gender issues related to AI is rather rich, we will not summarize it completely for reasons of space, but we wish to at least mention the well-known scholar Judy Wajcman, famous for the concept of "technofeminism" (Wajcman, 2006; Wajcman & Young, 2023.) For Wajcman the change of gender models is possible, but only on the condition that those who model and train AI introduce into the design different values from those introduced so far, especially with regard to the female gender.

Among the other scientific approaches to the relationship between gender and AI we include "intersectionality". According to Kimberlé Crenshaw (2013) "intersectionality" is the fundamental lens for analysing how AI creates not only gender discrimination but affects more strongly women of colour; working-class women; and non-binary people, operating an automated social exclusion (Benjamin, 2019).

Alongside these theories stands the traditional feminist contribution of Butler and Trouble (1990), who argue that gender is not something that we *are*, but something that we *do*. There is no "self" that decides to behave as a man or as a woman; it is the constant repetition of action (ways of walking, speaking, dressing) that creates the illusion of a natural inner substance. Gender is, therefore, an effect of power and language: we are "mentioned" as male or female, according to the scholar, even before being born and our entire life is a negotiation with this "performative label". If gender is a repeated act, which creates the illusion of an identity, AI is the "director" of this staging. In fact the algorithm forces us to declare our identity through a binary choice and, once this has been made, AI suggests contents that reinforce the performance, crystallizing stereotypes and prejudices.

A recent study (Sun, et al. 2024) has shown how AI highlights a tendency to underrepresent women in sectors dominated by the male gender and to overrepresent them in professions historically linked to roles of care, motherhood and education. Sun (2024) provides empirical evidence of how AI acts as an influential instrument of the social construction of gender through the "systematic underrepresentation" of women in STEM sectors; and the "stereotyping of care", confining women to subordinate roles in society, directing them toward assistance and education with images that communicate submission and emotional availability.

Among the most recent studies that have dealt with gender bias, we recall the *Bloomberg* research, which in 2023 analysed more than 5,000 images generated by artificial intelligence, highlighting the emphasis on certain stereotypes related to the male and female gender. Specifically AI showed, out of the total images, only 3% of women in the role of judges, while in the USA they are more than 34%; it likewise presented only 7% of female images associated with the medical profession, while in reality they are 39% of the total in the USA; and finally it proposed images of female lawyers equal to 15% while in reality they are 39%. The case has been classified as a case of "algorithmic masculinization", which contributes to vertical segregation.

The mitigation of biases in AI cannot be reduced to a simple technical correction: it requires a profoundly interdisciplinary initiative. Such a rethinking must also place at the centre the voices and experiences of the people, who directly suffer the harms of these systems. Sociology can provide the tools to analyse latent prejudices in data, understand the complexity of gender prejudice (Leavy, 2018) and analyse the phenomenon through its multiple manifestations both linguistic and visual.

THE MATERIALIZATION OF *GENDER*: THE IMPACT OF AI ON WELFARE SYSTEMS AND HUMANOID ROBOTICS.

Technoscience, today, is an essential component of society and it is impossible to address the welfare system mediated by AI, without embracing the different and numerous suggestions that come from the various political, social and cultural spheres. Studying welfare, correlating it with artificial intelligence, means intertwining social service studies with those of the sociology of science, engaging with *gender studies* and *feminist studies*, especially in the process of gender construction, which implies a construction of the body and identity in relation to technologies (Magaudda & Neresini, 2020). Technology and corporeality intertwine inexorably and shape each other through an open and continuous dialogue.

Examining biases more deeply becomes a source of critical discussions concerning not only the female dimension but also its representation with respect to the provision of welfare services. *Gender biases*, as highlighted in the previous chapters, remain highly present in our society and are, consciously or unconsciously, embedded within algorithmic languages (Nangia et al., 2020). This phenomenon tends to underrepresent women both in quantitative terms and in relation to the roles that women occupy across different productive sectors.

The radicalization of certain stereotypes may become even more profound and socially impactful if we consider the growing number of users who rely on Gemini or OpenAI (ChatGPT), which currently represent the most widespread artificial intelligences, and which today approach 750 million users for Gemini, and 800 million for OpenAI (ChatGPT). Lorentzen (2022) has demonstrated precisely how OpenAI is characterized by a dense presence of algorithmic bias in the representation of gender; and how the language addressed to the female gender remains anchored to, and preludes, the aestheticization of the female body. Even in humanoid robotics, a stereotyped male and female vision has emerged (Pasciuto, 2022). Feminized robots reproduce an aestheticized vision of the feminine, dictated above all by desirability or also by the functionality of the "machine" (Danaher & McArthur, 2017). We thus find robots with pleasant female features that are intended for the assistance of vulnerable subjects; for the care of the home and domestic environments; or even for sexuality (the so-called "sex robot"). The modelling of sex robots appears to converge toward standards of idealized and distorted beauty (Oleksy & Wnuk, 2021), oriented toward sexual functionalities, which could contribute to the perpetuation of inaccessible or harmful norms, producing increasing social and cultural pressure on the sexual dimension, and impacting the mental health and emotional well-being of those who make use of them (ibidem).

In our exploration at least three crucial issues emerge: the significant ethical question concerning data transparency; the responsibility involved in modelling;

as well as the inclusivity of languages and cultures in overcoming the gender gap. Technologies should reflect and incorporate a range of perspectives as broad as possible, useful for representing the complexity of contemporaneity, positioning themselves as a guide toward social equity and the minimization of gender disparities.

Gender biases can be overcome only by addressing a profound cultural transformation, directing the attention of designers, engineers, linguists and psychologists, who design and train AI, not so much toward technological development and the fascination that follows from it, but toward careful consideration of the construction of a society that takes into account the multidimensionality of social dynamics and their disparities. If technology, in fact, represents the reflection of our needs, aspirations, fashions and cultures, society is shaped through it, adapting and redefining itself.

ALGORITHMIC GOVERNANCE AND PREDICTIVE SYSTEMS: ETHICAL AND SOCIAL IMPLICATIONS OF THE DIGITALIZATION OF WELFARE

Some sociologists believe that we are witnessing the emergence of a new social order, founded on capitalism and digital surveillance (Damant et al., 2017). Big Tech companies have rapidly established themselves as necessary and indispensable infrastructures of contemporaneity across all existential sectors: from education to work; from health to politics, as well as welfare (Dencik & Kaun, 2020).

After reviewing the literature concerning processes of digitalization; the technological dimensions of socialization; the risks associated with global platformization and the categorization of the processes of individual action; as well as the possible distortions of thought underlying modelling and algorithmic training with particular attention to gender conditions; we will now attempt to define the complex relationship between artificial intelligence and digital welfare, focusing on the female condition.

Analyzing AI as a sociotechnical system, moving beyond the deterministic vision of the technological artifact, means considering the implications; the relationships and social impacts; the renewed services of digital welfare; social policies and the dimensions of action.

Today, among the numerous uses of AI, a widespread international use of predictive analytics emerges, for example in child protection and care services (Cuccaro-Alamin et al. 2017); in judicial services in cases concerning risks of recidivism to illegality (Završnik, 2021); within hospitals for cancer treatment (Coccia, 2020); for applications for social benefits (Velkova & Kaun, 2021); or also for employment services as in Austria (Allhutter et al., 2020).

The growing dependence on the algorithmic system of welfare services reveals a paradigm shift within public administrations, in which the citizen, holder of a single digital identity, no longer interacts with a human interface but with an information platform that provides information, stores sensitive data, and enables the direct management of welfare benefits. Government is transformed into a "platformized identity" through algorithms (Saiani, 2020), consequently altering public organization. If the provision of a digital service ensures an aseptic perception and an apparent decision-making procedure devoid of stereotypical judgments, on the other hand it renders the citizen more isolated in the relationship aimed at requesting the service. Beyond the aseptic automated dimension aimed at accelerating the delivery of welfare services, doubts remain, in light of the previous reflections on stereotyping and the presence of bias, regarding the actual neutrality of the service. The progressive dematerialization and dehumanization of the relationship between beneficiary and service risks distancing the citizen from the use of the service itself, both because of digital illiteracy and because of the impossibility of access (Deriu, 2020).

Let us consider the recent Australian case (Whelan, 2020). Australia, through the AI platform known as "*RoboDebt*", administered taxes and public debt; specifically, through *RoboDebt* it eliminated undue payments from taxpayers, minimizing human oversight, reducing the costs of public employees, and accelerating administrative management operations; until 2017, when the first economic inconsistencies began to emerge. *RoboDebt* had identified and labelled approximately 500 thousand Australian citizens as "undue recipients". The central welfare agency then asked citizens, who according to *RoboDebt* had unjustly received benefits not owed by the State, to return them: the recovery of the sums and the pressure exerted by the Central Agency were such that they caused the economic collapse of dozens of families and psychological crises, even leading to suicidal situations. A class action followed and the government was required to return approximately 1.7 billion dollars, after it was discovered that the *RoboDebt* AI system had been poorly designed and modelled, and contained numerous biases. In September 2025, another reimbursement amounting to 660 million dollars was announced.

This experience highlights several significant critical issues such as the risk of a loss of trust among individuals in the system of social security and governance; to which may be added the stigmatization and criminalization of need, which labelled citizens in need as "cheaters". The *Robodebt* experience has demonstrated how the use of opaque algorithms can create new forms of exclusion and asymmetry of power between citizens and public administration, because the former found themselves having to prove their own innocence. The opacity identified in different AI systems represents another emerging issue (Aragona, 2020); as does insufficient digital literacy which excludes women, vulnerable individuals and those experiencing economic and social poverty.

The massification of individuals and the process of datafication that transforms individual citizens into data, if not controlled and properly modelled, can lead to forms of social exclusion and increase deprivation.

AI risks perpetuating inequalities already evident in contemporary society: women, ethnic minorities, the poor and vulnerable subjects risk further marginalization (Broussard, 2018).

Some theorists (Alston, 2020) have also highlighted the risk of a "dystopian digital welfare" in which beneficiaries are punished for even the smallest irregularities, conditioning the autonomy and choices of individuals.

While automation and technological fascination present the most appealing aspects of innovation and generative intelligence, limits and critical issues are highlighted, as mentioned in this exploration, by numerous scholars in the field (Cohen, 2019).

DIGITAL WELFARE AND GENDER ALGORITHMS: SOME EXAMPLES

Digital welfare services are becoming increasingly widespread and, in light of our investigation, it may be useful to summarize here the Swedish experience known as "*Information-Driven Care*"(IDC). Halmstad University, in collaboration with the Government Agency for Innovation (Vinnova), had developed the IDC project, with specific attention to home care mediated by AI. The experimentation aimed to reduce the administrative burden of healthcare operators through automation, allowing them to dedicate more time to the relationship with the care recipient. It also provided that patients, family members and healthcare staff actively participated in the co-creation and validation of technological solutions. The benefits identified were numerous such as: diagnostic and predictive accuracy; the relative independence of patients under care; and the efficiency of public expenditure. However, several risks also emerged including: the complexity of adopting the care model itself; gender bias and biases related to design and training (Frennert, 2021); as well as issues connected to privacy, given the large amount of data that the system collected. The project had not been tailored to the user but was inspired by a "one-size-fits-all model", which did not take into account the diversity of patients and their different individual needs. In particular, the project managers had considered training activities necessary for Swedish women, who in the healthcare sector in Sweden occupy a larger share (about 80% of employees) compared to men who, however, occupy the top positions within healthcare institutions. The project managers considered it unproductive to train CEOs and executives, who were for the most part men. The managerial model therefore became consolidated by validating gender representations and hierarchies, excluding women from decision-making processes, and confirming vertical segregation. Frennert (2021) highlighted how, in this experimentation, pluralism was lacking and inequalities already present within the community were reinforced, consolidating not only vertical segregation but also horizontal segregation.

This case demonstrates how digitalization, if managed in a non-inclusive and unconscious manner, can perpetuate gender inequalities and marginalize women, even in sectors where they are more strongly represented.

Another interesting example for our investigation is the Swiss case. In Switzerland, active labour market policies provide for the publication of job vacancies for numerous employment positions on the portal "*work.swiss*", managed by SECO (State Secretariat for Economic Affairs). SECO is the federal government body responsible for economic policies and the labour market. Among the many functions it performs, it is responsible for supervising unemployment and managing the public employment service system; carrying out e-government policies; and dealing with worker protection and economic cooperation. The analysis conducted by Anna Maria De Cesare (2025) set out to explore state communication in the employment sector on the multilingual portal of the Swiss Confederation. From her investigation, conducted on 180 job advertisements, it emerged that the portal *work.swiss* uses a great heterogeneity of linguistic forms to refer to the masculine and feminine gender; whereas in a multilingual State it should be essential to use clear and effective language in order to guarantee all citizens access to services. De Cesare examined how the language used on the platform is not neutral, but reflects the activation strategies typical of the modern welfare state. The State no longer presents itself solely as an entity that pays subsidies but as a technological partner, guiding the user toward labour market reintegration. The scholar observed how Switzerland is transitioning from the inclusive masculine (using the form "*the male unemployed*" to indicate anyone) to more equitable forms that are more respectful of gender equality.

The prominent researcher, after analyzing the job advertisements, consulted nine LLM models to rewrite the job offers in a clear and inclusive manner, respecting gender equality, and it emerged that only three AI models, including ChatGPT, were able to do so, although not without distortions. They proposed, in fact, a reversed order of genders in the job offer, namely "female collaborator/male collaborator" instead of "male collaborate/female collaborator", as would be required by the grammatical convention of the Italian language, which uses the masculine as the "unmarked" gender for mixed groups. The majority of the LLM models returned the advertisements without any modification; while some others proposed grammatically incorrect forms, improperly applying the feminine morpheme "-a" to common-gender nouns.

The research has shown that LLMs can be useful for generating inclusive texts, but the quality of the results depends on the model used and on the type of prompt, and that grammatical formulations are often influenced by the English language. Also in the case of the adoption of AI in Swiss welfare services, gender bias emerges, as well as problematic training models that are insufficiently respectful of gender differences.

In Italy, the use of AI is still limited and, where present, it is concentrated mainly in the fields of care and education.

In recent years the care sector has faced significant challenges, including the growing demand for assistance and the increase in healthcare expenditure, both of which can be correlated with the phenomenon of aging. Several experiments mediated by AI have been conducted, including "smart home technology", which offers the opportunity for 24-hour assistance at low cost for the healthcare system.

AI has been employed to counteract the isolation of non-self-sufficient individuals or those who are simply alone (Christakis, 2019). In these latter two cases experimentation with humanoid robots capable of interacting, communicating and assisting has been particularly innovative. This proposal has profoundly modified the concept of socialization (Turkle, 2011). The advantage of these solutions lies in overcoming physical and psychological limitations. Among the many projects, we recall the project "*Veritas*", dedicated to the promotion of autonomy (Kuhlmann, 2023). Another increasingly widespread use concerns personnel recruitment and selection. AI, in fact, makes it possible to save time and automate the recruitment selection process (Azoulay et al., 2020).

We may recall the experience of the company L'Oreal, which by using AI reports saves approximately 90% of the time generally employed in recruitment processes, freeing human resources and reducing the costs of the process (Black & Van Esch, 2020). While many scholars identify AI as a valuable tool for easily processing curricula and applications for a wide range of job positions (Black & van Esch, 2020; Raghavan et al., 2020); others identify issues particularly related to the female gender (Cirillo et al., 2020) precisely because of gender bias, which excludes women from potential candidacy a priori.

Unilever has also adopted an artificial intelligence system to monitor employee well-being through the anonymous analysis of data (such as corporate emails, meetings and digital interactions). The objective is to detect signals of stress or decreased engagement and to propose targeted support activities, such as coaching or moments of decompression.

Vodafone, instead, has relied on a chatbot with a virtual assistant dedicated to its employees, which is able to respond in real time to various questions concerning holidays, leave, benefits and welfare initiatives.

The Italian proposal for the use of AI is still rather limited; in the public sector we may recall the CieID (Electronic Identity Card) and SPID (Public Digital Identity System), which has encountered several difficulties in its legitimization and use. However, pioneering initiatives are not lacking, including those specifically involving the female gender.

Beyond internal developments, many companies rely on external providers specializing in AI solutions for employee well-being, such as *Lifeed* or *Arianna.*

Lifeeed combines welfare and AI to give value to experiences such as those of caregivers: the competencies developed while caring for a child are "extracted" through a process known as *Life Based Learning* (LBL) by AI, transformed into algorithms and transliterated into value for the company. LBL is a corporate training project which aims to strengthen transversal competencies that develop during life transitions. Users participate in digital pathways, in which processes of metareflection on their daily responsibilities are stimulated. AI analyzes these reflections, transforms them into algorithms recognizable by the world of work, transliterating them into soft skills, such as empathy, resilience or problem-solving ability. In this model women are highly involved, since we know that they are much more engaged in caregiving tasks and in supporting the education of children. In Italy, unpaid care work represents 85% of unpaid labour; 71% of this value is produced by women's unpaid care work. Italy is the second country in the European Union, after Portugal, in the number of minutes (306 minutes, that is more than 6 hours) devoted daily by women to informal welfare.

Another interesting example that combines AI and welfare is *Arianna*: a digital assistant designed by Italian companies with the aim of supporting employees in accessing welfare services, managing benefits and booking various activities. Arianna also offers healthcare welfare systems and family assistance with *Arianna Care*; as well as assistance for the elderly in collaboration with the University of Genoa. The system uses modular devices, including wearable environmental sensors, namely "wearable nearables", useful for monitoring daily activities such as movement and posture; nutrition; and personal hygiene. Thanks to this technology, AI is able to localize, monitor and identify social actors in everyday life, processing habits and emergencies. Compared to other similar algorithmic systems, Arianna is more sophisticated thanks to a wide spectrum of ADL, adapting over time to the different needs of individuals. These innovative systems may also present critical issues such as:

-dependence on the device, in fact it is not suitable for use by those who present cognitive deficits and who, therefore, cannot guarantee its wearability;

-the ambiguity of the data, in fact *Arianna* might not be able to distinguish an accidental fall from a sitting, although it subsequently uses vocal interactions to resolve critical situations;

-technological limitations, particularly in cases where there are interruptions in network connectivity;

-acceptance of the system by its potential users. Not everyone may appreciate being monitored 24 hours a day by an algorithmic system.

With regard to women, bias-related limitations emerge, highlighting critical issues in identifying specific female needs, which are expressions of gendered physiology, such as posture or behavioral patterns, that may not be detected by the system and could cause serious risks. There is also the possibility, already mentioned, of training and design bias in the system with respect to complex and specific pathologies. Obviously, implementation solutions are currently being studied in order to address the issues just outlined.

Another example of AI applied to welfare, and specifically impacting women, is the *chatbot Viola*, designed through crowdfunding and made operational thanks to several private foundations that aim to develop the technological infrastructure and support the international expansion of the service. The *Viola* app, launched in the summer of 2024, offers a free video call service available 7 days a week, aimed at women who feel threatened in the street and seek support or assistance. *Viola* supporters virtually accompany users home through video calls thanks to geolocation. Large companies in the distribution, logistics and services sectors finance the system by joining the network of "Viola points", covering the costs of staff training and the management of physical support points across the territory. The operational sustainability of the virtual accompaniment service relies on voluntary solidarity, which helps reduce costs. There are also implementations of Viola such as, for example, *Viola IVG* (Judicial Sales Institute) of Cremona, which helps users navigate the complex world of legal procedures related to judicial real estate sales, making the possibility of purchasing a home more accessible.

Finally, we may cite the case of the strengthening of healthcare welfare in the Lombardy region, where AI aims to make the public system faster and more precise through large-scale oncological diagnostic imaging; predictive medicine; and high-precision surgery. The integration of AI into the healthcare and social system of Northern Italy represents the transition from a "redistributive welfare" model to a "predictive and personalized" model, based on risk management rather than damage management. The body, according to this welfare management model mediated by AI, is no longer classified according to statistical averages but becomes a unique biographical entity. The managerial and organizational model, therefore, seeks to orient itself toward the reduction of anomie and toward the provision of universal medical care. Despite the absolute novelty that certainly produces significant benefits, we identify at least one evident risk: that of algorithmic inequality, which runs across the various explorations examined here. In our view, there is in fact a concrete risk that a new hierarchy may emerge between those who have access to "AI-driven" hospitals and those who remain linked to technologically outdated structures.

As we have seen in several countries certain systems have been used for welfare services which, however, at the current state of the art have revealed a number of significant problems. Numerous critical issues concern the design and training of AI; and various complications arise during the modelling phase. Problems have been identified in the phases of monitoring the delivery of welfare services, just as the issue concerning the global dominance of a single geographical area in the production and provision of AI platforms remains crucial.

A highly complex multidimensional scenario emerges in its delineation, which requires the involvement of different disciplines in order to define the role and objectives of AI, as well as the goals that are intended to be achieved.

We might be tempted to think that the global world offers global opportunities, forgetting not only the pervasive *digital divide* between rich and poor countries, but also the *cognitive divide* that affects a large portion of the population even in the Global North. Technologies, even if they give us the impression of greater well-being, do not distribute it equally across the planet.

THREE EMBLEMATIC CASES: SYRI; CAF AND BOSCO

In our exploration, we encountered numerous international case studies that examined algorithmic systems applied to public welfare or the inequalities caused by bias. Among those investigated, using a "purposive sampling" strategy, we considered it decisive to select three: SYRI, CAF, and BOSCO because, in our view, they represent three symbolic cases that are particularly representative and comprehensive regarding the various types of bias that exclude women from welfare services. Comparing these cases allows us to isolate gender as a constant variable: the algorithm acts as a multiplier of marginalization, transforming the specific characteristics of single-parent households and female care networks into "systemic anomalies" or criteria for exclusion.

RESEARCH METHODOLOGY

The three case studies were selected using the "critical case selection" approach (Flyvbjerg, 2011). These three cases have already been examined individually in scientific research, but not from a gender perspective; furthermore, according to our exploratory findings, they have never been compared using a "qualitative comparative research" approach. We believe that comparing them is valuable for our research because it allows us to examine in practice what has been observed theoretically in platform-based welfare models.

By reaching a theoretical saturation that correlates the dimensions of the state, algorithms, and gender, these cases represent, in our view, "borderline cases" regarding the dimensions of surveillance, the issue of gender bias, and access to services.

Syri Case

In the Netherlands, the automation of the welfare system through algorithms and risk analysis systems has been gradually introduced since 2013–2014. The **SyRI** (System Risk Indicators) system was introduced in 2014 with the aim of profiling citizens and predicting the risk of fraud in social benefits. Through extensive use of administrative data, the system produced an automated classification of beneficiaries, identifying certain profiles as potential "fraudsters." Women—and in particular single mothers and women with immigrant backgrounds—were overrepresented among welfare recipients and, as a result, more exposed to monitoring mechanisms. After several years of testing, administrators realized that Syri disproportionately selected certain social groups, including women; so in 2019, they developed "Smart Check" (SC), a machine learning algorithm for assessing benefits based on "explainable boosting" techniques, to ensure greater transparency. SC excluded sensitive data such as ethnicity; age; or gender; focusing instead on factors like credit history, the number of registered addresses and previous welfare applications. In 2020, the Hague Court ruled that SyRI violated human rights and the right to privacy because it marginalized precisely those who needed help and services the most due to systemic biases.

Tests conducted in 2022 confirmed the persistence of systemic bias: the algorithm, in fact, disadvantaged migrants and single parents—particularly single mothers and women of North African origin—by marginalizing them relative to Dutch residents in applications for benefits. In 2023, Amsterdam abandoned AI, returning to manual case selection in the welfare sector.

This case is illustrative, as it demonstrates the shift from a welfare system based on redistribution and public trust to one focused on control and risk management. Far from being neutral, the algorithm tended to embed and amplify structural inequalities. Furthermore, the system's opacity made it difficult to challenge decisions, thereby reinforcing a dynamic of social exclusion.

This case thus highlights how the use of artificial intelligence in the welfare sector can lead to an asymmetrical redistribution of risk and control, with particularly severe consequences for women in vulnerable situations.

CAF Case

The Caisse d'Allocations Familiales (**CAF**) system is part of the French welfare system, which is characterized by a high degree of administrative digitalization and the progressive use of algorithmic tools. Starting in 2010 and intensifying to the present day, the agency has developed scoring models aimed at identifying beneficiaries considered at risk of fraud, operating on a national scale, with a particular focus on the most socially vulnerable areas. This constitutes a form of probability-based governance, in which beneficiaries are classified according to a risk score derived from administrative data such as income, job insecurity, and high housing costs. These socioeconomic factors disproportionately emphasize the female gender, which in France often faces job insecurity and lower income compared to men. In this context, the AI tends to monitor single mothers more closely due to the factors mentioned. Within this context, dynamics of institutional stigmatization emerge; in fact, single mothers are audited up to 25% more frequently than the average.

In this welfare system, artificial intelligence does not create new inequalities but rather institutionalizes and amplifies them, systematizing a selection process that disproportionately affects already vulnerable groups. AI contributes to shifting the welfare system toward a logic of permanent suspicion, creating tension between administrative efficiency and social justice, in which low-income women are particularly disadvantaged.

The result, therefore, is a welfare system that is increasingly focused on control, in which the logic of suspicion prevails over that of social protection.

Bosco Case

BOSCO was established in Belgium as an institutional response to the growing managerial complexity of the welfare system, in a context marked by fragmented services and social and political pressures aimed at improving administrative efficiency. The initial goal was to coordinate information flows among social agencies by creating an infrastructure capable of integrating data on unemployment; income; assistance; and family histories. This organizational core was later expanded to include a "predictive function" capable of transforming diverse information into "social risk" indicators designed to guide welfare monitoring and interventions.

Migrants, the unemployed, and vulnerable households—namely, the groups most exposed to precariousness—have become the primary targets of predictive surveillance in Belgium. According to BOSCO, women stand out among the "at-risk" groups in Belgium, as they are more likely to face housing insecurity and irregular income.

In this case, AI interprets socioeconomic data in a distorted way: it confuses vulnerability with "suspicion", transforming socially determined characteristics into "deviance".

The algorithm reproduces and exacerbates preexisting inequalities, disproportionately affecting those who are already marginalized, such as single women and widows (Wisner Glusko, 2025).

In the BOSCO system, therefore, managerial rationality takes precedence over the logic of care, giving rise to a welfare model focused on the administrative prevention of deviance rather than on providing support for precarious situations through welfare services.

Table 1. Case Studies: SYRI, CAF, and BOSCO. Source: Author's analysis (2026).

CASE	FOCUS	TARGET	WELFARE	BIAS	MISTAKE	LEGAL OUTCOME
SYRI (NL)	Welfare Fraud (Comprehensive Data Matching: Income; Employment; Housing; Family)	Low-income neighborhoods and vulnerable residents	Social assistance, housing, family benefits	Proxy discrimination based on social class (single mothers with intermittent employment histories); ethnicity (Moroccan, Turkish, and African)	Error in Geographic Profiling (Poverty + Female Gender = Risk)	Ruled illegal by the Hague Court (2020) because it violates privacy (ECHR)
CAF (FR)	Family benefits	Single mothers and low-income residents	Family benefits (child support, housing assistance, nursing homes)	Proxy discrimination based on social class (single mothers considered "high-risk")	Logical Error (Instability in Women's Life Paths)	Under Review (2024–2025): Amnesty International's Actions Regarding Systemic Discrimination
BOSCO (SP)	Energy poverty	Vulnerable female consumers at risk of energy poverty.	Unemployment, minimum income, family benefits	Discrimination against widows	Transparency Error (Code Opacity)	"Mandatory Transparency Ruling" (2025). The Supreme Court ordered the state to release the code.

Toward Digital Universalism and the Automation of Subsidiarity

Among the numerous critical issues illustrated, we also emphasize several positive aspects that can be identified within the "digital welfare state", such as: the elimination of physical or geographical barriers for those who are unable to reach the service location. AI-digitalized services allow certain marginalized groups to access benefits that would otherwise require prohibitive physical or economic efforts, transforming the old and pervasive "digital divide" into social capital, provided that behind the modelling of the service there is a "proper" design (Helsper, 2021, Ragnedda & Ruiu, 2020). Furthermore, there is the advantage of a form of "individual proactivism", which is expressed in state action that does not wait for the citizen's request for a service but anticipates it, configuring public administration as a 4.0 administration (Tang, 2021). For women, more generally, the advantage could consist of services that are more tailored and simplified in terms of timing and effective delivery, provided that the critical issues related to training and design bias are overcome. Digital welfare could potentially intervene in the process of the so-called "double presence" (Saraceno, 2021), namely the structural condition of women divided between production and social reproduction. The effect would be that of the "de-bureaucratization" of care work, which would reduce the overall burden that weighs on women. Platform welfare would be able to reduce the friction between everyday life and the administrative apparatus, thanks to an externalization of bureaucratic functions (Vecchi, 2020).

AI is transforming public work, proposing an "algorithmic bureaucracy" which, if correctly implemented, could be capable of reducing the informational asymmetry of the traditional welfare system. The advantage for women could lie in the minimization of "relational vulnerability", which some women have experienced in human interactions when requesting services. In the human dimension, in fact, subjectivity may give rise to prejudices and gender stereotypes. Automation shifts the provision of services onto algorithmic tracks which, if properly modelled, could reduce subjective arbitrariness (Casilli, 2020).

Moreover, the process of algorithmic datafication concerning care work and the management of family governance could stimulate the emergence of the invisible labour that women have carried out for decades in care and education, highlighting the importance and value of informal welfare, which would otherwise be difficult to quantify.

Digital welfare, by enabling service requests without intermediaries, would also allow women who live in contexts of strong social control direct access to the platform as well as decision-making autonomy.

Welfare systems, moreover, if interconnected, would allow the creation of a "proactive ecosystem" capable of ensuring the universalism of welfare, reducing phenomena of exclusion and social marginalization.

In light of the three cases analyzed, several policy recommendations emerge that are relevant for public decision-makers, particularly regarding the interplay between AI, welfare, and gender inequalities.

It is essential to introduce mechanisms for algorithmic transparency; ensuring that risk classification criteria are accessible, explainable, and contestable, while avoiding "opaque" models.

It is also crucial to integrate a gender perspective into system design, particularly for women—single mothers and migrant women—who are disproportionately subject to scrutiny. Particular attention must be paid to the quality and nature of the data used. Since many biases stem from proxy variables (income, family composition, geographic area), it is necessary to limit the use of indicators that reflect structural inequalities, or to correct them through fairness techniques and statistical rebalancing. It is also essential to strengthen institutional accountability mechanisms. Citizens must be able to challenge automated decisions quickly and using accessible tools, ensuring that technical complexity does not become a barrier to the exercise of their rights. Finally, governments should promote ongoing, independent evaluation of algorithmic systems, involving research institutions, regulatory authorities, and civil society organizations.

From our research, we have identified a new form of welfare, which we shall refer to here as "**universal digital welfare**", capable of guaranteeing women the bureaucratic restructuring of the female life course, which is rarely linear, both as a result of social reproduction and of caregiving responsibilities toward parents in later life, as well as due to the phenomenon of involuntary part-time work, which is very frequent in Italy. An integrated system in which individual data are able to reconstruct contributions; interruptions; part-time work; and benefits would also be capable of accounting for the "structural discontinuity" of female biographies.

The integration of systems would thus realize the automation of subsidiarity, freeing social time and transforming welfare from a reactive system into an environmental protection infrastructure, which intervenes automatically when a need arises.

CONCLUSION

In light of our reflections, we can affirm that technological architectures no longer represent merely possible cognitive frameworks for common sense, but act as genuine identity vectors within the dynamics of socialization and learning pathways. They reconfigure our ability to critically decode social phenomena and to process the flow of information.

The diffusion of AI, as shown in our empirical explorations, often leads to categorization and to the emergence of an artificial common sense. Among the numerous critical issues and the multiple doubts highlighted in our investigation, the concern repeatedly arises regarding the real capacity of these systems to capture the complexity of community contexts and of individual social actors.

The transition toward a model of a platformized society also raises crucial questions, which involve inequalities and the gender dimension.

If the danger, as Barrett (2019) suggests, lies in the potential slide toward reductionist "social ontologies", which attempt to map ethnicities, genders and human geographies through a superficial knowledge of the existential ecosystem, we should not forget to consider that this process is not without frictions such as: the diversity and resistance of environmental contexts; the irreducibility of human complexity; or individual agency.

From our observations, several social manifestations emerge, among which a phenomenon that we will refer to as "algorithmic ontological hegemony", which promotes global categorization and stimulates the crystallization of genders, ultimately leading to a form of "epistemological narcissism" (Tipaldo, 2019), that presents a partial dimension as a universal one.

A tendency toward the persistence of territorial asymmetries emerges, highlighting disparities between the Global North and the Global South, transforming the well-known phenomenon of the "digital divide" into a "cognitive divide".

Finally, a tendency emerges toward the underrepresentation of the female gender, particularly in the STEM sectors, and a certain propensity toward vertical segregation, which with AI transforms into "transversal segregation", further marginalizing women (Sun et al., 2024).

Numerous cases of AI-mediated welfare have not achieved the success expected by developers and gatekeepers, as we have illustrated in this contribution, however, there are also positive cases such as *Lifeed*, *Arianna* or *Viola*, which, being inspired by inclusive and transparent modelling, succeed in transforming technology into an ally of social justice. In these experiments, AI indeed opens spaces for mitigating gender differences, attempting to overcome social vulnerability and the phenomenon of the female "double presence".

We have repeatedly referred in our contribution to the numerous biases present in Italian and international welfare services, but some successful experiences show us that it is possible to overcome them by implementing a profound cultural transformation.

Technocrats, who play a significant role in the modelling work of AI, must be trained so that the algorithms they develop take into account the multidimensionality of human beings; social dynamics and their behavioral and expressive complexity, minimizing biases as much as possible.

The ethical issue, therefore, shifts our attention to data transparency and to social responsibility in algorithmic design, calling into question the need for inclusive languages and cultural structures capable of dismantling gender asymmetries. From this perspective, technologies should not be configured as monolithic structures but as open architectures, capable of integrating a pluralism of perspectives.

The evolution from traditional Welfare to Universal Digital Welfare thus marks a paradigm shift in the structure of public administrations. This transformation is reflected in the disintermediation of the relationship between the State and citizens (Tang, 2021). In this scenario, the platform does not represent a simple archive but becomes a genuine digital controller, governing access to fundamental rights through the management of sensitive data, guaranteeing democratic welfare processes beyond origin and social class; level of education; as well as gender.

Through a reconfiguration of cognitive paradigms and dominant cultural frames, it becomes possible to address ethical aporias and neutralize the structural biases intrinsic to these systems, thus enabling the transition toward platformized governance. From this perspective, Universal Digital Welfare would be configured as a proactive mechanism aimed at the systemic recomposition of female biographical trajectories, historically fragmented by the structural conflict between the sphere of production and that of social reproduction.

To achieve this goal it is necessary to undertake an epistemological repositioning, which restores centrality to the biographies and lived narratives of those who have directly experienced the negative externalities of AI architectures.

Within this perspective sociology emerges as an essential critical discipline, capable of activating a critical reading aimed at decoding the latent prejudices embedded in data (Wallach, 2014). Sociological research is indeed able to penetrate the dense web of gender biases; decode the complexity of logical structures, as well as the multifaceted discursive aesthetics, whether conveyed through linguistic codes or through the semantics of images.

In our view the challenge of the future lies precisely in the ability to model technologies, which are not merely aseptic automations, but instruments of social equity capable of representing the real complexity of contemporaneity.

REFERENCES

Airoldi, M. (2021). *Machine Habitus: Toward a Sociology of Algorithms*. Polity Press.

Allhutter, D., Cech, F., Fischer, F., Grill, G., & Mager, A. (2020). Algorithmic profiling of job seekers in Austria: How austerity politics are made effective. *Frontiers in Big Data, 3*, 5. DOI: 10.3389/fdata.2020.00005 PMID: 33693380

Alston, P. (2020). The committee on economic, social and cultural rights. *NYU Law and Economics Research Paper*, (20-24).

Alvarado, R. (2023). AI as an epistemic technology. *Science and Engineering Ethics, 29*(5), 32. DOI: 10.1007/s11948-023-00451-3 PMID: 37603120

Aragona, B. (2020). Sistemi di decisione algoritmica e disuguaglianze sociali: Le evidenze della ricerca, il ruolo della politica. *La Rivista delle Politiche Sociali, 2*(20), 213–226.

Arendt, H. (2019). [1958]). *La lingua materna: La condizione umana e il pensiero plurale. Mimesis.*

Armantier, O., ... (2024), "Nothing to hide? Gender and age differences in willingness to share data", *BIS Working Papers*, 1187: 1-33, available on: https://www.bis.org/publ/work1187.pdf

Azoulay, E., Lefebvre, P., & Marlin, R. (2020). Using artificial intelligence to diversify the recruitment process at L'Oréal. *Le journal de l'ecole de Paris du management, 142*(2), 16-22.

Bailey, S., Pierides, D., Brisley, A., Weisshaar, C., & Blakeman, T. (2020). Dismembering organisation: The coordination of algorithmic work in healthcare. *Current Sociology, 68*(4), 546–571. DOI: 10.1177/0011392120907638

Barrett, L. F., Adolphs, R., Marsella, S., Martinez, A. M., & Pollak, S. D. (2019). Emotional expressions reconsidered: Challenges to inferring emotion from human facial movements. *Psychological Science in the Public Interest, 20*(1), 1–68. DOI: 10.1177/1529100619832930 PMID: 31313636

Basta, C., Costa-Jussà, M. R., & Casas, N. (2019). Evaluating the underlying gender bias in contextualized word embeddings. In *Proceedings of the first workshop on gender bias in natural language processing* (pp. 33-39). DOI: 10.18653/v1/W19-3805

Bell, A., Sharma, D., & Britain, D. (2016). Labov in sociolinguistics: An introduction. *Journal of Sociolinguistics, 20*(4), 399–408. DOI: 10.1111/josl.12199

Bender, E. M., Gebru, T., McMillan-Major, A., & Shmitchell, S. (2021, March). On the dangers of stochastic parrots: Can language models be too big? In *Proceedings of the 2021 ACM conference on fairness, accountability, and transparency* (pp. 610-623). DOI: 10.1145/3442188.3445922

Benjamin, R. (Ed.). (2019). *Captivating technology: Race, carceral technoscience, and liberatory imagination in everyday life*. Duke University Press.

Bhambra, G. K. (2014). Introduction: Knowledge production in global context: Power and coloniality. *Current Sociology, 62*(4), 451–456. DOI: 10.1177/0011392114524504 PMID: 25418995

Black, J. S., & van Esch, P. (2020). AI-enabled recruiting: What is it and how should a manager use it? *Business Horizons, 63*(2), 215–226. DOI: 10.1016/j.bushor.2019.12.001

Bourdieu, P. (1983). *La distinzione: Critica sociale del gusto*. Il Mulino.

Boyd, R., & Holton, R. J. (2018). Technology, innovation, employment and power: Does robotics and artificial intelligence really mean social transformation? *Journal of Sociology (Melbourne, Vic.), 54*(3), 331–345. DOI: 10.1177/1440783317726591

Broussard, M. (2018). *Artificial unintelligence: How computers misunderstand the world*. mit Press.

Buolamwini, J., & Gebru, T. (2018, January). Gender shades: Intersectional accuracy disparities in commercial gender classification. In *Conference on fairness, accountability and transparency* (pp. 77-91). PMLR.

Burrell, J., & Fourcade, M. (2021). The society of algorithms. *Annual Review of Sociology, 47*(1), 213–237. DOI: 10.1146/annurev-soc-090820-020800

Butler, J., & Trouble, G. (1990). Feminism and the Subversion of Identity. *Gender trouble, 3*(1), 3-17.

Casilli, A. A. (2020). *Schiavi del clic: perché lavoriamo tutti per il nuovo capitalismo?* Feltrinelli Editore.

Christakis, N. A. (2019). *Blueprint: The evolutionary origins of a good society*. Little, Brown Spark.

Cirillo, D., Catuara-Solarz, S., Morey, C., Guney, E., Subirats, L., Mellino, S., Gigante, A., Valencia, A., Rementeria, M. J., Chadha, A. S., & Mavridis, N. (2020). Sex and gender differences and biases in artificial intelligence for biomedicine and healthcare. *NPJ Digital Medicine, 3*(1), 81. DOI: 10.1038/s41746-020-0288-5 PMID: 32529043

Clark, J. (1982). Catherine Hakim, Occupational Segregation: A comparative study of the degree and pattern of the differentiation between men and women's work in Britain, the United States and other countries, Research Paper No. 9, November 1979, Department of Employment, London, 1979. 65 pp. No price given. *Journal of Social Policy, 11*(1), 131–132. DOI: 10.1017/S004727940001151X

Coccia, M. (2020). Artificial intelligence technology in oncology: A new technological paradigm. *Technological Forecasting and Social Change*, 151, available on: https://arxiv.org/pdf/1905.06871

Cohen, J. E. (2019). Review of Zuboff's the age of surveillance capitalism. *Surveillance & Society, 17*(1/2), 240–245. DOI: 10.24908/ss.v17i1/2.13144

Correll, S. J. (2004). Constraints into preferences. Gender, status, and emerging career aspirations. *American Sociological Review, 69*(1), 93–113. DOI: 10.1177/000312240406900106

Couldry, N., & Mejias, U. A. (2019). *The Costs of Connection: How Data Is Colonizing Human Life and Appropriating It for Capitalism.* Stanford University Press.

Craciun, G., Zhou, W., & Shan, Z. (2020). Discrete emotions effects on electronic word-of-mouth helpfulness: The moderating role of reviewer gender and contextual emotional tone. *Decision Support Systems, 130*, 113226. DOI: 10.1016/j.dss.2019.113226

Crawford, K. (2017, December). The trouble with bias. In *Conference on Neural Information Processing Systems, invited speaker.*

Crawford, K. (2021). *Atlas of AI: Power, politics, and the planetary costs of artificial intelligence.* Yale University Press.

Crawford, K. (2024). World view. *Nature, 626*, 693. DOI: 10.1038/d41586-024-00478-x PMID: 38378831

Crenshaw, K. W. (2013). Mapping the margins: Intersectionality, identity politics, and violence against women of color. In *The public nature of private violence* (pp. 93–118). Routledge.

Cuccaro-Alamin, S., Foust, R., Vaithianathan, R., & Putnam-Hornstein, E. (2017). Risk assessment and decision making in child protective services: Predictive risk modeling in context. *Children and Youth Services Review, 79*, 291–298. DOI: 10.1016/j.childyouth.2017.06.027

Damant, J., Knapp, M., Freddolino, P., & Lombard, D. (2017). Effects of digital engagement on the quality of life of older people. *Health & Social Care in the Community*, *25*(6), 1679–1703. DOI: 10.1111/hsc.12335 PMID: 26919220

Danaher, J., & McArthur, N. (Eds.). (2017). *Robot sex: Social and ethical implications*. MIT press. DOI: 10.7551/mitpress/9780262036689.001.0001

De Cesare, A. M. (2025). L'intelligenza artificiale generativa al servizio della parità di genere: uno studio esplorativo sugli annunci di lavoro della Confederazione svizzera. *Inclusione ed elaborazione del linguaggio naturale nell'era dell'intelligenza artificiale generativa*, 59.

De las Cuevas, P., García-Arenas, M., & Rico, N. (2022). Why not STEM? A study case on the influence of gender factors on students' higher education choice. *Mathematics*, *10*(2), 239. DOI: 10.3390/math10020239

De Simone, A. (2020). Essere e politica: Dialettica dell'umano. *Mimesis.*

Dencik, L., & Kaun, A. (2020). Datafication and the welfare state. *Global Perspectives*, *1*(1), 12912. DOI: 10.1525/gp.2020.12912

Deriu, F. (2020). Luci e ombre dell'innovazione digitale nel welfare dei servizi alla persona in Italia. *La Rivista delle Politiche sociali, 3*, 255-271.

England, P. (2010). The gender revolution. Uneven and Stalled. *Gender & Society*, *24*(2), 149–166. DOI: 10.1177/0891243210361475

Esposito, E. (2022). Does explainability require transparency? *Sociologica*, *16*(3), 17–27.

Eubanks, V. (2018). *Automating inequality: How high-tech tools profile, police, and punish the poor.* Macmillan+ ORM.

Fahse, A., Karimi, F., & Kunegis, J. (2021). The structure of bias in human-generated data. *Journal of Computational Social Science*, *4*(2), 645–663.

Floridi, L. (2015). The new grey power. *Philosophy & Technology*, *28*(3), 329–332. DOI: 10.1007/s13347-015-0206-y

Foucault, M. (1996). *Archivio Foucault. Interventi, colloqui, interviste* (Vol. 3). Feltrinelli Editore.

Frennert, S. (2021). Gender blindness: On health and welfare technology, AI and gender equality in community care. [Wiley.]. *Nursing Inquiry*, *28*(4), e12411. DOI: 10.1111/nin.12419 PMID: 33979011

Garrido-Muñoz, A., Montejo-Ráez, A., Martínez-Camara, E., Almeida-Cruz, Y., Frenda, S., García-Vega, M., & Sánchez, D. (2021). A normative definition of cognitive bias for computational applications. *arXiv preprint arXiv:2305.09281.*

Gebru, T. (2020). Race and gender. *The Oxford handbook of ethics of AI, 4,* 253.

Gehl Sampath, P. (2021). Governing artificial intelligence in an age of inequality. *Global Policy, 12*(S6), 21–31. DOI: 10.1111/1758-5899.12940

Gillespie, T. (2024). Generative AI and the politics of visibility. *Big Data & Society, 11*(2), 20539517241252131. DOI: 10.1177/20539517241252131

Gmyrek, P., Berg, J., & Bescond, D. (2023). Generative AI and jobs: A global analysis of potential effects on job quantity and quality.

Gray, M. L., & Suri, S. (2019). *Ghost Work: How to Stop Silicon Valley from Building a New Global Underclass.* Houghton Mifflin Harcourt.

Green, B., & Viljoen, S. (2020). Algorithmic realism: Expanding the boundaries of algorithmic thought. *Philosophy & Technology, 33*(1), 1–23.

Grieve, J., Bartl, S., & Fuoli, M.. (2025). The sociolinguistic foundations of language modeling. *Frontiers.* PMID: 39871863

Guo, W., & Caliskan, A. (2021). Detecting emergent intersectional biases: Contextualized word embeddings contain a distribution of human-like biases. *In Proceedings of the 2021 AAAI/ACM Conference on AI, Ethics, and Society* (pp. 122-133).

Hakim, C. (1992). Explaining trends in occupational segregation: The measurement, causes, and consequences of the sexual division of labour. *European Sociological Review,* 8(2), 127–152. DOI: 10.1093/oxfordjournals.esr.a036628

Hans, J. (2009). *Il principio responsabilità. Un'etica per la civiltà tecnologica.* Einaudi.

Hansen, M. J., Palakal, M. J., & White, L. J. (2024). The importance of STEM sense of belonging and academic hope in enhancing persistence for low-income, underrepresented STEM students. *Journal for STEM Education Research,* 7(2), 155–180. DOI: 10.1007/s41979-023-00096-8

Helsper, E. J. (2021). Digital world: from divides to socio-digital inequalities. *The digital disconnect. The social causes and consequences of digital inequalities. SAGE Publications,* 27-45.

Huang, J., Saleh, S., & Liu, Y. (2021). A review on artificial intelligence in education. *Academic Journal of Interdisciplinary Studies, 10*(3), 3. DOI: 10.36941/ajis-2021-0077

James, A., & Whelan, A. (2022). 'Ethical' artificial intelligence in the welfare state: Discourse and discrepancy in Australian social services. [Sage.]. *Critical Social Policy, 42*(1), 22–42. DOI: 10.1177/0261018320985463

Joyce, K., & Cruz, T. M. (2024). A Sociology of Artificial Intelligence: Inequalities, Power, and Data Justice. *Socius: Sociological Research for a Dynamic World, 10*, 10. DOI: 10.1177/23780231241275393

Kristensen, D. B., & Prigge, C. (2017). Human/technology associations in self-tracking practices. In *Self-tracking: Empirical and philosophical investigations* (pp. 43–59). Springer International Publishing.

Kuhlmann, R. (2023). Assistive technologies for people with disabilities, available on: https://www.veritas-project.eu/assistive-technologienfuer-menschen-mit-behinderungen/

Lamont, M. (2000). *The dignity of working men: Morality and the boundaries of race, class, and immigration*. Harvard University Press. DOI: 10.4159/9780674039889

Leavy, S. (2018, May). Gender bias in artificial intelligence: The need for diversity and gender theory in machine learning. In *Proceedings of the 1st international workshop on gender equality in software engineering* (pp. 14-16). DOI: 10.1145/3195570.3195580

Longworth, J. (2021). Benjamin Ruha (2019) Race After Technology: Abolitionist Tools for the New Jim Code. Medford: Polity Press. *Science & Technology Studies, 34*(2), 92–94. DOI: 10.23987/sts.102639

Lorentzen, A. C. R. (2022). Digital transformation as distributed leadership: Firing the change agent. *Procedia Computer Science, 196*, 245–254. DOI: 10.1016/j.procs.2021.12.011

Magaudda, P., & Neresini, F. (2020). *Gli studi sociali sulla scienza e la tecnologia, il Mulino.*

McCarthy, J. (2022). Artificial intelligence, logic, and formalising common sense. *Machine Learning and the City: Applications in Architecture and Urban Design*, 69-90.

Miano, F. (2013). *Günther Anders, Sulla vergogna prometeica, Etica & Politica / Ethics & Politics*, XV, 2013, 2, pp. 246-257, available on: https://www.openstarts.units.it/server/api/core/bitstreams/9a045474-1f61-4f37-9013-75a62a663f1d/content

Miragoli, M. (2025). Conformism, ignorance & injustice: AI as a tool of epistemic oppression. *Episteme (Edinburgh)*, *22*(2), 522–540. DOI: 10.1017/epi.2024.11

Murru, M. F., & Selva, D. (2025). Senso comune artificiale: Egemonia culturale e intelligenza artificiale generativa. *COMUNICAZIONI SOCIALI*, 1-18.

Nangia, N., Vania, C., Bhalerao, R., & Bowman, S. (2020). CrowS-pairs: A challenge dataset for measuring social biases in masked language models. *In Proceedings of the 2020 Conference on Empirical Methods in Natural Language Processing (EMNLP)* (pp. 1953-1967). DOI: 10.18653/v1/2020.emnlp-main.154

Newell, A., & Simon, H. A. (1976). Computer science as empirical inquiry: Symbols and search. *Communications of the ACM*, *19*(3), 113–126. DOI: 10.1145/360018.360022

Noble, S. U. (2018). Algorithms of oppression: How search engines reinforce racism. In *Algorithms of oppression*. New York university press.

Oleksy, T., & Wnuk, A. (2021). Do women perceive sex robots as threatening? The role of political views and presenting the robot as a female-vs male-friendly product. *Computers in Human Behavior*, *117*, 106664. DOI: 10.1016/j.chb.2020.106664

Park, S., & Humphry, J. (2019). Exclusion by design: Intersections of social, digital and data exclusion. [Taylor & Francis.]. *Information Communication and Society*, *22*(7), 934–953. DOI: 10.1080/1369118X.2019.1606266

Parsons, T. (2021). *La struttura dell'azione sociale: Uno studio di teoria sociale con particolare riferimento a un gruppo di autori europei recenti* (Vol. I e II). Mimesis.

Pascale, C. M. (2013). Social inequality & the politics of representation. *Sage (Atlanta, Ga.)*.

Pasciuto, F. (2022). *L'algoritmo della cultura: Processi di produzione e consumo nell'era digitale*. FrancoAngeli.

Piccone Stella, S., & Saraceno, C. (1996). *Genere. La costruzione sociale del femminile e del maschile*. Il Mulino.

Pronzato, R. (2024). *Algoritmi, strutture e agire sociale: Un'analisi sociologica*

Raghavan, M., Barocas, S., Kleinberg, J., & Levy, K. (2020, January). Mitigating bias in algorithmic hiring: Evaluating claims and practices. In *Proceedings of the 2020 conference on fairness, accountability, and transparency* (pp. 469-481). DOI: 10.1145/3351095.3372828

Ragnedda, M., & Ruiu, M. L. (2020). *Digital capital: A Bourdieusian perspective on the digital divide.* Emerald Group Publishing. DOI: 10.1108/9781839095504

Report, I. (2025). Livelli di Istruzione e ritorni occupazionali. Anno 2024. Available on: https://www.istat.it/wp-content/uploads/2025/12/Report-Livelli-di-istruzione-e-ritorni-occupazionali-Anno-2024.pdf

Report, O. E. C. D. (2022). The Effects of AI on the Working Lives of Women, available on: https://www.oecd.org/en/publications/the-effects-of-ai-on-the-working-lives-of-women_14e9b92c-en.html

Report, W. E. F. World Economic Forum (2024). Global Gender Gap. Insight Report, available on: https://www3.weforum.org/docs/WEF_GGGR_2024.pdf

Rubin, G. (1975). The traffic in women: Notes on the "political economy" of sex. In Reiter, R. R. (Ed.), *Toward an anthropology of women* (pp. 157–210). Monthly Review Press.Ruble, D. N., Martin, C. L., & Berenbaum, S. A. (2006). Gender development. In *Damon W., R. M. Lerner R. M. e Eisenberg John N. a cura di* (pp. 858–932). Handbook of Child Psychology. John Wiley & Sons, Inc.

Sadowski, J. (2020). *Too Smart: How Digital Capitalism is Extracting Data, Controlling Our Lives, and Transforming the World.* The MIT Press. DOI: 10.7551/mitpress/12240.001.0001

Saguy, A. C. (2025, November). The Social Constructions of Gender. *Sociological Forum, 40*(S1), S17–S28. DOI: 10.1111/socf.70007

Saiani, P. P. (2020). Verso un welfare state digitale? L'intelligenza artificiale tra politiche sociali e apparati di controllo. *la Rivista delle Politiche Sociali, 237.*

Santosuosso, A. (2020). *Intelligenza artificiale e diritto*. Mondadori Università.

Saraceno, C. (2021). *Il welfare: tra vecchie e nuove disuguaglianze*. Il Mulino.

Shelby, R., Rismani, S., Henne, K., Moon, A., Rostamzadeh, N., Nicholas, P., & Virk, G. (2023, August). Sociotechnical harms of algorithmic systems: Scoping a taxonomy for harm reduction. In *Proceedings of the 2023 AAAI/ACM Conference on AI, Ethics, and Society* (pp. 723-741). DOI: 10.1145/3600211.3604673

Silberg, J., & Manyika, J. (2019). Notes from the AI frontier: Tackling bias in AI (and in humans). *McKinsey Global Institute, 1*(6), 1–31.

Solferino, N., Biondo, A., Alessio E., & D'Agostino, M. (2025). *Sfide etiche dell'Intelligenza Artificiale*. TAB edizioni.

Sorice, M. (2021). *Partecipazione disconnessa. Innovazione democratica e illusione digitale al tempo del neoliberismo*. Carocci editore.

Spencer, S. J., Steele, C. M., & Quinn, D. M. (1999). Stereotype threat and women's math performance. *Journal of Experimental Social Psychology, 35*(1), 4–28. DOI: 10.1006/jesp.1998.1373

Sun, L., Wei, M., Sun, Y., Suh, Y. J., Shen, L., & Yang, S. (2024). Smiling women pitching down: Auditing representational and presentational gender biases in image-generative AI. *Journal of Computer-Mediated Communication, 29*(1), zmad045. DOI: 10.1093/jcmc/zmad045

Suresh, H., & Guttag, J. V. (2020). A framework for understanding unintended consequences of machine learning. ArXiv E-Prints. *arXiv preprint arXiv:1901.10002.*

Tang, C. (2021). *Data capital: How data is reinventing capital for globalization.* Springer Nature. DOI: 10.1007/978-3-030-60192-8

Tipaldo, G. (2019). *La società della post-verità: Dieci tesi su matti, impostori e mentitori seriali*. Il Mulino.

Toupin, S. (2024). Shaping feminist artificial intelligence. [Sage.]. *New Media & Society, 26*(1), 580–595. DOI: 10.1177/14614448221150776

Turing, A. M. (1956). Can a machine think. *The world of mathematics, 4*, 2099-2123.

Turk, V. (2023). How AI reduces the world to stereotypes. *Rest of world, 10.*

Turkle, S. (2011). Insieme ma soli. *Perché ci aspettiamo sempre più dalla tecnologia e sempre meno dagli altri*, 23-27.

Tversky, A., & Kahneman, D. (1974). Judgment under Uncertainty: Heuristics and Biases: Biases in judgments reveal some heuristics of thinking under uncertainty. *science, 185*(4157), 1124-1131.

Van Dijk, J. A. (2006). Digital divide research, achievements and shortcomings. *Poetics, 34*(4-5), 221–235. DOI: 10.1016/j.poetic.2006.05.004

Vantin, S. (2018). *L'eguaglianza di genere tra mutamenti sociali e nuove tecnologie: Percorsi di diritto antidiscriminatorio*. Pacini Editore.

Vecchi, B. (2020). *Il capitalismo delle piattaforme*. Manifestolibri.

Velkova, J., & Kaun, A. (2021). Algorithmic resistance: Media practices and the politics of repair. *Information Communication and Society*, *24*(4), 523–540. DOI: 10.1080/1369118X.2019.1657162

Veneziano, M. (2020). José van Dijck, Thomas Poell, Martijn de Waal, Platform society. Valori pubblici e società connessa. *Quaderni di Sociologia*, (84-LXIV), 168-170.

Vermilyea, M., Hall, J. M. M., Diakiw, S. M., Johnston, A., Nguyen, T., Perugini, D., Miller, A., Picou, A., Murphy, A. P., & Perugini, M. (2020). Development of an artificial intelligence-based assessment model for prediction of embryo viability using static images captured by optical light microscopy during IVF. *Human Reproduction (Oxford, England)*, *35*(4), 770–784. DOI: 10.1093/humrep/deaa013 PMID: 32240301

Vicsek, L. (2021). Artificial intelligence and the future of work–lessons from the sociology of expectations. *The International Journal of Sociology and Social Policy*, *41*(7-8), 842–861. DOI: 10.1108/IJSSP-05-2020-0174

Vogel, B., Avecedo, M., Appelman, Y., & Noel, B. M.. (2021). The Lancet women and cardiovascular disease Commission: Reducing the global burden by 2030. *Lancet*, *397*(10292), 2385–2438. DOI: 10.1016/S0140-6736(21)00684-X PMID: 34010613

Wajcman, J. (2006). Technocapitalism meets technofeminism: women and technology in a wireless world. *Labour & Industry: a journal of the social and economic relations of work*, *16*(3), 7-20.

Wajcman, J. (2017). Automation: Is it really different this time? *The British Journal of Sociology*, *68*(1), 119–127. DOI: 10.1111/1468-4446.12239 PMID: 28321856

Wajcman, J., & Young, E. (2023). Feminism confronts AI. *Feminist AI: Critical perspectives on algorithms, data, and intelligent machines, 47*.

Wallach, H. (2014, December). Big data, machine learning, and the social sciences: Fairness, accountability, and transparency. In *NIPS workshop on fairness, accountability, and transparency in machine learning*.

Wang, M. T., & Degol, J. L. (2017). Gender gap in science, technology, engineering, and mathematics (STEM): Current knowledge, implications for practice, policy, and future directions. *Educational Psychology Review*, *29*(1), 119–140. DOI: 10.1007/s10648-015-9355-x PMID: 28458499

Weizenbaum, J. (1976). *Computer power and human reason: From judgment to calculation*. W. H. Freeman.

Whelan, A. (2020). "Ask for more time": Big data chronopolitics in the Australian welfare bureaucracy. *Critical Sociology, 46*(6), 867–880. DOI: 10.1177/0896920519866004

Women, U. N. (2025). *Advancing gender equality through partnerships for gender-responsive artificial intelligence.* https://www.unwomen.org/sites/default/files/2025-01/partnering-for-gender-responsive-ai-003.pdf

Young, E., Wajcman, J. e Sprejer, L. (2021), *Where are the women? mapping the gender job gap in AI policy briefing* – full report, The Alan Turing Institute, Londra.

Zajko, M. (2022). Artificial intelligence, algorithms, and social inequality: Sociological contributions to contemporary debates. [Wiley.]. *Sociology Compass, 16*(3), e12962. DOI: 10.1111/soc4.12962

Završnik, A. (2021). Algorithmic justice: Algorithms and big data in criminal justice settings. *European Journal of Criminology, 18*(5), 623–642. DOI: 10.1177/1477370819876762

Compilation of References

Abarna, S., Sheeba, J. I., Jayasrilakshmi, S., & Devaneyan, S. P. (2022). Identification of cyber harassment and intention of target users on social media platforms. *Engineering Applications of Artificial Intelligence*, *115*, 105283. DOI: 10.1016/j.engappai.2022.105283 PMID: 35968532

Abramovitz, M., & Zelnik, J. (2026). Managerialism on steroids. The rise of Artificial Intelligence. In Ottman, G., & Noble, C. (Eds.), *AI and the Disruption of Welfare* (pp. 11–28). Routledge., DOI: 10.4324/9781003673675-2

Aceto, G., Persico, V., & Pescapé, A. (2018). The role of information and communication technologies in healthcare: Taxonomies, perspectives, and challenges. *Journal of Network and Computer Applications*, *107*, 125–154. DOI: 10.1016/j.jnca.2018.02.008

Adams, V., Murphy, M., & Clarke, A. E. (2009). Anticipation: Technoscience, life, affect, temporality. *Subjectivity*, *28*(1), 246–265. DOI: 10.1057/sub.2009.18

Addeo, F., & Masullo, G. (2021). Research Methods in the Digital Society: Challenges and opportunities. *Italian Sociological Review*, 11(4S), 153- 369. https://doi.org/DOI: 10.13136/isr.v11i4S.428

Agardh, E., Allebeck, P., Hallqvist, J., Moradi, T., & Sidorchuk, A. (2011). Type 2 diabetes incidence and socio-economic position: A systematic review and meta-analysis. *International Journal of Epidemiology*, *40*(3), 804–818. DOI: 10.1093/ije/dyr029 PMID: 21335614

AgID. (2024). *Piano Triennale per l'Informatica nella Pubblica Amministrazione 2024–2026*. Agenzia per l'Italia Digitale.

Ahmed, S. F., Sharmin, S., Kuldeep, S. A., & Gandomi, A. H. (2025). Transformative impacts of the Internet of Medical Things on modern healthcare. [CoLab]. *Results in Engineering*, *25*, 103787. DOI: 10.1016/j.rineng.2024.103787

Airoldi, M. (2021). *Machine Habitus: Toward a Sociology of Algorithms*. Polity Press.

Al Khatib, I., Shamayleh, A., & Ndiaye, M. (2024). Healthcare and the Internet of Medical Things: Applications, trends, key challenges, and proposed resolutions. [MDPI]. *Informatics (MDPI), 11*(3), 47. DOI: 10.3390/informatics11030047

Albertini, M., & Pavolini, E. (2017). Unequal Inequalities: The Stratification of the Use of Formal Care Among Older Europeans. *The Journals of Gerontology. Series B, Psychological Sciences and Social Sciences, 72*(3), 510–521. DOI: 10.1093/geronb/gbv038 PMID: 26224754

Alexopoulou, S. (2024). Paradigm shift: Exploring the impact of digital technologies on the welfare state through a systematic literature review. *Social Policy and Administration, 59*(1), 135–157. DOI: 10.1111/spol.13054

Alexopoulou, S., Åström, J., & Karlsson, M. (2022). The grey digital divide and welfare state regimes: A comparative study of European countries. *Information Technology & People, 35*(8), 273–291. DOI: 10.1108/ITP-11-2020-0803

Allhutter, D., Cech, F., Fischer, F., Grill, G., & Mager, A. (2020). Algorithmic profiling of job seekers in Austria: How austerity politics are made effective. *Frontiers in Big Data, 3*, 5. DOI: 10.3389/fdata.2020.00005 PMID: 33693380

Alshallaqi, M. (2024). The complexities of digitization and street-level discretion: A socio-materiality perspective. *Public Management Review, 26*(1), 25–47. DOI: 10.1080/14719037.2022.2042726

Alston, P. (2019). *Digital welfare states and human rights: Report of the Special Rapporteur on extreme poverty and human rights* (A/74/493). United Nations General Assembly.

Alston, P. (2020). The committee on economic, social and cultural rights. *NYU Law and Economics Research Paper*, (20-24).

Alvarado, R. (2023). AI as an epistemic technology. *Science and Engineering Ethics, 29*(5), 32. DOI: 10.1007/s11948-023-00451-3 PMID: 37603120

Amato, R. (2025). *Collecting Data on Technology-Facilitated Violence Against Women: Challenges and Ways Forward*. Council of Europe.

Amaturo, E., & Punziano, G. (2013). *Content analysis tra comunicazione e politica*. Ledizioni.

Amnesty International. (2017, 20 November). *Amnesty reveals alarming impact of online abuse against women*. https://www.amnesty.org/en/latest/press-release/2017/11/amnesty-reveals-alarming-impact-of-online-abuse-against-women/

Amnesty International. (2022, 20 April). *Black and Asian women MPs abused more online.* https://www.amnesty.org.uk/knowledge-hub/all-resources/online-violence-women-mps/

Ananny, M., & Crawford, K. (2018). Seeing without knowing: Limitations of the transparency ideal and its application to algorithmic accountability. *New Media & Society*, *20*(3), 973–989. DOI: 10.1177/1461444816676645

Anderson, D. R. (2008). *Model based inference in the life sciences: a primer on evidence*. Springer New York. DOI: 10.1007/978-0-387-74075-1

Andrade, A. N., Cabral, A. T., Bellini, B., Facco Rodrigues, V., da Rosa Righi, R., André da Costa, C., & Barbosa, J. L. V. (2024). IoT-based vital sign monitoring: A literature review. *Smart Health (Amsterdam, Netherlands)*, *32*, 100462. Advance online publication. DOI: 10.1016/j.smhl.2024.100462

Andreassen, H. K., & Trondsen, M. (2010). The empowered patient and the sociologist. *Social Theory & Health*, *8*(3), 280–287. DOI: 10.1057/sth.2010.9

Andrejevic, M. (2014). The big data divide. *International Journal of Communication*, *8*, 1673–1689.

Arab-Borzu, Z., Keikha, L., & Shahraki-Mohammadi, A. (2025). Knowledge, Readiness, and Perception of Medical Students Toward Medical Artificial Intelligence: A Cross-Sectional Study. *Journal of Medical Education and Curricular Development*, *12*, 23821205251407758. Bandura, A. (2004). Health promotion by social cognitive means. *Health Education & Behavior*, *31*(2), 143–164.

Aragona, B. (2020). Sistemi di decisione algoritmica e disuguaglianze sociali: Le evidenze della ricerca, il ruolo della politica. *La Rivista delle Politiche Sociali*, *2*(20), 213–226.

Arendt, H. (2019). [1958]). *La lingua materna: La condizione umana e il pensiero plurale. Mimesis.*

Armantier, O., ... (2024), “Nothing to hide? Gender and age differences in willingness to share data”, *BIS Working Papers*, 1187: 1-33, available on: https://www.bis.org/publ/work1187.pdf

Aroldi, P., Fortunati, L., Gebhardt, J., & Vincent, J. (2011). Generational Belonging Between Media Audiences and ICT Users. *Broadband Society and Generational Changes*, *5*(3), 51–67.

Azoulay, E., Lefebvre, P., & Marlin, R. (2020). Using artificial intelligence to diversify the recruitment process at L'Oréal. *Le journal de l'ecole de Paris du management, 142*(2), 16-22.

Azzopardi-Muscat, N., & Sorensen, K. (2019). Towards an equitable digital public health era: Promoting equity through a health literacy perspective. *European Journal of Public Health, 29*(3, Supplement_3), 13–17. DOI: 10.1093/eurpub/ckz166

Badr, J., Motulsky, A., & Denis, J. (2024). Digital health technologies and inequalities: A scoping review of potential impacts and policy recommendations. *Health Policy (Amsterdam), 146*, 105122. DOI: 10.1016/j.healthpol.2024.105122 PMID: 38986333

Bailey, S., Pierides, D., Brisley, A., Weisshaar, C., & Blakeman, T. (2020). Dismembering organisation: The coordination of algorithmic work in healthcare. *Current Sociology, 68*(4), 546–571. DOI: 10.1177/0011392120907638

Bakardjieva, M. (2005). *Internet Society: The Internet in Everyday Life*. Sage Academic Books.

Barillà, L., & Locatelli, N. (2013). Welfare, tecnologie digitali e imprese sociali. *WelfareOggi, 3*, 85–89.

Barocas, S., Hardt, M., & Narayanan, A. (2019). *Fairness and Machine Learning: Limitations and Opportunities*. fairmlbook.org.

Barocas, S., & Selbst, A. D. (2016). Big data's disparate impact. *California Law Review, 104*(3), 671–732.

Barrett, A., Consolandi, M., Fattorini, E., & Vecchione, K. (2026). Altruistic Ageing: How Age Inequality Contributes to Care Work's Construction as a Burden. *Ageing and Society, 46*, e4. DOI: 10.1017/S0144686X25100342

Barrett, L. F., Adolphs, R., Marsella, S., Martinez, A. M., & Pollak, S. D. (2019). Emotional expressions reconsidered: Challenges to inferring emotion from human facial movements. *Psychological Science in the Public Interest, 20*(1), 1–68. DOI: 10.1177/1529100619832930 PMID: 31313636

Basta, C., Costa-Jussà, M. R., & Casas, N. (2019). Evaluating the underlying gender bias in contextualized word embeddings. In *Proceedings of the first workshop on gender bias in natural language processing* (pp. 33-39). DOI: 10.18653/v1/W19-3805

Bast, J., Oschatz, C., & Renner, A. M. (2022). Successfully overcoming the "double bind"? A mixed-method analysis of the self-presentation of female right-wing populists on Instagram and the impact on voter attitudes. *Political Communication, 39*(3), 358–382. DOI: 10.1080/10584609.2021.2007190

Batalden, M., Batalden, P., Margolis, P., Seid, M., Armstrong, G., Opipari-Arrigan, L., & Hartung, H. (2016). Coproduction of healthcare service. *BMJ Quality & Safety, 25*(7), 509–517. DOI: 10.1136/bmjqs-2015-004315

Battista, D., & Coppola, M. (2025). Gender-Based Violence and Cyber-Helping: The Affordance of Dedicated Apps Between Opportunities and Obstacles. *Welfare e Ergonomia, 2*, 169–180.

Battisti, D. (2020). The digital transformation of Italy's public sector: government cannot be left Behind!. *JeDEM-eJournal of eDemocracy and Open Government, 12*(1), 25-39.

Beaunoyer, E., Dupéré, S., & Guitton, M. J. (2020). COVID-19 and digital inequalities: Reciprocal impacts and mitigation strategies. *Computers in Human Behavior, 111*, 106424. DOI: 10.1016/j.chb.2020.106424 PMID: 32398890

Beer, D. (2009). Power through the algorithm? Participatory web cultures and the technological unconscious. *New Media & Society, 11*(6), 985–1002. DOI: 10.1177/1461444809336551

Bell, A., Sharma, D., & Britain, D. (2016). Labov in sociolinguistics: An introduction. *Journal of Sociolinguistics, 20*(4), 399–408. DOI: 10.1111/josl.12199

Belle, A., Thiagarajan, R., Soroushmehr, S. M. R., Navidi, F., Beard, D. A., & Najarian, K. (2015). Big data analytics in healthcare. *BioMed Research International, 2015*, 1–16. DOI: 10.1155/2015/370194 PMID: 26229957

Bender, E. M., Gebru, T., McMillan-Major, A., & Shmitchell, S. (2021, March). On the dangers of stochastic parrots: Can language models be too big? In *Proceedings of the 2021 ACM conference on fairness, accountability, and transparency* (pp. 610-623). DOI: 10.1145/3442188.3445922

Benjamin, R. (2019). Race After Technology: Abolitionist Tools for the New Jim Code. *Polity.*

Benjamin, R. (Ed.). (2019). *Captivating technology: Race, carceral technoscience, and liberatory imagination in everyday life*. Duke University Press.

Bhambra, G. K. (2014). Introduction: Knowledge production in global context: Power and coloniality. *Current Sociology*, *62*(4), 451–456. DOI: 10.1177/0011392114524504 PMID: 25418995

Birhane, A. (2021). Algorithmic injustice: Data poverty and social inequality in AI. *Patterns (New York, N.Y.)*, *2*(2), 1–9.

Birkinshaw, J., & Mol, M. J. (2006). How Management Innovation Happens. *Sloan Management Review*, *47*(4), 81–88.

Birkland, J. L. (2024). How Older Adult Information and Communication Technology Users Are Impacted by Aging Stereotypes: A Multigenerational Perspective. *New Media & Society*, *26*(7), 3967–3988. DOI: 10.1177/14614448221108959

Bjelajac, Ž., & Filipović, A. (2021). Specific characteristics of digital violence and digital crime. *Pravo-teorija i praksa, 38*(4), 16-32.

Black, J. S., & van Esch, P. (2020). AI-enabled recruiting: What is it and how should a manager use it? *Business Horizons*, *63*(2), 215–226. DOI: 10.1016/j.bushor.2019.12.001

Blei, D. M., Ng, A. Y., & Jordan, M. I. (2003). Latent dirichlet allocation. *Journal of Machine Learning Research*, *3*(Jan), 993–1022.

Blumer, H. (1954). What is wrong with social theory? *American Sociological Review*, *19*(1), 3–10. DOI: 10.2307/2088165

Boddington, G. (2021). The Internet of Bodies—alive, connected and collective: The virtual physical future of our bodies and our senses. *AI & Society*, *38*(5), 1897–1913. DOI: 10.1007/s00146-020-01137-1 PMID: 33584018

Bodewitz, H. J. H. W., Buurma, H., & de Vries, G. H. (1987). Regulatory science and the social management of trust in medicine. In Bijker, W. E., Hughes, T. P., & Pinch, T. (Eds.), *The social construction of technological systems* (pp. 243–259). MIT Press.

Boethius, S., Åkerström, M., & Hydén, M. (2022). The double-edged sword – abused women's experiences of digital technology. *European Journal of Social Work*, *26*(3), 506–518. DOI: 10.1080/13691457.2022.2040437

Bonina, C., López-Berzosa, D., & Scarlata, M. (2021). Social, commercial, or both? An exploratory study of the identity orientation of digital social innovations. *Information Systems Journal*, *31*(5), 695–716. DOI: 10.1111/isj.12290

Bottari, C. (2017). L'inquadramento costituzionale del Fascicolo Sanitario Elettronico. *Salute e Società*, *2*(2), 65–70. DOI: 10.3280/SES2017-002005

Boumans, J. W., & Trilling, D. (2018). Taking stock of the toolkit: An overview of relevant automated content analysis approaches and techniques for digital journalism scholars. *Rethinking research methods in an age of digital journalism*, 8-23.

Bourdieu, P. (1983). *La distinzione: Critica sociale del gusto*. Il Mulino.

Bovens, M., & Zouridis, S. (2002). From street-level to system-level bureaucracies: How information and communication technology is transforming administrative discretion and constitutional control. *Public Administration Review*, *62*(2), 174–184. DOI: 10.1111/0033-3352.00168

Bowker, G. C. (2014). The theory/data thing. *International Journal of Communication*, *8*, 1795–1799.

Bowker, G. C., & Star, S. L. (1999). *Sorting things out: Classification and its consequences*. MIT Press. DOI: 10.7551/mitpress/6352.001.0001

Bowker, G. C., & Star, S. L. (1999). *Sorting things out: Classification and its consequences*. MIT Press. boyd, d., & Crawford, K. (2012). Critical questions for big data. *Information Communication and Society*, *15*(5), 662–679.

Bowker, G. C., & Star, S. L. (2000). Invisible mediators of action: Classification and the ubiquity of standards. *Mind, Culture, and Activity*, *7*(1-2), 147–163. DOI: 10.1080/10749039.2000.9677652

Bowles, T., Trentino, K. M., Lloyd, A., Trentino, L., Jones, G., Murray, K., Thompson, A., Halpin, S., & Waterer, G. (2024). Outcomes in patients receiving continuous monitoring of vital signs on general wards: A systematic review and meta-analysis of randomised controlled trials. *Digital Health*, *10*, 20552076241288826. DOI: 10.1177/20552076241288826 PMID: 39398891

Boyatzis, R. E. (1998). *Transforming Qualitative Information*. Sage.

boyd, d., & Crawford, K. (2012). Critical questions for big data: Provocations for a cultural, technological, and scholarly phenomenon. Information, Communication & Society, 15(5), 662–679. DOI: 10.1080/1369118X.2012.678878

Boyd, D. (2010). Social network sites as networked publics: Affordances, dynamics, and implications. In *A networked self* (pp. 47–66). Routledge.

Boyd, R., & Holton, R. J. (2018). Technology, innovation, employment and power: Does robotics and artificial intelligence really mean social transformation? *Journal of Sociology (Melbourne, Vic.)*, *54*(3), 331–345. DOI: 10.1177/1440783317726591

Bramer, W. M., De Jonge, G. B., Rethlefsen, M. L., Mast, F., & Kleijnen, J. (2018). A systematic approach to searching: An efficient and complete method to develop literature searches. *Journal of the Medical Library Association: JMLA, 106*(4), 531. DOI: 10.5195/jmla.2018.283 PMID: 30271302

Braun, V., & Clarke, V. (2006). Using thematic analysis in psychology. *Qualitative Research in Psychology, 3*(2), 77–101. DOI: 10.1191/1478088706qp063oa

Braun, V., & Clarke, V. (2017). Thematic analysis. *The Journal of Positive Psychology, 12*(3), 297–298. DOI: 10.1080/17439760.2016.1262613

Bria, F. (2015). *Growing a digital social innovation ecosystem for Europe, Digital Social Innovation Final Report*

Broussard, M. (2018). *Artificial unintelligence: How computers misunderstand the world.* mit Press.

Brown, W. (2015). *Undoing the demos: Neoliberalism's stealth revolution.* Zone Books. DOI: 10.2307/j.ctt17kk9p8

Brynjolfsson, E., & McAfee, A. (2014). *The second machine age: Work, progress, and prosperity in a time of brilliant technologies.* W. W. Norton.

Buchert, U., Kemppainen, L., Olakivi, A., Wrede, S., & Kouvonen, A. (2023). Is digitalisation of public health and social welfare services reinforcing social exclusion? The case of Russian-speaking older migrants in Finland. *Critical Social Policy, 43*(3), 375–400. DOI: 10.1177/02610183221105035

Büchi, M. (2021). Digital well-being as a dynamic capability. *New Media & Society, 23*(11), 3281–3301.

Buck, C., Krombacher, A., Röglinger, M., & Körner-Wyrtki, K. (2023). Doing good by going digital: A taxonomy of digital social innovation in the context of incumbents. *The Journal of Strategic Information Systems*, 32(4), 101806. https:// doi.org/ s.2023.101806DOI: 10.1016/j.jsi

Buolamwini, J., & Gebru, T. (2018, January). Gender shades: Intersectional accuracy disparities in commercial gender classification. In *Conference on fairness, accountability and transparency* (pp. 77-91). PMLR.

Burawoy, M. (2005). For public sociology. *American Sociological Review, 70*(1), 4–28. DOI: 10.1177/000312240507000102 PMID: 15926908

Bureau of European Policy Advisers. (2011). *Empowering people, driving change: Social innovation in the European Union.* Publications Office of the European Union.

Burrell, J., & Fourcade, M. (2021). The society of algorithms. *Annual Review of Sociology*, *47*(1), 213–237. DOI: 10.1146/annurev-soc-090820-020800

Burton, J., & van den Broek, D. (2008). Accountable and Countable: Information Management Systems and the Bureaucratization of Social Work. *British Journal of Social Work*, *26*, 1–17. DOI: 10.1093/bjsw/bcn027

Busacca, M. (2022). Imprese sociali e transizione digitale [Social Enterprises and Digital Transition]. *Impresa sociale*, 4, 27-28

Busch, P. A., & Henriksen, H. Z. (2018). Digital discretion: A systematic literature review of ICT and street-level discretion. *Information Polity*, *23*(1), 3–28. DOI: 10.3233/IP-170050

Busch, P. A., Henriksen, H. Z., & Sæbø, Ø. (2018). Opportunities and challenges of digitized discretionary practices: A public service worker perspective. *Government Information Quarterly*, *35*(4), 547–556. DOI: 10.1016/j.giq.2018.09.003

Butler, J., & Trouble, G. (1990). Feminism and the Subversion of Identity. *Gender trouble, 3*(1), 3-17.

Cahill, E., Lewis, L. M., Barg, F. K., & Bogner, H. R. (2009). "You Don't Want to Burden Them": Older Adults' Views on Family Involvement in Care. *Journal of Family Nursing*, *15*(3), 295–317. DOI: 10.1177/1074840709337247 PMID: 19474397

CALP Network. (2012). *E-payments in Emergency Cash Transfer Programming*. CALP Network.

Camera dei Deputati. (2024). *Il nuovo Fascicolo Sanitario Elettronico*. https://temi.camera.it/leg19/post/il-nuovo-fascicolo-sanitario-elettronico.html

Campedelli, M., & Vesan, P. (2023). Welfare digitalizzato, welfare digitale e i nuovi rischi sociali digitali: Un'introduzione. Politiche Sociali/Social Policies, 10(2), 169–192. DOI: 10.7389/108019

Cardoso, L. F., Sorenson, S. B., Webb, O., & Landers, S. (2019). Recent and emerging technologies: Implications for women's safety. *Technology in Society*, *58*, 101108. DOI: 10.1016/j.techsoc.2019.01.001

Carlo, S., & Sourbati, M. (2020). Age and Technology in Digital Inclusion Policy: A Study of Italy and the UK. *ESSACHESS–Journal for Communication Studies*, 13.2 (26), 107-127.

Carlo, S., & Diodati, F. (2026). Ageing and Mobile Phones: Tactical Uses/Nonuses in Postpandemic Italy. *Mobile Media & Communication*, *14*(1), 89–107. DOI: 10.1177/20501579251359072

Carswell, G., & De Neve, G. (2022). Transparency, exclusion and mediation: How digital and biometric technologies are transforming social protection in Tamil Nadu, India. *Oxford Development Studies*, *50*(2), 126–141. DOI: 10.1080/13600818.2021.1904866

Casilli, A. A. (2020). *Schiavi del clic: perché lavoriamo tutti per il nuovo capitalismo?* Feltrinelli Editore.

Castells, M. (2009). *Communication power*. Oxford University Press.

Castells, M. (2010). *The rise of the network society* (2nd ed.). Wiley-Blackwell.

Cataldi, S. (2009). *Come si analizzano i focus group* [How to Analyze Focus Groups]. Franco Angeli.

Cavotta, V., Grassi, E., & Toschi, L. (2022). Uso delle tecnologie digitali da parte degli imprenditori e innovatori sociali: Potenzialità e limiti. *Impresa Sociale*, *4*, 29–35.

Chalovska Dimovska, N. (2024). *Analysis of Technology facilitated Gender-Based Violence*. United Nations Development Programme.

Chang, J., Gerrish, S., Wang, C., Boyd-Graber, J., & Blei, D. (2009). Reading tea leaves: How humans interpret topic models. *Advances in Neural Information Processing Systems*, •••, 22.

Charmaz, K. (2003). Grounded theory: Objectivist and constructivist methods. In Denzin, N. K., & Lincoln, Y. S. (Eds.), *Strategies for Qualitative Inquiry* (pp. 249–291). Sage.

Chatterjee, B., Mohseni, P., & Sen, S. (2022). Bioelectronic sensor nodes for Internet of Bodies. arXiv. https://arxiv.org/abs/2212.11370

Cheney-Lippold, J. (2011). A new algorithmic identity: Soft biopolitics and the modulation of control. *Theory, Culture & Society*, *28*(6), 164–181. DOI: 10.1177/0263276411424420

Chen, I. Y., Pierson, E., Rose, S., Joshi, S., Ferryman, K., & Ghassemi, M. (2023). Ethical machine learning in healthcare. *Annual Review of Biomedical Data Science*, *6*(1), 123–144. DOI: 10.1146/annurev-biodatasci-092820-114757 PMID: 34396058

Christakis, N. A. (2019). *Blueprint: The evolutionary origins of a good society*. Little, Brown Spark.

Chung, Y., Shin, H., Kim, H., & Kim, J. S. (2024). The role of health empowerment on digital health technology literacy by generation. *American Journal of Health Behavior*, *48*(4), 967–978. DOI: 10.5993/AJHB.48.4.8

Cirillo, D., Catuara-Solarz, S., Morey, C., Guney, E., Subirats, L., Mellino, S., Gigante, A., Valencia, A., Rementeria, M. J., Chadha, A. S., & Mavridis, N. (2020). Sex and gender differences and biases in artificial intelligence for biomedicine and healthcare. *NPJ Digital Medicine*, *3*(1), 81. DOI: 10.1038/s41746-020-0288-5 PMID: 32529043

Ciurleo, E., Ceraso, D., Iaquinta, P., & Comite, U. (2025). Digitalizzazione e disuguaglianze: Un'analisi empirica sulle regioni italiane. *Regional Economy*, *9*, 15–31.

Civitarese Matteucci, S. (2016). Digitalisation and reforms of public administration in Italy. *Italian J. Pub. L.*, *8*, 127.

Clarke, A. E., & Shim, J. (2010). Medicalization and biomedicalization revisited: technoscience and transformations of health, illness and American medicine. In *Handbook of the sociology of health, illness, and healing: A blueprint for the 21st century* (pp. 173–199). Springer New York.

Clark, J. (1982). Catherine Hakim, Occupational Segregation: A comparative study of the degree and pattern of the differentiation between men and women's work in Britain, the United States and other countries, Research Paper No. 9, November 1979, Department of Employment, London, 1979. 65 pp. No price given. *Journal of Social Policy*, *11*(1), 131–132. DOI: 10.1017/S004727940001151X

Coccia, M. (2020). Artificial intelligence technology in oncology: A new technological paradigm. *Technological Forecasting and Social Change*, 151, available on: https://arxiv.org/pdf/1905.06871

Cochoy, F., Hagberg, J., McIntyre, M. P., & Sörum, N. (2017). Digitalizing consumption: Introduction. In *Digitalizing consumption*. Routledge. DOI: 10.4324/9781315647883-1

Cockerham, W. C. (2005). Health lifestyle theory and the convergence of agency and structure. *Journal of Health and Social Behavior*, *46*(1), 51–67. DOI: 10.1177/002214650504600105 PMID: 15869120

Cohen, J. E. (2019). Review of Zuboff's the age of surveillance capitalism. *Surveillance & Society*, *17*(1/2), 240–245. DOI: 10.24908/ss.v17i1/2.13144

Collington, R. (2022). Disrupting the Welfare State? Digitalisation and the Retrenchment of Public Sector Capacity. *New Political Economy*, *27*(2), 312–328. DOI: 10.1080/13563467.2021.1952559

Colombo, F., Aroldi, P., & Carlo, S. (2018). 'I Use it Correctly!': The Use of ICTs among Italian Grandmothers in a Generational Perspective. *Human Technology*, *14*(3), 343–365. DOI: 10.17011/ht/urn.201811224837

Corbetta, (2003). *Social Research Theory, Methods and Techniques*, Londra. *Sage (Atlanta, Ga.).*

Cordella, A. (2005). Actor Network Theory per lo studio dei sistemi informativi. *Sinergie Rapporti di Ricerca, 19*, 71–86.

Corradi, C., & Stöckl, H. (2016). The lessons of history: The role of the nation-states and the EU in fighting violence against women in 10 European countries. *Current Sociology, 64*(4), 671–688. DOI: 10.1177/0011392116640457

Corrao, S. (2002). *I focus group* [Focus Groups]. Franco Angeli.

Correll, S. J. (2004). Constraints into preferences. Gender, status, and emerging career aspirations. *American Sociological Review, 69*(1), 93–113. DOI: 10.1177/000312240406900106

Couldry, N., & Mejias, U. A. (2019). *The Costs of Connection: How Data Is Colonizing Human Life and Appropriating It for Capitalism*. Stanford University Press.

Coutu, F.-A., Iorio, O. C., & Ross, B. A. (2023). Remote patient monitoring strategies and wearable technology in chronic obstructive pulmonary disease. *Frontiers in Medicine, 10*, 1236598. DOI: 10.3389/fmed.2023.1236598 PMID: 37663662

Craciun, G., Zhou, W., & Shan, Z. (2020). Discrete emotions effects on electronic word-of-mouth helpfulness: The moderating role of reviewer gender and contextual emotional tone. *Decision Support Systems, 130*, 113226. DOI: 10.1016/j.dss.2019.113226

Crawford, K. (2017, December). The trouble with bias. In *Conference on Neural Information Processing Systems, invited speaker.*

Crawford, K. (2021). *Atlas of AI: Power, politics, and the planetary costs of artificial intelligence*. Yale University Press.

Crawford, K. (2024). World view. *Nature, 626*, 693. DOI: 10.1038/d41586-024-00478-x PMID: 38378831

Crawford, K., Gray, M. L., & Miltner, K. (2014). Critiquing big data: Politics, ethics, epistemology. *International Journal of Communication, 8*, 1663–1672.

Crenshaw, K. W. (2013). Mapping the margins: Intersectionality, identity politics, and violence against women of color. In *The public nature of private violence* (pp. 93–118). Routledge.

Cresswell, K., Papoutsi, C., Simon, G. E., Bates, D. W., & Sheikh, A. (2025). Advancing learning health systems: Leveraging routine data for improvement and research. *NPJ Digital Medicine*, *8*, 12. DOI: 10.1038/s41746-024-01045-4

Cruz, T. M. (2022). The social life of biomedical data: Capturing, obscuring, and envisioning care in the digital safety-net. *Social Science & Medicine*, *294*, 114670. Advance online publication. DOI: 10.1016/j.socscimed.2021.114670 PMID: 35114488

Cuccaro-Alamin, S., Foust, R., Vaithianathan, R., & Putnam-Hornstein, E. (2017). Risk assessment and decision making in child protective services: Predictive risk modeling in context. *Children and Youth Services Review*, *79*, 291–298. DOI: 10.1016/j.childyouth.2017.06.027

D'Alessandro, F., Landoni, P., & Marocchi, G. (2022). Le imprese sociali di inserimento lavorativo: Che rapporto hanno con le tecnologie [Work Integration Social Enterprises: Their Relationship with Technologies]. *Impresa Sociale*, *4*, 36–44. DOI: 10.7425/IS.2022.04.06

D'Ancona, G., Massussi, M., Savardi, M., Signoroni, A., Di Bacco, L., Farina, D., Metra, M., Maroldi, R., Muneretto, C., Ince, H., Costabile, D., Murero, M., Chizzola, G., Curello, S., & Benussi, S. (2023). Deep learning to detect significant coronary artery disease from plain chest radiographs (AI4CAD). *International Journal of Cardiology*, *370*, 435–441. DOI: 10.1016/j.ijcard.2022.10.154 PMID: 36343794

D'ignazio, C., & Klein, F., L. (. (2020). Seven intersectional feminist principles for equitable and actionable COVID-19 data. *Big Data & Society*, *7*(2), 2053951720942544. DOI: 10.1177/2053951720942544 PMID: 32802347

Dadà, S. (2022). Autonomia in telemedicina. L'e-patient tra indipendenza e coinvolgimento. *Teoria*, *42*(2), 33–51.

Dahlgren, G., & Whitehead, M. (2021). The Dahlgren–Whitehead model of health determinants: 30 years on. *Public Health*, *199*, 20–24. DOI: 10.1016/j.puhe.2021.08.009 PMID: 34534885

Damant, J., Knapp, M., Freddolino, P., & Lombard, D. (2017). Effects of digital engagement on the quality of life of older people. *Health & Social Care in the Community*, *25*(6), 1679–1703. DOI: 10.1111/hsc.12335 PMID: 26919220

Damschroder, L. J., Aron, D. C., Keith, R. E., Kirsh, S. R., Alexander, J. A., & Lowery, J. C. (2009). Fostering implementation of health services research findings into practice: A consolidated framework for advancing implementation science. *Implementation Science : IS*, *4*(1), 50. DOI: 10.1186/1748-5908-4-50 PMID: 19664226

Danaher, J., & McArthur, N. (Eds.). (2017). *Robot sex: Social and ethical implications*. MIT press. DOI: 10.7551/mitpress/9780262036689.001.0001

Dash, S., Shakyawar, S. K., Sharma, M., & Kaushik, S. (2019). Big data in healthcare: Management, analysis and future prospects. *Journal of Big Data*, *6*(1), 54. DOI: 10.1186/s40537-019-0217-0

Datta, A., & Sen, S. (2023). Invited: IoB: The vision of the Internet of Bodies. *Proceedings of the IEEE Midwest Symposium on Circuits and Systems (MWSCAS)*, 444–448. DBLPDOI: 10.1109/MWSCAS57524.2023.10405903

Davies, B. (2021). Personal health surveillance: The use of mHealth in healthcare responsibilisation. *Public Health Ethics*, *14*(3), 268–280. DOI: 10.1093/phe/phab013 PMID: 34899983

De Cesare, A. M. (2025). L'intelligenza artificiale generativa al servizio della parità di genere: uno studio esplorativo sugli annunci di lavoro della Confederazione svizzera. *Inclusione ed elaborazione del linguaggio naturale nell'era dell'intelligenza artificiale generativa*, 59.

De las Cuevas, P., García-Arenas, M., & Rico, N. (2022). Why not STEM? A study case on the influence of gender factors on students' higher education choice. *Mathematics*, *10*(2), 239. DOI: 10.3390/math10020239

De Lathauwer, I. L. J., Nieuwenhuys, W. W., Hafkamp, F., Regis, M., Brouwers, R. W. M., Funk, M., & Kemps, H. M. C. (2025). Remote patient monitoring in heart failure: A comprehensive meta-analysis of effective programme components for hospitalization and mortality reduction. *European Journal of Heart Failure*, *27*(9), 1670–1685. Advance online publication. DOI: 10.1002/ejhf.3568 PMID: 39834044

De Simone, A. (2020). Essere e politica: Dialettica dell'umano. *Mimesis.*

de Waal, C.. (2025). Accuracy of vital sign monitoring using a photoplethysmography upper arm wearable in hospitalised patients. *Journal of Clinical Monitoring and Computing*. Advance online publication. DOI: 10.1007/s10877-025-01358-z

Dècina, M. M. (2016). *Digital divide et impera: Il ritardo del digitale è un caso?* Editori Riuniti.

Demurtas, P., & Mangone, E. (2025). Ripensare il welfare per prevenire e contrastare la violenza di genere: Sfide e opportunità per un sistema integrato. *Welfare e Ergonomia*, *2*, 7–26.

Dencik, L. (2022). The datafied welfare state: A perspective from the UK. In Hepp, A., Jarke, J., & Kramp, L. (Eds.), *New perspectives in critical data studies* (pp. 145–165). Palgrave Macmillan., DOI: 10.1007/978-3-030-96180-0_7

Dencik, L., & Kaun, A. (2020). Datafication and the welfare state. *Global Perspectives, 1*(1), 12912. DOI: 10.1525/gp.2020.12912

Deriu, F. (2020). Luci e ombre dell'innovazione digitale nel welfare dei servizi alla persona in Italia. *La Rivista delle Politiche sociali, 3*, 255-271.

Devlieghere, J., Roose, R., & Evans, T. (2020). Managing the electronic turn. *European Journal of Social Work, 23*(5), 767–778. DOI: 10.1080/13691457.2019.1582009

Di Viggiano, P. (2014). Sanità digitale e Welfare elettronico. *Rivista Elettronica di Diritto, Economia. Management, 3*, 74–95.

Diao, J. A., Wu, G. J., Taylor, H. A., Tucker, J. K., Powe, N. R., & Kohane, I. S. (2021). Clinical implications of removing race from estimates of kidney function. *Journal of the American Medical Association, 325*(2), 184–186. PMID: 33263721

Díaz Gorfinkiel, M., Díaz Gandasegui, V., & Gómez García, M. V. (2021). New technology proposals for tackling intimate partner violence: Challenges and opportunities. *Technology in Society, 67*, 101714. DOI: 10.1016/j.techsoc.2021.101714

Dominici, P. (2019). *Dentro la società interconnessa: La cultura della complessità per abitare i confini e le tensioni della civiltà ipertecnologica*. Franco Angeli.

Donato, S., Eslen-Ziya, H., & Mangone, E. (2022). From offline to online violence: New challenges for the contemporary society. *International Review of Sociology, 32*(3), 400–412. DOI: 10.1080/03906701.2022.2133405

Doshi-Velez, F., & Kim, B. (2017). Towards a rigorous science of interpretable machine learning. *arXiv preprint arXiv:1702.08608.*

Duan, S., Liu, C., Rong, T., Zhao, Y., & Liu, B. (2025). Integrating AI in medical education: A comprehensive study of medical students' attitudes, concerns, and behavioral intentions. *BMC Medical Education, 25*(1), 599. DOI: 10.1186/s12909-025-07177-9 PMID: 40269824

Dubey, R., & Tiwari, A. (2023). Artificial intelligence and remote patient monitoring in US healthcare market: A literature review. *Journal of Market Access & Health Policy, 11*(1), 2205618. DOI: 10.1080/20016689.2023.2205618 PMID: 37151736

Duguet, A. M., Dubruel, N., & Sebbag, E. R. (2025). Digital Health, Health Data Base and Artificial Intelligence in France: What Benefits for Patients and Society Interests. *Medicine and Law*, •••, 201. DOI: 10.63776/CHMT7934

Duncombe, C. (2020). Social media and the visibility of horrific violence. *International Affairs*, *96*(3), 609–629. DOI: 10.1093/ia/iiaa055

Dunleavy, P., Margetts, H., Bastow, S., & Tinkler, J. (2006). *Digital era governance*. Oxford University Press. DOI: 10.1093/acprof:oso/9780199296194.001.0001

Edelson, D. P., Churpek, M. M., Carey, K. A., Lin, Z., Huang, C., Siner, J. M., Johnson, J., Krumholz, H. M., & Rhodes, D. J. (2024). Early warning scores with and without artificial intelligence. *JAMA Network Open*, *7*(10), e2438986. DOI: 10.1001/jamanetworkopen.2024.38986 PMID: 39405061

Eder, M., & Sjøvaag, H. (2024). Artificial intelligence and the dawn of an algorithmic divide. *Frontiers in Communication*, *9*, 1453251. DOI: 10.3389/fcomm.2024.1453251

Ehrenstein, V., Kharrazi, H., Lehmann, H., & Taylor, R. J. (2019). Obtaining data from electronic health records. In Gliklich, R. E., Dreyer, N. A., & Leavy, M. B. (Eds.), *Registries for evaluating patient outcomes: A user's guide* (3rd ed.). Agency for Healthcare Research and Quality., https://www.ncbi.nlm.nih.gov/books/NBK551878/

EIGE. (2018). *Gender equality and youth: opportunities and risks of digitalisation*. Publications Office of the European Union., DOI: 10.2839/148393

El-deep, S. E., Abohany, A. A., Sallam, K. M., & Abd El-Mageed, A. A. (2025). A comprehensive survey on impact of applying various technologies on the Internet of Medical Things. [SpringerLink]. *Artificial Intelligence Review*, *58*(3), 86. DOI: 10.1007/s10462-024-11063-z

Elish, M. C., & Boyd, D. (2018). Situating methods in the magic of Big Data and AI. *Communication Monographs*, *85*(1), 57–80. DOI: 10.1080/03637751.2017.1375130

El-Khoury, M., & Arikan, C. L. (2021). From the Internet of Things toward the Internet of Bodies: Ethical and legal considerations. Journal of Strategic Contracting and Negotiation, 7(2), 307–314. doi:10.1002/jsc.2411 RSD Journal

England, P. (2010). The gender revolution. Uneven and Stalled. *Gender & Society*, *24*(2), 149–166. DOI: 10.1177/0891243210361475

Epifani, S. (2020). *Sostenibilità digitale: Perché la sostenibilità non può fare a meno della trasformazione digitale*. Digital Transformation Institute.

Epiphanio, F., & Oms, C. (2025). The use of digital technology to prevent violence against women: A scoping review of recent literature. *International Journal of Technological Learning. Innovation and Development*, *16*(2), 134–152. DOI: 10.1504/IJTLID.2025.146723

Erickson, R. J., & Grove, W. J. (2008). Emotional labor and health care. *Sociology Compass, 2*(2), 704–733. DOI: 10.1111/j.1751-9020.2007.00084.x

Esping-Andersen, G. (1990). The three worlds of welfare capitalism.

Esping-Andersen, G. (1990). *The three words of welfare capitalism.* Princeton University Press.

Esping-Andersen, G. (1990). *The three worlds of welfare capitalism.* Polity Press.

Esposito, E. (2022). Does explainability require transparency? *Sociologica, 16*(3), 17–27.

Eubanks, V. (2018). *Automating inequality: How high-tech tools profile, police, and punish the poor.* Macmillan+ ORM.

Eubanks, V. (2018). *Automating Inequality: How High-Tech Tools Profile, Police, and Punish the Poor.* St. Martin's Press.

Eurofound (2025). *Europe's Digital Welfare Revolution: Progress at What Price?* European Foundation for the Improvement of Living and Working Conditions.

European Commission. (2022). *EUROSHIP project: Closing gaps in social citizenship.* https://euroship-research.eu/

European Commission. (2025). *Digital decade 2025: eHealth indicator study.* Publications Office of the European Union. https://digital-strategy.ec.europa.eu/en/library/digital-decade-2025-ehealth-indicator-study

European Commission. *Digital Economy and Society Index (DESI) 2022, Thematic chapters,* https://digital-strategy.ec.europa.eu/en/policies/desi

European Commission. Directorate-General for Communications Networks, Content and Technology & Capgemini Invent. (2025). *2025 digital decade ehealth indicator study: final report.* Publications Office of the European Union. https://data.europa.eu/doi/10.2759/2737039

Eurostat (2025). *Individuals' Level of Digital Skills by Sex and Age* https://ec.europa.eu/eurostat/databrowser/view/eq_dskl07/default/table?lang=en

Eurostat. (2023). *Digitalisation in Europe – level of digital skills in 2023.* Eurostat News Release. https://ec.europa.eu/eurostat/web/interactive-publications/digitalisation-2024

Evans, R. S. (2016). Electronic health records: then, now, and in the future. *Yearbook of medical informatics, 25*(S 01), S48-S61.

Ewoh, P., & Vartiainen, T. (2024). Vulnerability to cyberattacks and sociotechnical solutions for health care systems: Systematic review. Journal of Medical Internet Research, 26, e46904. 10.2196/46904

Fahim, Y. A., Hasani, I. W., Kabba, S., & Ragab, W. M. (2025). Artificial intelligence in healthcare and medicine: Clinical applications, therapeutic advances, and future perspectives. *European Journal of Medical Research, 30*(1), 848. Advance online publication. DOI: 10.1186/s40001-025-03196-w PMID: 40988064

Fahse, A., Karimi, F., & Kunegis, J. (2021). The structure of bias in human-generated data. *Journal of Computational Social Science, 4*(2), 645–663.

Feickert, S., Ewertsen, C., Rother, W., Ince, H., & D'Ancona, G. (2024). Pulsed field ablation and ultra-high-density mapping for PVI: Use of machine learning and data augmentation to guide procedure and identify recurrent tachycardia mechanisms at one-year follow-up. European Heart Journal, 45(Suppl. 1), Article ehae666.577. DOI: 10.1093/eurheartj/ehae666.577

Felix, F. A. S., & Martins, L. E. G. (2024). IoT devices in use in healthcare applications: A systematic literature review. [SpringerLink]. *Research on Biomedical Engineering, 40*(3-4), 547–561. DOI: 10.1007/s42600-024-00356-5

Ferguson, C. J. (2007). The good, the bad and the ugly: A meta-analytic review of positive and negative effects of violent video games. *The Psychiatric Quarterly, 78*(4), 309–316. DOI: 10.1007/s11126-007-9056-9

Fernández-Ardèvol, M. (2016). An Exploration of Mobile Telephony Non-Use among Older People. In E., Domínguez-Rué, & L.E., Nierling. (Eds.). *Ageing and Technology: Perspectives from the Social Sciences* (pp. 47-66). Transcript Verlag. DOI: 10.14361/9783839429570-003

Fiscella, K., Franks, P., Gold, M., & Clancy, C. (2000). Inequality in quality: Addressing socioeconomic disparities in health care. *Journal of the American Medical Association, 283*(19), 2579–2584. DOI: 10.1001/jama.283.19.2579 PMID: 10815125

Floridi, L. (2015). The new grey power. *Philosophy & Technology, 28*(3), 329–332. DOI: 10.1007/s13347-015-0206-y

Floridi, L. (2015). *The Onlife Manifesto. Being Human in a Hyperconnected Era.* Sprnger.

Floridi, L., Cowls, J., Beltrametti, M., Chatila, R., Chazerand, P., Dignum, V., Luetge, C., Madelin, R., Pagallo, U., Rossi, F., Schafer, B., Valcke, P., & Vayena, E. (2018). AI4People—An ethical framework for a good AI society: Opportunities, risks, principles, and recommendations. *Minds and Machines*, *28*(4), 689–707. DOI: 10.1007/s11023-018-9482-5 PMID: 30930541

Fornari, S., & Masullo, G. (2023). Ripensare il fenomeno della violenza nella digital society. In S. Fornari, & G. Masullo (Eds.), *Forme di violenza e rischi per le persone* (monographic issue). *Sicurezza e scienze sociali*, 3, 7-10. DOI: 10.3280/SISS2023-003001

Foster, L., & Walker, A. (2021). Active Ageing across the Life Course: Towards a Comprehensive Approach to Prevention. *BioMed Research International*, *2021*(1), 6650414. DOI: 10.1155/2021/6650414 PMID: 33623785

Foucault, M. (1996). *Archivio Foucault. Interventi, colloqui, interviste* (Vol. 3). Feltrinelli Editore.

Fourcade, M., & Healy, K. (2017). Classification situations: Life-chances in the neoliberal era. *Historical Social Research. Historische Sozialforschung*, *42*(1), 23–51.

FRA. (2020). *A long way to go for LGBTI equality*. Publications Office of the European Union., DOI: 10.2811/7746

Frasca, M., La Torre, D., Pravettoni, G., & Cutica, I. (2024). Explainable and interpretable artificial intelligence in medicine: A systematic bibliometric review. *Discover Artificial Intelligence*, *4*(1), 15. DOI: 10.1007/s44163-024-00114-7

Freidson, E. (1970). *Professional dominance: The social structure of medical care*. Transaction Publishers.

Frennert, S. (2021). Gender blindness: On health and welfare technology, AI and gender equality in community care. [Wiley.]. *Nursing Inquiry*, *28*(4), e12411. DOI: 10.1111/nin.12419 PMID: 33979011

Friemel, T. N. (2016). The Digital Divide Has Grown Old: Determinants of a Digital Divide Among Seniors. *New Media & Society*, *18*(2), 313–331. DOI: 10.1177/1461444814538648

Fudim, M., Feldman, D. I., & Sayed, A. (2025). Digital health: From remote monitoring to remote care. *Journal of Cardiac Failure*, *31*(2), 489–491. DOI: 10.1016/j.cardfail.2024.08.033

Gallistl, V., Rohner, R., Hengl, L., & Kolland, F. (2021). Doing Digital Exclusion – Technology Practices of Older Internet Non-Users. *Journal of Aging Studies, 59*, 100973. DOI: 10.1016/j.jaging.2021.100973 PMID: 34794717

Gallistl, V., Seifert, A., & Kolland, F. (2021). COVID-19 as a "digital push?" Research experiences from long-term care and recommendations for the post-pandemic era. *Frontiers in Public Health, 9*, 660064. DOI: 10.3389/fpubh.2021.660064 PMID: 34041216

Garavaglia, E., Caliandro, A., Melis, G., Sala, E., & Zaccaria, D. (2023). Contrasting ageism in research on older adults and digital technologies: A methodological reflection. In Rosales, A., Fernández-Ardèvol, M., & Svensson, J. (Eds.). *Digital ageism: How it operates and approaches to tackling it.* (pp. 248-265). Routledge.

Garrido-Muñoz, A., Montejo-Ráez, A., Martínez-Camara, E., Almeida-Cruz, Y., Frenda, S., García-Vega, M., & Sánchez, D. (2021). A normative definition of cognitive bias for computational applications. *arXiv preprint arXiv:2305.09281.*

Gebru, T. (2020). Race and gender. *The Oxford handbook of ethics of AI, 4*, 253.

Gehl Sampath, P. (2021). Governing artificial intelligence in an age of inequality. *Global Policy, 12*(S6), 21–31. DOI: 10.1111/1758-5899.12940

Georgantopoulos, A., & Lamnisos, D. (2025). Associations of Health and Digital Health Literacy with Health-Related Quality of Life: A Cross-Sectional Study in Greece and Cyprus. *Journal of Health Literacy, 11*(1), 64–79.

Gershon, I. (2010). Media Ideologies: An Introduction. *Journal of Linguistic Anthropology, 20*(2), 283–293. DOI: 10.1111/j.1548-1395.2010.01070.x

Ghanem, S., Moraleja, M., Gravesande, D., & Rooney, J. (2025). Integrating health equity in artificial intelligence for public health in Canada: A rapid narrative review. *Frontiers in Public Health, 13*, 1524616. DOI: 10.3389/fpubh.2025.1524616 PMID: 40171421

Giarelli, G., Genova, A., & Moretti, V. (Eds.). (2023). *Personalizzazione della cura e partecipazione dei cittadini nella società digitale sindemica.* Franco Angeli.

Gillespie, T. (2014). The relevance of algorithms. In *Media technologies*. MIT Press. DOI: 10.7551/mitpress/9042.003.0013

Gillespie, T. (2024). Generative AI and the politics of visibility. *Big Data & Society, 11*(2), 20539517241252131. DOI: 10.1177/20539517241252131

Gitelman, L. (2013). *"Raw data" is an oxymoron.* MIT Press. DOI: 10.7551/mitpress/9302.001.0001

Gmyrek, P., Berg, J., & Bescond, D. (2023). Generative AI and jobs: A global analysis of potential effects on job quantity and quality.

Goldkind, L., Ming, J., & Fink, A. (2025). AI in the Nonprofit Human Services: Distinguishing Between Hype, Harm, and Hope. *Human Service Organizations, Management, Leadership & Governance*, *49*(3), 225–236. DOI: 10.1080/23303131.2024.2427459

Goldzweig, C., Orshansky, G., Paige, N., Towfigh, A. A., Haggstrom, D. A., Miake-Lye, I., Beroes, J. M., & Shekelle, P. G. (2013). Electronic patient portals. *Annals of Internal Medicine*, *159*(10), 677–687. DOI: 10.7326/0003-4819-159-10-201311190-00006 PMID: 24247673

Gonzales, A., Guruswamy, G., & Smith, S. R. (2023). Synthetic data in health care: A narrative review. *PLOS Digital Health*, *2*(1), e0000082. Advance online publication. DOI: 10.1371/journal.pdig.0000082 PMID: 36812604

Goswami, M. R. (2025). The Algorithmic Citizen: How AI is Rewriting Rights, Representation and Responsibility. [ISRN]. *International Social Research Nexus*, *1*(3), 1–14. DOI: 10.63539/isrn.2025022

Gough, I. (1979). *The political economy of the welfare state*. Red Globe Press London. DOI: 10.1007/978-1-349-16122-5

Gray, M. L., & Suri, S. (2019). *Ghost Work: How to Stop Silicon Valley from Building a New Global Underclass*. Houghton Mifflin Harcourt.

Green, B., & Viljoen, S. (2020). Algorithmic realism: Expanding the boundaries of algorithmic thought. *Philosophy & Technology*, *33*(1), 1–23.

Greenhalgh, T. (2017). *How to implement evidence-based healthcare*. John Wiley & Sons.

Greenhalgh, T., Wherton, J., & Papoutsi, C.. (2017). Beyond adoption of health technologies. *Journal of Medical Internet Research*, *19*(11), e367. DOI: 10.2196/jmir.8775 PMID: 29092808

Grieve, J., Bartl, S., & Fuoli, M.. (2025). The sociolinguistic foundations of language modeling. *Frontiers*. PMID: 39871863

Gui, M., Fasoli, M., & Carradore, R. (2017). “Digital Well-Being”: Developing a new theoretical tool for media literacy research. *Italian Journal of Sociology of Education*, *9*(1), 155–173.

Guo, W., & Caliskan, A. (2021). Detecting emergent intersectional biases: Contextualized word embeddings contain a distribution of human-like biases. *In Proceedings of the 2021 AAAI/ACM Conference on AI, Ethics, and Society* (pp. 122-133).

Guven, M., Yeachuri, A., & Almenfi, M. (2025). *Global Insights on Social Registries: Coverage and Beyond*. World Bank. DOI: 10.1596/43585

Guy, M. E., Newman, M. A., & Mastracci, S. H. (2014). *Emotional labor: Putting the service in public service*. Routledge. DOI: 10.4324/9781315704852

Guzzo, M. del R. (2026). The Multiple Faces of Warm Experts. In V. G., Duffy, Q., Gao, & J. Zhou. (Eds.). *HCI International 2025* – Late Breaking Papers (pp. 52–68). Springer Nature Switzerland. DOI: 10.1007/978-3-032-13022-8_5

Haase, M., Bosse, M., Sackmann, S., & Meyer, G. (2025). IT Skills of Young and Older People: A Qualitative Study. *International Journal of Human-Computer Interaction*, *41*(4), 2301–2311. DOI: 10.1080/10447318.2024.2319916

Haddon, L. (2011). Domestication Analysis, Objects of Study, and the Centrality of Technologies in Everyday Life. *Canadian Journal of Communication*, *36*(2), 311–324. DOI: 10.22230/cjc.2011v36n2a2322

Haddon, L., & Mante-Meijer, E. (2016). *Generational Use of New Media*. Routledge. DOI: 10.4324/9781315584270

Hakim, C. (1992). Explaining trends in occupational segregation: The measurement, causes, and consequences of the sexual division of labour. *European Sociological Review*, *8*(2), 127–152. DOI: 10.1093/oxfordjournals.esr.a036628

Hanna, N. (2018). A role for the state in the digital age. *Journal of Innovation and Entrepreneurship*, *7*(1), 5. DOI: 10.1186/s13731-018-0086-3

Hänninen, R., Taipale, S., & Luostari, R. (2021). Exploring Heterogeneous ICT Use among Older Adults: The Warm Experts' Perspective. *New Media & Society*, *23*(6), 1584–1601. DOI: 10.1177/1461444820917353

Hansen, M. J., Palakal, M. J., & White, L. J. (2024). The importance of STEM sense of belonging and academic hope in enhancing persistence for low-income, underrepresented STEM students. *Journal for STEM Education Research*, *7*(2), 155–180. DOI: 10.1007/s41979-023-00096-8

Hans, J. (2009). *Il principio responsabilità. Un'etica per la civiltà tecnologica*. Einaudi.

Hardey, M., Loader, B. D., & Keeble, L. (2009). Introduction. In *Digital welfare for the third age*. Routledge.

Hargittai, E., & Dobransky, K. (2017). Old Dogs, New Clicks: Digital Inequality in Skills and Uses Among Older Adults. *Canadian Journal of Communication, 42*(2), 195–212. DOI: 10.22230/cjc.2017v42n2a3176

He, P., Huang, D., Wu, D., He, H., Wei, Y., Cui, Y., Wang, R., & Peng, L. (2024). A survey of Internet of Medical Things: Technology, application and future directions. Digital Communications and Networks. Advance online publication. sciencedirect. comDOI: 10.1016/j.dcan.2024.11.013

Hearn, J., Strid, S., Humbert, A. L., Balkmar, D., & Delaunay, M. (2022). From Gender Regimes to Violence Regimes: Re-thinking the Position of Violence. *Social Politics, 29*(2), 682–705. DOI: 10.1093/sp/jxaa022

Helsper, E. (2021). The digital disconnect: The social causes and consequences of digital inequalities.

Helsper, E. J. (2021). Digital world: from divides to socio-digital inequalities. *The digital disconnect. The social causes and consequences of digital inequalities. SAGE Publications*, 27-45.

Henman, P. (2010). *Governing Electronically: E-Government and the Reconfiguration of Public Administration, Policy and Power*. Palgrave Macmillan. DOI: 10.1057/9780230248496

Henriksen, L. S., Smith, S. R., & Zimmer, A. (2012). At the Eve of Convergence? Transformations of Social Service Provision in Denmark, Germany, and the United States. *Voluntas, 23*(2), 458–501. DOI: 10.1007/s11266-011-9221-5

Henry, N., & Powell, A. (2018). Technology-facilitated sexual violence: A literature review of empirical research. *Trauma, Violence & Abuse, 19*(2), 195–208. DOI: 10.1177/1524838016650189 PMID: 27311818

Hicks, M. H., Tore, M., Michard, F., & Khanna, A. K. (2025). Portable wireless monitoring of vital signs in hospital wards. *BJA Education, 25*(7), 265–272. DOI: 10.1016/j.bjae.2025.04.004 PMID: 40575591

Higgs, P., & Gilleard, C. (2022). Techno-Fixes for an Ageing Society. *Aging & Mental Health, 26*(7), 1303–1305. DOI: 10.1080/13607863.2021.2008308 PMID: 34823393

Hinduja, S., & Patchin, J. W. (2010). Bullying, cyberbullying, and suicide. *Archives of Suicide Research, 14*(3), 206–221. DOI: 10.1080/13811118.2010.494133 PMID: 20658375

Hochschild, A. R. (1979). Emotion work, feeling rules, and social structure. *American Journal of Sociology, 85*(3), 551–575. DOI: 10.1086/227049

Hochschild, A. R. (1983). *The Managed Heart: Commercialization Of Human Feeling*. University of California Press.

Hogle, L. F. (2016). Data-intensive resourcing in healthcare. *Biosocieties, 11*(3), 372–393. DOI: 10.1057/s41292-016-0004-5

Hsieh, H. F., & Shannon, S. E. (2005). Three approaches to qualitative content analysis. *Qualitative Health Research, 15*(9), 1277–1288. DOI: 10.1177/1049732305276687 PMID: 16204405

Huang, B., Gan, W., & Li, Z. (2021). Application of medical material inventory model under deep learning in supply planning of public emergency. *IEEE Access : Practical Innovations, Open Solutions, 9*, 44128–44138. DOI: 10.1109/ACCESS.2021.3057869

Huang, J., Saleh, S., & Liu, Y. (2021). A review on artificial intelligence in education. *Academic Journal of Interdisciplinary Studies, 10*(3), 3. DOI: 10.36941/ajis-2021-0077

Huang, Y., Wang, J., Wang, S., & Zhang, Y. (2023). Internet of medical things: A systematic review. *Neurocomputing, 557*, 126719. Advance online publication. DOI: 10.1016/j.neucom.2023.126719

Hunsaker, A., Nguyen, M. H., Fuchs, J., Djukaric, T., Hugentobler, L., & Hargittai, E. (2019). "He Explained It to Me and I Also Did It Myself": How Older Adults Get Support with Their Technology Uses. *Socius: Sociological Research for a Dynamic World, 5*, 2378023119887866. DOI: 10.1177/2378023119887866

Iliadis, A., & Russo, F. (2016). Critical data studies: An introduction. *Big Data & Society, 3*(2), 2053951716674238. DOI: 10.1177/2053951716674238

Institute of Medicine. (2004). *Health literacy: A prescription to end confusion*. National Academies Press.

Isin, E. F., & Ruppert, E. (2015). *Being digital citizens*. Rowman & Littlefield.

Istat (2025). *Rapporto annuale 2025*. Roma

ISTAT. (2022). *Censimento permanente. Struttura e profili del terzo settore in Italia* [Permanent Census: Structure and Profiles of Italy's Third Sector], https://www.istat.it/files//2022/10/Report-Non-Profit-2022.pdf

Italia non profit. (2021). *L'impatto della Riforma sugli enti non profit* [The Impact of the Reform on Non-profit Organizations]. https://italianonprofit.it/riforma-in-movimento/risultati/#intro

Italia non profit. (2024). *Terzo Settore & Digitale, Verso un futuro digitale* [Third Secor and Digital, towards a Digital Future]. https://italianonprofit.it/riforma-in-movimento/risultati/#intro

Italian Government. (2021) «*PNRR - Piano Nazionale di Ripresa e Resilienza. Presidency of the Council of Ministers.*» https://www.governo.it/sites/governo.it/files/PNRR.pdf

ITC. (2023). *Bridging the gender divide* (last Update November). https://www.itu.int/en/mediacentre/backgrounders/Pages/bridging-the-gender-divide.aspx

Ivan, L., & Nimrod, G. (2021). Family Conflicts and Technology Use: The Voices of Grandmothers. *Family Relations*, *70*(1), 104–119. DOI: 10.1111/fare.12530

James, A., & Whelan, A. (2022). 'Ethical' artificial intelligence in the welfare state: Discourse and discrepancy in Australian social services. [Sage.]. *Critical Social Policy*, *42*(1), 22–42. DOI: 10.1177/0261018320985463

Jane, E. A. (2017). 'Dude... stop the spread': Antagonism, agonism, and# manspreading on social media. *International Journal of Cultural Studies*, *20*(5), 459–475. DOI: 10.1177/1367877916637151

Jasanoff, S. (2004). The idiom of co-production. In *States of knowledge* (pp. 1–12). Routledge. DOI: 10.4324/9780203413845-6

Ji, H., Dong, J., Pan, W., & Yu, Y. (2024). Associations between digital literacy, health literacy, and digital health behaviors among rural residents: Evidence from Zhejiang, China. *International Journal for Equity in Health*, *23*(1), 68. DOI: 10.1186/s12939-024-02150-2 PMID: 38594723

Johansson, J. (2025). Research on digital discretion—The subjectification of street-level work in public administration. *The Review of Policy Research*, *42*(1), 122–148. DOI: 10.1111/ropr.12637

Jokisch, M. R., Schmidt, L. I., & Doh, M. (2022). Acceptance Of Digital Health Services Among Older Adults: Findings on Perceived Usefulness, Self-Efficacy, Privacy Concerns, ICT Knowledge, and Support Seeking. *Frontiers in Public Health*, *10*, 1073756. DOI: 10.3389/fpubh.2022.1073756 PMID: 36582385

Joshi, M., Iqbal, F. M., Sharabiani, M., Ashrafian, H., Arora, S., McAndrew, K., Khan, S., Cooke, G., & Darzi, A. (2025). Performance of continuous digital monitoring of vital signs with a wearable sensor in acute hospital settings. *Sensors (Basel)*, *25*(9), 2644. DOI: 10.3390/s25092644 PMID: 40363083

Joyce, K., & Cruz, T. M. (2024). A Sociology of Artificial Intelligence: Inequalities, Power, and Data Justice. *Socius: Sociological Research for a Dynamic World, 10*, 10. DOI: 10.1177/23780231241275393

Jurėnienė, V. (2026). Technology-Driven Gender Violence. In Shaw, S. M., Santos, X. M., Mayilsamy, J., Veni, K., Pallarés Ameneiro, L., Rosaline, Z., & Lockhart, J. (Eds.), *Resisting Gender Violence* (pp. 159–179). Oregon State University.

Kabir, M. R., Shishir, F. S., Shomaji, S., & Ray, S. (2025). Digital twins in healthcare IoT: A systematic review. *High-Confidence Computing*, *5*(3), 100340. DOI: 10.1016/j.hcc.2025.100340

Kakhi, K., Jagatheesaperumal, S. K., Khosravi, A., Alizadehsani, R., & Acharya, U. R. (2025). Fatigue monitoring using wearables and AI: Trends, challenges, and future opportunities. *Computers in Biology and Medicine*, *195*, 110461. DOI: 10.1016/j.compbiomed.2025.110461 PMID: 40580618

Kaun, A., & Forsman, M. (2024). Digital Care Work at Public Libraries: Making Digital First Possible. *New Media & Society*, *26*(7), 3751–3766. DOI: 10.1177/14614448221104234

Kaun, A., & Liminga, A. (2023). Welfare service centres: Maintenance, repair, and care at the analogue interfaces of the digital welfare state. *New Media & Society*, *27*(5), 3039–3054. DOI: 10.1177/14614448231220362

Khan, S., & Alam, M. (2021). Wearable Internet of Things for personalized healthcare: Study of trends and latent research. In Das, H. (Eds.), *Health informatics: A computational perspective in healthcare* (pp. 43–60). Springer., DOI: 10.1007/978-981-15-9735-0_3

Kharisma, D. B., Hernoko, A. Y., & Thalib, P. (2026). Artificial intelligence in healthcare: Risk analysis and regulatory issues. *The Theory and Practice of Legislation*, *14*(1), 46–62. DOI: 10.1080/20508840.2025.2576415

Kirubakaran, D. (2025). Review on emerging frontiers in medical sensing: Innovations shaping the future of healthcare. *Biomedical Materials & Devices*, *3*, 385. DOI: 10.1007/s44174-025-00385-3

Kitchin, R. (2014). Big Data, new epistemologies and paradigm shifts. *Big Data & Society*, *1*(1), 2053951714528481. DOI: 10.1177/2053951714528481

Kitchin, R. (2014). The data revolution. *Sage (Atlanta, Ga.)*.

Kitchin, R. (2014). *The data revolution: Big data, open data, data infrastructures and their consequences*. SAGE Publications., DOI: 10.4135/9781473909472

Kleinman, A., Eisenberg, L., & Good, B. (1978). Culture, illness, and care: Clinical lessons from anthropologic and cross-cultural research. *Annals of Internal Medicine, 88*(2), 251–258. DOI: 10.7326/0003-4819-88-2-251

König, L., Kuhlmey, A., & Suhr, R. (2024). Digital health literacy of the population in Germany and its association with physical health, mental health, life satisfaction, and health behaviors: Nationally representative survey study. *JMIR Public Health and Surveillance, 10*(1), e48685. DOI: 10.2196/48685 PMID: 38381497

Korpela, V., Pajula, L., & Hänninen, R. (2023). Older Adults Learning Digital Skills Together: Peer Tutors' Perspectives on Non-Formal Digital Support. *Media and Communication, 11*(3), 53–62. DOI: 10.17645/mac.v11i3.6742

Korpela, V., Pajula, L., & Hänninen, R. (2024). Investigating the multifaceted role of warm experts in enhancing and hindering older adults' digital skills in Finland. *International Journal of Lifelong Education, 43*(5), 509–522. DOI: 10.1080/02601370.2024.2353176

Krieger, N. (2011). *Epidemiology and the people's health: Theory and context.* Oxford University Press. DOI: 10.1093/acprof:oso/9780195383874.001.0001

Krippendorff, K. (2018). *Content analysis: An introduction to its methodology.* Sage publications.

Kristensen, D. B., & Prigge, C. (2017). Human/technology associations in self-tracking practices. In *Self-tracking: Empirical and philosophical investigations* (pp. 43–59). Springer International Publishing.

Kroll, J. A., Huey, J., Barocas, S., Felten, E. W., Reidenberg, J. R., Robinson, D. G., & Yu, H. (2017). Accountable algorithms. *University of Pennsylvania Law Review, 165*(3), 633–705.

Kruse, C. S., Bolton, K., & Freriks, G. (2015). The effect of patient portals on quality outcomes. *Journal of Medical Internet Research, 17*(2), e44. DOI: 10.2196/jmir.3171 PMID: 25669240

Kruse, C. S., Goswamy, R., Raval, Y., & Marawi, S. (2016). Big data in health care. *JMIR Medical Informatics, 4*(4), e38. DOI: 10.2196/medinform.5359 PMID: 27872036

Kruse, C. S., Pesek, B., Anderson, M., Brennan, K., & Comfort, H. (2019). Telemonitoring for COPD. *JMIR Medical Informatics.*

Kuhlmann, R. (2023). Assistive technologies for people with disabilities, available on: https://www.veritas-project.eu/assistive-technologienfuer-menschen-mit-behinderungen/

Kumar, R., Singh, A., Kassar, A. S. A., Humaida, M. I., Joshi, S., & Sharma, M. (2025). Adoption challenges to artificial intelligence literacy in public healthcare: An evidence based study in Saudi Arabia. *Frontiers in Public Health, 13*, 1558772. DOI: 10.3389/fpubh.2025.1558772 PMID: 40371275

Lamont, M. (2000). *The dignity of working men: Morality and the boundaries of race, class, and immigration.* Harvard University Press. DOI: 10.4159/9780674039889

Lancia, F. (2004). *Strumenti per l'analisi dei testi.* Franco Angeli.

Larrazabal, A. J., Nieto, N., Peterson, V., Milone, D., & Ferrante, E. (2020). Gender imbalance in medical imaging datasets. *Proceedings of the National Academy of Sciences of the United States of America, 117*(23), 12592–12594. DOI: 10.1073/pnas.1919012117 PMID: 32457147

Laukka, E., Lakoma, S., Harjumaa, M., Hiltunen, S., Härkönen, H., Jansson, M., Leskelä, R., Martikainen, S., Pennanen, P., Verho, A., & Torkki, P. (2024). Older Adults' Preferences in the Utilisation of Digital Health and Social Services: A Qualitative Analysis of Responses to Open-Ended Questions. *BMC Health Services Research, 24*(1), 1184. DOI: 10.1186/s12913-024-11564-1 PMID: 39367429

Layne, K., & Lee, J. (2001). Developing Fully Functional E-Government: A Four Stage Model. *Government Information Quarterly, 18*(2), 122–136. DOI: 10.1016/S0740-624X(01)00066-1

Leavy, S. (2018, May). Gender bias in artificial intelligence: The need for diversity and gender theory in machine learning. In *Proceedings of the 1st international workshop on gender equality in software engineering* (pp. 14-16). DOI: 10.1145/3195570.3195580

LegaCoop. (2023). *Indagine sulla digitalizzazione nelle imprese cooperative* [Survey on the Social Enterprises Digitalization].

Leidner, R. (1999). Emotional labor in service work. *The Annals of the American Academy of Political and Social Science, 561*(1), 81–95. DOI: 10.1177/000271629956100106

Levy, K., Chasalow, K. E., & Riley, S. (2021). Algorithms and decision-making in the public sector. *Annual Review of Law and Social Science, 17*(1), 309–334. DOI: 10.1146/annurev-lawsocsci-041221-023808

Lincoln, Y. C., & Guba, E. G. (1985). Naturalistic Inquiry. *Sage (Atlanta, Ga.)*.

Lipsky, M. (2010). *Street-Level Bureaucracy, 30th Anniversary Edition: Dilemmas of the Individual in Public Service*. Russell Sage Foundation.

Litchfield, I., Shukla, D., & Greenfield, S. (2021). Impact of COVID-19 on the digital divide: A rapid review. *BMJ Open*, *11*(10), e053440. DOI: 10.1136/bmjopen-2021-053440 PMID: 34642200

Liu, J., & Liu, H. (2025). Research on flexible sensors for wearable devices: A review. *Nanomaterials (Basel, Switzerland)*, *15*(7), 520. DOI: 10.3390/nano15070520 PMID: 40214565

Li, Y. (2025). Vlogging as mediated mobility: Warm Experts 3.0 engaging in peer production and digital labor in the era of short videos. *International Journal of Cultural Studies*, *28*(3), 562–579. DOI: 10.1177/13678779241298707

Lo Schiavo, L., & Giumelli, R. (2021). Dal sociale al social: Società in trasformazione. Una mappatura del campo analitico. *Sociologie*, *2*(1), 5–18.

Loe, M. (2010). Doing It My Way: Old Women, Technology and Wellbeing. *Sociology of Health & Illness*, *32*(2), 319–334. DOI: 10.1111/j.1467-9566.2009.01220.x PMID: 20149150

Longworth, J. (2021). Benjamin Ruha (2019) Race After Technology: Abolitionist Tools for the New Jim Code. Medford: Polity Press. *Science & Technology Studies*, *34*(2), 92–94. DOI: 10.23987/sts.102639

Loos, E. F. (2012). Senior Citizens: Digital Immigrants in their Own Country? *Observatorio (OBS*). Journal*, *6*, 1–23.

Loos, E., & Ivan, L. (2024). Not Only People Are Getting Old, the New Media Are Too: Technology Generations and the Changes in New Media Use. *New Media & Society*, *26*(6), 3588–3613. DOI: 10.1177/14614448221101783

Lorentzen, A. C. R. (2022). Digital transformation as distributed leadership: Firing the change agent. *Procedia Computer Science*, *196*, 245–254. DOI: 10.1016/j.procs.2021.12.011

Lorenz, W. (2025). Re-positioning the social mandate of social work. *Nordic Social Work Research*, 1–13. DOI: 10.1080/2156857X.2025.2478838

Lowe, C. (2022). *The Digitalisation of Social Protection Before and Since the Onset of COVID-19: Opportunities, Challenges and Lessons*. ODI Working Paper. ODI.

Lupton, D. (2013). The digitally engaged patient. *Social Theory & Health, 11*(3), 256–270. DOI: 10.1057/sth.2013.10

Lupton, D. (2014). *Digital sociology*. Routledge. DOI: 10.4324/9781315776880

Lupton, D. (2016). *The quantified self*. Polity Press.

Lupton, D. (2018). *Digital health: Critical and cross-disciplinary perspectives*. Routledge., DOI: 10.4324/9781315648835

Magaudda, P., & Neresini, F. (2020). *Gli studi sociali sulla scienza e la tecnologia, il Mulino*.

Malakhov, K. (2023). Insight into the digital health system of Ukraine. *International Journal of Telerehabilitation, 15*(2). Advance online publication. DOI: 10.5195/ijt.2023.6599 PMID: 38162941

Mangone, E. (2016). Implicazioni normative e istituzionali nello sviluppo integrato del welfare. In Del Forno, M. (Ed.), *Nel complesso mondo del welfare. Idee, metodi e pratiche* (pp. 93–104). FrancoAngeli.

Mangone, E., Masullo, G., & Gallego, M. (Eds.). (2018). *Gender and Sexuality in the Migration Trajectories. Studies between the Northern and Southern Mediterranean Shores*. Information Age Publishing.

Marent, B., & Henwood, F. (2021). Digital health. In *Routledge international handbook of critical issues in health and illness* (pp. 261–275). Routledge. DOI: 10.4324/9781003185215-24

Marent, B., & Henwood, F. (2023). Digital health: A sociomaterial approach. *Sociology of Health & Illness, 45*(1), 37–53. DOI: 10.1111/1467-9566.13538 PMID: 36031756

Margetts, H., & Dunleavy, P. (2013). The second wave of digital-era governance: a quasi-paradigm for government on the Web. *Philosophical transactions of the royal society A: mathematical, physical and engineering sciences, 371*(1987).

Marinescu, M.-R., Ionescu, O. N., Pachiu, C. I., Dinescu, M. A., Muller, R., & uchea, M. P. (2025). Next-gen healthcare devices: Evolution of MEMS and BioMEMS in the era of the Internet of Bodies for personalized medicine. *Micromachines, 16*(10), 1182. DOI: 10.3390/mi16101182 PMID: 41156428

Markert, C., Sasangohar, F., Mortazavi, B., & Fields, S. (2021). Telehealth technology for older adults. *JMIR Human Factors*. Advance online publication. DOI: 10.2196/23796 PMID: 33512322

Marshall, T. H. (1950). *Citizenship and social class and other essays*. Cambridge University Press.

Martines, F. (2019). La digitalizzazione della pubblica amministrazione. *Medicine and Law*, *2*, 146–161.

Martinez, C., & Olsson, T. (2022). The Warm Expert – A Warm Teacher? Learning about Digital Media in Intergenerational Interaction. *Convergence (London)*, *28*(6), 1861–1877. DOI: 10.1177/13548565211070409

Marwick, A. E., & Caplan, R. (2018). Drinking male tears: Language, the manosphere, and networked harassment. *Feminist Media Studies*, *18*(4), 543–559. DOI: 10.1080/14680777.2018.1450568

Masiero, S., & Shakthi, S. (2020). Grappling with Aadhaar: Biometrics, social identity and the Indian state. *South Asia Multidisciplinary Academic Journal*, *23*(23). Advance online publication. DOI: 10.4000/samaj.6279

Massanari, A. (2017). # Gamergate and The Fappening: How Reddit's algorithm, governance, and culture support toxic technocultures. *New Media & Society*, *19*(3), 329–346. DOI: 10.1177/1461444815608807

Masullo, G., & Picarella, L. (2025). Men's involvement in preventing gender violence: Socio-educational and cultural strategies for an integrated welfare. *Welfare e Ergonomia*, *2*, 39–50.

Matthew, A. J., Dhanalakshmi, R., & Vimal, S. (2025). A systematic review of Internet of Medical Things (IoMT) in healthcare. *Sci*, *7*(2), 36. DOI: 10.3390/sci7020036

Mayer-Schönberger, V., & Cukier, K. (2013). *Big data*. Houghton Mifflin Harcourt.

Mayer-Schönberger, V., & Cukier, K. (2013). *Big data: A revolution that will transform how we live, work, and think*. Eamon Dolan/Houghton Mifflin Harcourt.

Mazzeo, A. E. P., & dos Santos, L. W. (2025). Integration of biomedical devices and the internet of bodies revolution. Research. *Social Development*, *14*(5), e48921. DOI: 10.33448/rsd-v14i5.48921

Mazzucato, M. (2021). *Mission economy: A moonshot guide to changing capitalism*. Penguin.

McCarthy, J. (2022). Artificial intelligence, logic, and formalising common sense. *Machine Learning and the City: Applications in Architecture and Urban Design*, 69-90.

McCray, A. T. (2005). Promoting health literacy. *Journal of the American Medical Informatics Association : JAMIA*, *12*(2), 152–163. DOI: 10.1197/jamia.M1687 PMID: 15561782

Meijer, A., & Bolívar, M. P. R. (2016). Governing the smart city: A review of the literature on smart urban governance. *International Review of Administrative Sciences*, *82*(2), 392–408. DOI: 10.1177/0020852314564308

Melis, G., Sala, E., & Zaccaria, D. (2021). Remote recruiting and video-interviewing older people: a research note on a qualitative case study carried out in the first Covid-19 Red Zone in Europe. *International Journal of Social Research Methodology*, *25*(4), 477-482.

Melis, G., Sala, E., & Zaccaria, D. (2022). The Role of Information and Communication Technologies in Researching Older People During the Covid-19 Pandemic: The Case of the Italian Longitudinal Study on Older People's Quality of Life During the Covid-19 Pandemic (ILQA-19). In *International Conference on Human-Computer Interaction* (pp. 53-68). Cham: Springer International Publishing.

Meyer, S. (2016). Examining women's agency in managing intimate partner violence and the related risk of homelessness: The role of harm minimisation. *Global Public Health: An International Journal for Research, Policy and Practice*, *11*(1-2), 198–210. DOI: 10.1080/17441692.2015.1047390 PMID: 26110781

Miano, F. (2013). *Günther Anders, Sulla vergogna prometeica, Etica & Politica / Ethics & Politics*, XV, 2013, 2, pp. 246-257, available on: https://www.openstarts.units.it/server/api/core/bitstreams/9a045474-1f61-4f37-9013-75a62a663f1d/content

Michard, F., & Saugel, B. (2025). New sensors for the early detection of clinical deterioration on general wards and beyond – A clinician's perspective. *Journal of Clinical Monitoring and Computing*, *39*(2), 435–442. DOI: 10.1007/s10877-024-01235-1 PMID: 39546216

Miller, D. (1987). *Material Culture and Mass Consumption*. Blackwell.

Millward, P. (2003). The 'Grey Digital Divide': Perception, Exclusion and Barriers of Access to the Internet for Older People. *First Monday*, *8*(7). Advance online publication. DOI: 10.5210/fm.v8i7.1066

Ministero della Salute. (2021). *Fascicolo Sanitario Elettronico: stato di attuazione e prospettive*. https://www.salute.gov.it/portale/temi/p2_6.jsp?id=5323&area=fascicoloSanitarioElettronico&menu=vuoto

Mintzberg, H. (1978). Patterns in Strategy Formation Author. *Management Science*, *24*(9), 934–948. DOI: 10.1287/mnsc.24.9.934

Miragoli, M. (2025). Conformism, ignorance & injustice: AI as a tool of epistemic oppression. *Episteme (Edinburgh)*, *22*(2), 522–540. DOI: 10.1017/epi.2024.11

Mishler, E. G. (1984). *The discourse of medicine: Dialectics of medical interviews*. Bloomsbury Academic.

Mittelstadt, B., Allo, P., Taddeo, M., Wachter, S., & Floridi, L. (2016). The ethics of algorithms. *Big Data & Society*, *3*(2), 2053951716679679. DOI: 10.1177/2053951716679679

Mocellin, S. (2023). Il lavoro nel framework del capability approach: L'interpretazione di A. Sen. *Lavoro Diritti Europa*, *1*, 1–18.

Mol, A. (2008). *The logic of care: Health and the problem of patient choice*. Routledge. DOI: 10.4324/9780203927076

Mori, L. (2019). Il flebile bisbiglio degli organi. Datificazione della salute e processi di costruzione identitaria. *Rassegna Italiana di Sociologia*, *60*(3), 531–558.

Morley, J., & Floridi, L. (2020). The limits of empowerment. *Science and Engineering Ethics*, *26*(3), 1159–1183. DOI: 10.1007/s11948-019-00115-1 PMID: 31172424

Morozov, E. (2014). *To save everything, click here: The folly of technological solutionism*. PublicAffairs.

Morris, A., & Brading, H. (2007). E-Literacy and the Grey Digital Divide: A Review with Recommendations. *Journal of Information Literacy*, *1*(3), 1–13. DOI: 10.11645/1.3.14

Morris, T., Aspinal, F., Ledger, J., Li, K., & Gomes, M. (2023). The impact of digital health interventions for the management of type 2 diabetes on health and social care utilisation and costs: A systematic review. *PharmacoEconomics Open*, *7*(2), 163–173. DOI: 10.1007/s41669-022-00377-9 PMID: 36495462

Mossberger, K., Tolbert, C., & McNeal, R. (2008). *Digital citizenship*. MIT Press.

Mulgan, G., Tucker, S., Ali, R., & Sanders, B. (2007). *Social Innovation. What it is, why it matters and how it can be accelerated*, The Young Foundation Working Paper, The Young Foundation

Muralidharan, K., Niehaus, P., & Sukhtankar, S. (2022). Integrating biometric authentication in India's welfare programs: Lessons from a decade of reforms. *India Policy Forum : [Papers]. India Policy Forum. Conference*, *18*(1), 139–172.

Murru, M. F., & Selva, D. (2025). Senso comune artificiale: Egemonia culturale e intelligenza artificiale generativa. *COMUNICAZIONI SOCIALI*, 1-18.

Naghib, M., Chalechale, A., & Gharehchopogh, F. S. (2025). A comprehensive and systematic literature review on intrusion detection systems in the Internet of Medical Things: Current status, challenges, and opportunities. *Artificial Intelligence Review, 58*(4), 114. Advance online publication. DOI: 10.1007/s10462-024-11101-w

Naldini, M., & Saraceno, C. (2022). Changes in the Italian Work-Family System and the Role of Social Policies in the Last Forty Years. *Stato e Mercato, 42*(1), 87–115.

Nangia, N., Vania, C., Bhalerao, R., & Bowman, S. (2020). CrowS-pairs: A challenge dataset for measuring social biases in masked language models. *In Proceedings of the 2020 Conference on Empirical Methods in Natural Language Processing (EMNLP)* (pp. 1953-1967). DOI: 10.18653/v1/2020.emnlp-main.154

Nash, J. C. (2021). Intersectionality. In The Keywords Feminist Editorial Collective (Ed.), *Keywords for gender and sexuality* (pp. 128-133). New York University Press.

Ndikumana, F., Izabayo, J., Kalisa, J., Nemerimana, M., Nyabyenda, E. C., Muzungu, S. H., Komezusenge, I., Uwase, M., Ndagijimana, S., Twizere, C., & Sezibera, V. (2025). Machine learning-based predictive modelling of mental health in Rwandan Youth. *Scientific Reports, 15*(1), 16032. DOI: 10.1038/s41598-025-00519-z PMID: 40341215

Neale, B. (2020). *Qualitative Longitudinal Research: Research Methods*. Bloomsbury Publishing.

Neittaanmäki, N. (2025, February). Swedish medical students' attitudes toward artificial intelligence and effects on career plans: A survey. [). Frontiers Media SA.]. *Frontiers in Education, 10*, 1517116. DOI: 10.3389/feduc.2025.1517116

Newell, A., & Simon, H. A. (1976). Computer science as empirical inquiry: Symbols and search. *Communications of the ACM, 19*(3), 113–126. DOI: 10.1145/360018.360022

Nilsen, P., Svedberg, P., Nygren, J., Frideros, M., Johansson, J., & Schueller, S. (2022). Accelerating the impact of artificial intelligence in mental healthcare through implementation science. *Implementation Research and Practice, 3*, 26334895221112033. DOI: 10.1177/26334895221112033 PMID: 37091110

Ning, L., Zheng, Z., Liu, M., Gao, S., Yang, X., Bi, J., Yu, X., & Yi, D. (2024). Profiles of digital health literacy among university students and its association with mental health during the COVID-19 pandemic: A latent profile analysis. *Digital Health, 10*, 20552076231224596. DOI: 10.1177/20552076231224596 PMID: 38205038

Noble, S. U. (2018). Algorithms of oppression: How search engines reinforce racism. In *Algorithms of oppression*. New York university press.

Noble, S. U. (2018). *Algorithms of Oppression: How Search Engines Reinforce Racism*. New York University Press. DOI: 10.18574/nyu/9781479833641.001.0001

Norman, C. D., & Skinner, H. A. (2006). eHEALS: The eHealth literacy scale. *Journal of Medical Internet Research*, *8*(4), 1–7. DOI: 10.2196/jmir.8.4.e27

Norman, C. D., & Skinner, H. A. (2006). eHealth literacy. *Journal of Medical Internet Research*, *8*(2), e9. DOI: 10.2196/jmir.8.2.e9 PMID: 16867972

Norori, N., Hu, Q., Aellen, F. M., Faraci, F. D., & Tzovara, A. (2021). Addressing bias in big data and AI for health care: A call for open science. *Patterns (New York, N.Y.)*, *2*(10), 100347. Advance online publication. DOI: 10.1016/j.patter.2021.100347 PMID: 34693373

Norris, P. (2001). Digital divide: Civic engagement, information poverty, and the Internet worldwide.

Novello, M., & Garavaglia, E. (2026). Ageing and technology in the policy discourse on public services digitalisation: a missed opportunity?. *Ageing & Society*, *46*, e6.

Nussbaum, M. C. (2011). *Creating capabilities: The human development approach*. Harvard University Press. DOI: 10.4159/harvard.9780674061200

Nyanjom, J., & Naylor, D. (2021). Performing emotional labour while teaching online. *Educational Research*, *63*(2), 147–163. DOI: 10.1080/00131881.2020.1836989

O'Neil, C. (2017). *Armi di distruzione matematica*. Bompiani.

Obermeyer, Z., & Emanuel, E. J. (2016). Predicting the future-big data, machine learning, and clinical medicine. *The New England Journal of Medicine*, *375*(13), 1216–1219. DOI: 10.1056/NEJMp1606181 PMID: 27682033

Obermeyer, Z., Powers, B., Vogeli, C., & Mullainathan, S. (2019). Dissecting racial bias in an algorithm used to manage the health of populations. *Science*, *366*(6464), 447–453. DOI: 10.1126/science.aax2342

OECD. (2016). *Digital government strategies for transforming public services in welfare areas*. OECD.

Oleksy, T., & Wnuk, A. (2021). Do women perceive sex robots as threatening? The role of political views and presenting the robot as a female-vs male-friendly product. *Computers in Human Behavior*, *117*, 106664. DOI: 10.1016/j.chb.2020.106664

Olsson, T., & Viscovi, D. (2023). Digitalised Welfare: Access, Usage, and Outcomes Among Older Adults. *Media and Communication*, *11*(3), 18–28. DOI: 10.17645/mac.v11i3.6694

Ong, A. (2006). *Neoliberalism as exception*. Duke University Press.

Organisation for Economic Co-operation and Development. (2023). *Health at a glance 2023: OECD indicators*. OECD Publishing. https://doi.org/.DOI: 10.1787/7a7afb35-en

Orlikowski, W. (1992). Rethinking the concept of technology in organizations. *Organization Science*, *3*(3), 398–427. DOI: 10.1287/orsc.3.3.398

Orlikowski, W. J. (2000). Using technology and constituting structures: A practice lens for studying technology in organizations. *Organization Science*, *11*(4), 404–428. DOI: 10.1287/orsc.11.4.404.14600

Orlikowski, W. J. (2007). Sociomaterial Practices: Exploring Techology at Work. *Organization Studies*, *28*(09), 1435–1448. DOI: 10.1177/0170840607081138

Orlikowski, W. J., & Scott, S. V. (2008). Sociomateriality: Challenging the Separation of Technology, Work and Organization. *The Academy of Management Annals*, *2*(2), 433–474. DOI: 10.5465/19416520802211644

Otte-Trojel, T., de Bont, A., Rundall, T., & van de Klundert, J. (2014). Developing patient portals. *Journal of the American Medical Informatics Association : JAMIA*. PMID: 26335985

Oz, M., Zheng, P., & Chen, G. M. (2018). Twitter versus Facebook: Comparing incivility, impoliteness, and deliberative attributes. *New Media & Society*, *20*(9), 3400–3419. DOI: 10.1177/1461444817749516

Page, M. J., McKenzie, J. E., Bossuyt, P. M., Boutron, I., Hoffmann, T. C., Mulrow, C. D., ... & Moher, D. (2021). The PRISMA 2020 statement: an updated guideline for reporting systematic reviews. *bmj, 372*.

Papacharissi, Z. (2015). We have always been social. *Social Media + Society*, *1*(1), 2056305115581185. DOI: 10.1177/2056305115581185

Parihar, A., Prajapati, J. B., Prajapati, B. G., Trambadiya, B., Thakkar, A., & Engineer, P. (2024). Role of IoT in healthcare: Applications, security & privacy concerns. *Intelligent Pharmacy*, *2*(5), 707–714. DOI: 10.1016/j.ipha.2024.01.003

Park, S., & Humphry, J. (2019). Exclusion by design: Intersections of social, digital and data exclusion. [Taylor & Francis.]. *Information Communication and Society*, *22*(7), 934–953. DOI: 10.1080/1369118X.2019.1606266

Parsons, T. (1991). *The social system*. Routledge.

Parsons, T. (2021). *La struttura dell'azione sociale: Uno studio di teoria sociale con particolare riferimento a un gruppo di autori europei recenti* (Vol. I e II). Mimesis.

Pascale, C. M. (2013). Social inequality & the politics of representation. *Sage (Atlanta, Ga.).*

Pasceri, E. (2025). Knowledge Organization Systems come strumenti di sorveglianza sanitaria. L'applicazione della ICD in Italia. *AIDA Informazioni: Rivista di Scienze dell'informazione*, 43(1-2), 45–62.

Pasciuto, F. (2022). *L'algoritmo della cultura: Processi di produzione e consumo nell'era digitale.* FrancoAngeli.

Pasquale, F. (2015). *The black box society: The secret algorithms that control money and information.* Harvard University Press. DOI: 10.4159/harvard.9780674736061

Pasqualotto, L. (2014). Disabilità e inclusione secondo il capability approach. *L'integrazione Scolastica e Sociale, 13*(3), 278–284.

Pastorelli, G. (2022). L'economia Sociale Digitale e la sfida dell'interoperatiblità. Verso una prossima economia sociale [The Social Digital Economy and the Interoperability Challenge. Toward a Further Social Economi]. *Impresa Sociale, 1*, 87–91. DOI: 10.7425/IS.2022.01.12

Paul, M. M., Khera, N., Elugunti, P. R., Ruff, K. C., Hommos, M. S., Thomas, L. F., Nagaraja, V., Garrett, A. L., Pantoja-Smith, M., Delafield, N. L., Lizaola-Mayo, B. C., Kresin, M. M., Seetharam, M., Nagarakanti, S. R., & Kaur, M. (2025). The state of remote patient monitoring for chronic disease management in the United States. *Journal of Medical Internet Research, 27*, e70422. DOI: 10.2196/70422 PMID: 40570326

Peine, A., & Neven, L. (2019). From Intervention to Co-constitution: New Directions in Theorizing about Aging and Technology. *The Gerontologist, 59*(1), 15–21. DOI: 10.1093/geront/gny050 PMID: 29850812

Petersen, A. (2018). *Digital health and technological promise: A sociological inquiry.* Routledge. DOI: 10.4324/9781315200880

Petticrew, M., & Roberts, H. (2008). Systematic reviews–do they 'work' in informing decision-making around health inequalities? *Health Economics, Policy, and Law, 3*(2), 197–211. DOI: 10.1017/S1744133108004453 PMID: 18634627

Pew Research Center. (2021). *The State of Online Harassment.* https://www.pewresearch.org/internet/2021/01/13/the-state-of-online-harassment/

Pezoulas, V. C., Zaridis, D. I., Mylona, E., Androutsos, C., Apostolidis, K., Tachos, N. S., & Fotiadis, D. I. (2024). Synthetic data generation methods in healthcare: A review on open-source tools and methods. *Computational and Structural Biotechnology Journal, 23*, 2892–2910. DOI: 10.1016/j.csbj.2024.07.005 PMID: 39108677

Piccone Stella, S., & Saraceno, C. (1996). *Genere. La costruzione sociale del femminile e del maschile*. Il Mulino.

Polanyi, K. (1944). *The Great Transformation*. Farrar and Rinehart.

Pope, N. D., Riley, J. E., Haberkorn, J., & Ely, G. E. (2016). Being "Easy": Women's Desire to Accept Help in Later Life. *Journal of Women & Aging, 28*(5), 352–362. DOI: 10.1080/08952841.2014.962863 PMID: 26933929

Powell, J., & Deetjen, U. (2019). Characterizing the digital health citizen. *Journal of Medical Internet Research, 21*(3), e11279. DOI: 10.2196/11279 PMID: 30835238

Powell, W. W., & DiMaggio, P. J. (Eds.). (1991). *The new instituzionalism in organizational analysis*. The University of Chicago Press. DOI: 10.7208/chicago/9780226185941.001.0001

Pravettoni, G., & Triberti, S. (2019). *Il medico 4.0: Come cambia la relazione medico-paziente nell'era delle nuove tecnologie*. Edra.

Prior, L. (2020). *Using documents in social research. Qualitative Research* (5th ed.). Sage.

Pronzato, R. (2024). *Algoritmi, strutture e agire sociale: Un'analisi sociologica*

Punziano, G., & Acampa, S. (2023). Reti, digitale e processi di innovazione tra profili di resilienza e mutamento: i pilastri del fronteggiamento alla doppia transizione. [Networks, Digital and Innovation Processes between Resilience and Change: the Pillars to Cope with the Double Transition] In Punziano, G., Cicellin, M., & Zito, E. (Eds.), *Nuove risposte organizzative, innovazioni e impatti sociali del Covid-19 sul Terzo Settore* [New Organizational Responses, Innovations, and Social Impact of Covid-19 on Third Sector Organizations]. (pp. 110–123). Franco Angeli.

Punziano, G., Cicellin, M., Zito, E., Acampa, S., & Sorrentino, R. (2023). Role of the Digital for the Third Sector in the Campania Region (Italy): From the Side of Research to the Side of the Objects in the Aftermath of the COVID-19 Pandemic. *Italian Sociological Review, 13*(X), 279–296. DOI: 10.13136/isr.v13i2.638

Raghavan, M., Barocas, S., Kleinberg, J., & Levy, K. (2020, January). Mitigating bias in algorithmic hiring: Evaluating claims and practices. In *Proceedings of the 2020 conference on fairness, accountability, and transparency* (pp. 469-481). DOI: 10.1145/3351095.3372828

Ragnedda, M., & Ruiu, M. L. (2017). Social Capital and the Three Levels of Digital Divide. In G., Muschert & M., Ragnedda (Eds.). *Theorizing Digital Divides* (pp. 21-34). Routledge. DOI: 10.4324/9781315455334-3

Ragnedda, M. (2018). Conceptualizing Digital Capital. *Telematics and Informatics, 35*(8), 2366–2375. DOI: 10.1016/j.tele.2018.10.006

Ragnedda, M. (2020). *Enhancing digital equity: Connecting the digital underclass.* PalgraveMacmillan., DOI: 10.1007/978-3-030-49079-9

Ragnedda, M., & Ruiu, M. L. (2020). *Digital capital: A Bourdieusian perspective on the digital divide.* Emerald Group Publishing. DOI: 10.1108/9781839095504

Rashid, S., & Nemati, A. (2024). Human-centered IoT-based health monitoring in the Healthcare 5.0 era: Literature descriptive analysis and future research guidelines. *Discover Internet of Things, 4*(1), 26. DOI: 10.1007/s43926-024-00082-5

Rebergen, M., Swart, J., & Broersma, M. (2025). Directing digital citizenship: How librarians mediate the Dutch digital welfare state. *Social Inclusion (Lisboa), 13,* 9949. DOI: 10.17645/si.9949

Recuero, R. (2024). The platformization of violence: Toward a concept of discursive toxicity on social media. *Social Media + Society, 10*(1), 20563051231224264. DOI: 10.1177/20563051231224264

Reed, M., Huang, J., & Brand, R.. (2019). Patient portal use and health outcomes. *Journal of Medical Internet Research, 21*(7). PMID: 31593546

Rejeb, A., Rejeb, K., Treiblmaier, H., Appolloni, A., Alghamdi, S., Alhasawi, Y., & Iranmanesh, M. (2023). The Internet of Things (IoT) in healthcare: Taking stock and moving forward. *Internet of Things : Engineering Cyber Physical Human Systems, 22,* 100721. DOI: 10.1016/j.iot.2023.100721

Report, I. (2025). Livelli di Istruzione e ritorni occupazionali. Anno 2024. Available on: https://www.istat.it/wp-content/uploads/2025/12/Report-Livelli-di-istruzione-e-ritorni-occupazionali-Anno-2024.pdf

Report, O. E. C. D. (2022). The Effects of AI on the Working Lives of Women, available on: https://www.oecd.org/en/publications/the-effects-of-ai-on-the-working-lives-of-women_14e9b92c-en.html

Report, W. E. F. World Economic Forum (2024). Global Gender Gap. Insight Report, available on: https://www3.weforum.org/docs/WEF_GGGR_2024.pdf

Risling, T., Martinez, J., Young, J., & Thorp-Froslie, N. (2017). Evaluating patient empowerment in eHealth. *Journal of Medical Internet Research, 19*(9), e329. DOI: 10.2196/jmir.7809 PMID: 28963090

Roberts, M. E., Stewart, B. M., Tingley, D., Lucas, C., Leder-Luis, J., Gadarian, S. K., Albertson, B., & Rand, D. G. (2014). Structural topic models for open-ended survey responses. *American Journal of Political Science*, *58*(4), 1064–1082. DOI: 10.1111/ajps.12103

Robinson, L., Cotten, S., Ono, H., Quan-Haase, A., Mesch, G., Chen, W., Schulz, J., Hale, T. M., & Stern, M. J. (2015). Digital inequalities and why they matter. *Information Communication and Society*, *18*(5), 569–582. DOI: 10.1080/1369118X.2015.1012532

Rogers, E. M. (1983). *Diffusion of Innovation*. The Free Press.

Romaniuk, O. O., Kozak, L. M., & Kovalenko, O. S. (2021). Formation oF interoperable Digital meDicine inFormation environment: personal meDical Data. *Science and innovation*, (17,N° 5), 50-62.

Ross, A. R., Chadwick, A., & Vaccari, C. (2021). Digital media and the proliferation of public opinion cues online: Biases and vulnerabilities in the new attention economy. In *The Routledge companion to political journalism* (pp. 241–251). Routledge. DOI: 10.4324/9780429284571-22

Rothstein, B., & Stolle, D. (2008). The state and social capital: An institutional theory of generalized trust. *Comparative Politics*, *40*(4), 441–459. DOI: 10.5129/001041508X12911362383354

Rowe, I. (2015). Civility 2.0: A comparative analysis of incivility in online political discussion. *Information Communication and Society*, *18*(2), 121–138. DOI: 10.1080/1369118X.2014.940365

Rowland, B., Saha, A., Motamedi, V., Bundy, R., Winsor, S., McNavish, D., Lippert, W., & Khanna, A. K. (2025). Impact on patient outcomes of continuous vital sign monitoring on medical wards: Propensity-matched analysis. *Journal of Medical Internet Research*, *27*, e66347. DOI: 10.2196/66347 PMID: 40068153

Rubin, G. (1975). The traffic in women: Notes on the "political economy" of sex. In Reiter, R. R. (Ed.), *Toward an anthropology of women* (pp. 157–210). Monthly Review Press.Ruble, D. N., Martin, C. L., & Berenbaum, S. A. (2006). Gender development. In *Damon W., R. M. Lerner R. M. e Eisenberg John N. a cura di* (pp. 858–932). Handbook of Child Psychology. John Wiley & Sons, Inc.

Ruckenstein, M., & Schüll, N. D. (2017). The datafication of health. *Annual Review of Anthropology*, *46*(1), 261–278. DOI: 10.1146/annurev-anthro-102116-041244

Sadowski, J. (2020). *Too Smart: How Digital Capitalism is Extracting Data, Controlling Our Lives, and Transforming the World*. The MIT Press. DOI: 10.7551/mitpress/12240.001.0001

Saeed, S. A., & Masters, R. M. (2021). Disparities in health care and the digital divide. *Current Psychiatry Reports*, *23*(9), 61. DOI: 10.1007/s11920-021-01274-4 PMID: 34297202

Saguy, A. C. (2025, November). The Social Constructions of Gender. *Sociological Forum*, *40*(S1), S17–S28. DOI: 10.1111/socf.70007

Saiani, P. P. (2020). Verso un welfare state digitale? L'intelligenza artificiale tra politiche sociali e apparati di controllo. *la Rivista delle Politiche Sociali, 237*.

Sala, E., & Kochergina, E. (2025). Is E-Government an Opportunity for All? Identifying Barriers and Enablers of E-Government Use Among Older Adults in Europe. *Social Sciences & Humanities Open*, *12*, 102158. DOI: 10.1016/j.ssaho.2025.102158

Salganik, M. J. (2019). *Bit by bit: Social research in the digital age*. Princeton University Press.

Sameh, A., Rostami, M., Oussalah, M., Korpelainen, R., & Farrahi, V. (2025). Digital phenotypes and digital biomarkers for health and diseases: A systematic review of machine learning approaches utilizing passive non-invasive signals collected via wearable devices and smartphones. *Artificial Intelligence Review*, *58*(2), 66. DOI: 10.1007/s10462-024-11009-5

Santana, A. D. (2014). Virtuous or vitriolic: The effect of anonymity on civility in online newspaper reader comment boards. *Journalism Practice*, *8*(1), 18–33. DOI: 10.1080/17512786.2013.813194

Santosuosso, A. (2020). *Intelligenza artificiale e diritto*. Mondadori Università.

Saraceni, G. (2019). Digital divide e povertà. *Dirittifondamentali.it*, 2, 1–19.

Saraceno, C. (2021). *Il welfare: tra vecchie e nuove disuguaglianze*. Il Mulino.

Saraceno, C., & Keck, W. (2010). Can we Identify Intergenerational Policy Regimes in Europe? *European Societies*, *12*(5), 675–696. DOI: 10.1080/14616696.2010.483006

Sauerborn, E., Eisenhut, K., Ganguli-Mitra, A., & Wild, V. (2022). Digitally supported public health interventions through the lens of structural injustice: The case of mobile apps responding to violence against women and girls. *Bioethics, 36*(1), 71–76. DOI: 10.1111/bioe.12965 PMID: 34668600

Schein, E. H. (1999). *The Corporate Culture Survival Guide*. Jossey-Bass and Wiley & Sons.

Schmidt, E., & Cohen, J. (2013). *The new digital age*. John Murray.

Schou, J., & Hjelholt, M. (2017). Digitalizing the welfare state. *Critical Policy Studies, 13*(1), 3–22. DOI: 10.1080/19460171.2017.1333441

Schou, J., & Pors, A. S. (2019). Digital by Default? A Qualitative Study of Exclusion in Digitalised Welfare. *Social Policy and Administration, 53*(3), 464–477. DOI: 10.1111/spol.12470

Schreurs, K., Quan-Haase, A., & Martin, K. (2017). Problematizing the Digital Literacy Paradox in the Context of Older Adults' ICT Use: Aging, Media Discourse, and Self-Determination. *Canadian Journal of Communication, 42*(2), 359–377. DOI: 10.22230/cjc.2017v42n2a3130

Schultz, C. (2023). Telehealth and remote patient monitoring innovations in nursing practice: State of the science. Online Journal of Issues in Nursing, 28(2). *Online Journal of Issues in Nursing, 1*(2). Advance online publication. DOI: 10.3912/OJIN.Vol28No02ST01

Selbst, A. D., Boyd, D., Friedler, S. A., Venkatasubramanian, S., & Vertesi, J. (2019). Fairness and abstraction in sociotechnical systems. In *Proceedings of the Conference on Fairness, Accountability, and Transparency* (pp. 59–68). Association for Computing Machinery. DOI: 10.1145/3287560.3287598

Sen, A. (1999). *Development as freedom*. Knopf.

Shajari, M., Kuruvinashetti, K., Komeili, A., & Sundararaj, U. (2023). The emergence of AI-based wearable sensors for digital health technology: A review. *Sensors (Basel), 23*(23), 9498. DOI: 10.3390/s23239498 PMID: 38067871

Sharon, T. (2016). La Googleizzazione della ricerca sanitaria: Dall'innovazione dirompente all'etica dirompente. *Medicina Personalizzata, 13*(6), 563–574.

Sharon, T. (2016). The Googlization of health research. *Personalized Medicine, 13*(6), 563–574. DOI: 10.2217/pme-2016-0057 PMID: 29754546

Sharon, T. (2017). Self-tracking for health and the quantified self: Re-articulating autonomy, solidarity, and authenticity in an age of personalized healthcare. *Ethics and Information Technology, 19*(2), 93–106.

Sharon, T. (2018). Quando la salute digitale incontra il capitalismo digitale, quanti beni comuni sono in gioco? *Big Data & Society, 5*(2).

Sharon, T. (2018). When digital health meets digital capitalism, how many common goods are at stake? *Big Data & Society, 5*(2), 2053951718819032. DOI: 10.1177/2053951718819032

Shelby, R., Rismani, S., Henne, K., Moon, A., Rostamzadeh, N., Nicholas, P., & Virk, G. (2023, August). Sociotechnical harms of algorithmic systems: Scoping a taxonomy for harm reduction. In *Proceedings of the 2023 AAAI/ACM Conference on AI, Ethics, and Society* (pp. 723-741). DOI: 10.1145/3600211.3604673

Shen, S., Qi, W., Zeng, J., Li, S., Liu, X., Zhu, X., & Lou, X. (2025). Passive sensing for mental health monitoring using machine learning with wearables and smartphones: Scoping review. *Journal of Medical Internet Research, 27*, e77066. DOI: 10.2196/77066 PMID: 40811794

Shigekawa, E., Fix, M., Corbett, G., Roby, D., & Coffman, J. (2018). Telehealth evidence review. *Health Affairs*. Advance online publication. DOI: 10.1377/hlthaff.2018.05132 PMID: 30633674

Shimizu, M., Perinpanayagam, S., & Namoano, B. (2022). A real-time fault detection framework based on unsupervised deep learning for prognostics and health management of railway assets. *IEEE Access : Practical Innovations, Open Solutions, 10*, 96442–96458. DOI: 10.1109/ACCESS.2022.3205352

Siala, H., & Wang, Y. (2022). SHIFTing artificial intelligence to be responsible in healthcare: A systematic review. *Social Science & Medicine, 296*, 114782. DOI: 10.1016/j.socscimed.2022.114782 PMID: 35152047

Signorelli, S., Torrecillas Jodar, J., Papazoglou, M., & López Cobo, M. (2024). *Mapping EU Level Funding Instruments 2021-2027 to Digital Decade Targets*. European Commission, Joint Research Centre. Publication Office of the European Union. https://data.europa.eu/doi/10.2760/45054

Silberg, J., & Manyika, J. (2019). Notes from the AI frontier: Tackling bias in AI (and in humans). *McKinsey Global Institute, 1*(6), 1–31.

Silverstone, R., & Hirsch, E. (Eds.). (1992). *Consuming Technologies: Media and Information in Domestic Spaces*. Routledge.

Singh, B., Lopez, D., & Ramadan, R. (2023). Internet of things in healthcare: A conventional literature review. *Health and Technology*, *13*(5), 699–719. Advance online publication. DOI: 10.1007/s12553-023-00771-1

Si, Y., Du, J., Li, Z., Jiang, X., Miller, T., Wang, F., Jim Zheng, W., & Roberts, K. (2021). Deep representation learning of patient data from electronic health records (EHR): A systematic review. *Journal of Biomedical Informatics*, *115*, 103671. Advance online publication. DOI: 10.1016/j.jbi.2020.103671 PMID: 33387683

SkyQuest Technology Consulting. (2024). *Global digital health market size, share and industry report, 2032*. SkyQuest Technology Consulting.

Smokovski, I., Steinle, N., Behnke, A., Bhaskar, S. M. M., Grech, G., Richter, K., Niklewski, G., Birkenbihl, C., Parini, P., Andrews, R. J., Bauchner, H., & Golubnitschaja, O. (2024). Digital biomarkers: 3PM approach revolutionizing chronic disease management—EPMA 2024 position. *The EPMA Journal*, *15*(2), 149–162. DOI: 10.1007/s13167-024-00364-6 PMID: 38841615

Snyder, I., Jones, A., & Lo Bianco, J. (2005). *Using information and communication technologies in adult literacy education: New practices, new challenges (Report)*. National Centre for Vocational Education Research.

Solferino, N., Biondo, A., Alessio E., & D'Agostino, M. (2025). *Sfide etiche dell'Intelligenza Artificiale*. TAB edizioni.

Sørensen, K., Van den Broucke, S., Fullam, J., Doyle, G., Pelikan, J., Slonska, Z., & Brand, H. (2012). Health literacy and public health: A systematic review and integration of definitions and models. *BMC Public Health*, *12*(1), 80. DOI: 10.1186/1471-2458-12-80

Sorice, M. (2021). *Partecipazione disconnessa. Innovazione democratica e illusione digitale al tempo del neoliberismo*. Carocci editore.

Sourbati, M. (2009). 'It Could be Useful, but not for me at the Moment': Older People, Internet Access and E-Public Service Provision. *New Media & Society*, *11*(7), 1083–1100. DOI: 10.1177/1461444809340786

Sourbati, M. (2015). Age(ism) in Digital Information Provision: The Case of Online Public Services for Older Adults. In Zhou, J., & Salvendy, G. (Eds.), *Human Aspects of IT for the Aged Population. Design for Aging* (pp. 376–386). Springer International Publishing., DOI: 10.1007/978-3-319-20892-3_37

Southern, R., & Harmer, E. (2021). Twitter, incivility and "everyday" gendered othering: An analysis of tweets sent to UK members of parliament. *Social Science Computer Review*, *39*(2), 259–275. DOI: 10.1177/0894439319865519

Spencer, S. J., Steele, C. M., & Quinn, D. M. (1999). Stereotype threat and women's math performance. *Journal of Experimental Social Psychology*, *35*(1), 4–28. DOI: 10.1006/jesp.1998.1373

Srnicek, N. (2017). *Platform capitalism*. John Wiley & Sons.

Stark, G. F., Hart, G. R., Nartowt, B. J., & Deng, J. (2019). Predicting breast cancer risk using personal health data and machine learning models. *PLoS One*, *14*(12), e0226765. DOI: 10.1371/journal.pone.0226765 PMID: 31881042

Star, S. L. (1999). The ethnography of infrastructure. *The American Behavioral Scientist*, *43*(3), 377–391. DOI: 10.1177/00027649921955326

Star, S. L., & Ruhleder, K. (1996). Steps toward an ecology of infrastructure: Design and access for large information spaces. *Information Systems Research*, *7*(1), 111–134. DOI: 10.1287/isre.7.1.111

Strid, S., Humbert, A. L., Hearn, J., & Balkmar, D. (2021). States of violence: Exploring welfare state regimes as violence regimes by developing a violence regimes index. *Journal of European Social Policy*, *31*(3), 321–336. DOI: 10.1177/09589287211002370

Sun, K., Chen, J., & Viboud, C. (2020). Early epidemiological analysis of the coronavirus disease 2019 outbreak based on crowdsourced data: A population-level observational study. *The Lancet. Digital Health*, *2*(4), e201–e208. DOI: 10.1016/S2589-7500(20)30026-1 PMID: 32309796

Sun, L., Wei, M., Sun, Y., Suh, Y. J., Shen, L., & Yang, S. (2024). Smiling women pitching down: Auditing representational and presentational gender biases in image-generative AI. *Journal of Computer-Mediated Communication*, *29*(1), zmad045. DOI: 10.1093/jcmc/zmad045

Sun, S., Simonsson, O., McGarvey, S., Torous, J., & Goldberg, S. B. (2024). Mobile phone interventions to improve health outcomes among patients with chronic diseases: An umbrella review and evidence synthesis from 34 meta-analyses. *The Lancet. Digital Health*, *6*(11), e857–e870. DOI: 10.1016/S2589-7500(24)00119-5 PMID: 39332937

Suresh, H., & Guttag, J. V. (2020). A framework for understanding unintended consequences of machine learning. ArXiv E-Prints. *arXiv preprint arXiv:1901.10002*.

Tabaie, Z., & Omidvar, A. (2023). Human body heat-driven thermoelectric generators as a sustainable power supply for wearable electronic devices: Recent advances, challenges, and future perspectives. *Heliyon*, *9*(4), e14707. DOI: 10.1016/j.heliyon.2023.e14707 PMID: 37025803

Taherdoost, H. (2024). Wearable healthcare and continuous vital sign monitoring with IoT integration. *Computers, Materials & Continua, 81*(1), 79–104. DOI: 10.32604/cmc.2024.054378

Taipale, S. (2019). *Intergenerational Connections in Digital Families.* Springer International Publishing. DOI: 10.1007/978-3-030-11947-8

Taipale, S., Wilska, T. A., & Gilleard, C. J. (Eds.). (2017). *Digital Technologies and Generational Identity*. Routledge. DOI: 10.4324/9781315398624

Tang, C. (2021). *Data capital: How data is reinventing capital for globalization.* Springer Nature. DOI: 10.1007/978-3-030-60192-8

Tapuria, A., Kalra, D., & Kobayashi, S.. (2021). Patients' access to electronic health records. *BMJ Open.*

Taylor, L., & Broeders, D. (2015). In the name of development: Power, profit and the datafication of the Global South. *Geoforum, 64*, 229–237. DOI: 10.1016/j.geoforum.2015.07.002

Teo, Z. L., Jin, L., Liu, N., Li, S., Miao, D., Zhang, X., Ng, W. Y., Tan, T. F., Lee, D. M., Chua, K. J., Heng, J., Liu, Y., Goh, R. S. M., & Ting, D. S. W. (2024). Federated machine learning in healthcare: A systematic review on clinical applications and technical architecture. *Cell Reports Medicine, 5*(2), 101419. DOI: 10.1016/j.xcrm.2024.101419 PMID: 38340728

Terzi, L. (2013). Disabilità e uguaglianza civica: La prospettiva del capability approach. *Italian Journal of Disability Studies, 1*(1), 41–58.

The Young Foundation. (2012). *Social Innovation overview: A deliverable of the project: "The theoretical, empirical and policy foundations for building social innovation in Europe" (TEPSIE).* European Commission.

Timmermans, S., & Berg, M. (2003). The practice of medical technology. *Sociology of Health & Illness, 25*(3), 97–114. DOI: 10.1111/1467-9566.00342 PMID: 14498932

Tipaldo, G. (2019). *La società della post-verità: Dieci tesi su matti, impostori e mentitori seriali.* Il Mulino.

Tirado-Morueta, R., Rodríguez-Martín, A., Álvarez-Arregui, E., Ortíz-Sobrino, M. Á., & Aguaded-Gómez, J. I. (2023). The Digital Inclusion of Older People in Spain: Technological Support Services for Seniors as Predictor. *Ageing and Society, 43*(6), 1409–1435. DOI: 10.1017/S0144686X21001173

Tomasello, F. (2022). From industrial to digital citizenship: Rethinking social rights in cyberspace. *Theory and Society, 52*(3), 463–486. DOI: 10.1007/s11186-022-09480-6 PMID: 35676929

Topol, E. (2012). *The creative destruction of medicine*. Basic Books.

Topol, E. J. (2019). *Deep medicine: How artificial intelligence can make healthcare human again*. Basic Books.

Topol, E. J. (2019). High-performance medicine: The convergence of human and artificial intelligence. *Nature Medicine, 25*(1), 44–56. DOI: 10.1038/s41591-018-0300-7 PMID: 30617339

Toupin, S. (2024). Shaping feminist artificial intelligence. [Sage.]. *New Media & Society, 26*(1), 580–595. DOI: 10.1177/14614448221150776

Tracey, P., & Stott, N. (2017). Social innovation: A window on alternative ways of organizing and innovating. *Innovation (North Sydney, N.S.W.), 19*(1), 51–60. DOI: 10.1080/14479338.2016.1268924

Trapani, M. (2022). *L'impatto della digitalizzazione negli enti del terzo settore* [The Impact of Digitalization on Third Sector Organizations]. I Quaderni, Cesvot Edizioni.

Treu, T. (2021). *La digitalizzazione del lavoro: Proposte europee e piste di ricerca, conversazioni sul lavoro a distanza*. Cacucci Editore.

Trindade Pereira, I., & Zaba, M. (2026, 19 January). *How is cyberviolence against women and girls spreading across Europe?* https://www.euronews.com/my-europe/2026/01/19/how-is-cyberviolence-against-women-and-girls-spreading-across-europe

Tung, L. T., Thang, P. N., & Tram, N. H. M. (2025). Impact of technological development on national competitiveness: Empirical evidence from developing countries. *Competitiveness Review*, •••, 1–23.

Turing, A. M. (1956). Can a machine think. *The world of mathematics, 4*, 2099-2123.

Turk, V. (2023). How AI reduces the world to stereotypes. *Rest of world, 10.*

Turkle, S. (2011). Insieme ma soli. *Perché ci aspettiamo sempre più dalla tecnologia e sempre meno dagli altri*, 23-27.

Tversky, A., & Kahneman, D. (1974). Judgment under Uncertainty: Heuristics and Biases: Biases in judgments reveal some heuristics of thinking under uncertainty. *science, 185*(4157), 1124-1131.

van der Horst, A. Y., Kelders, S. M., Bohlmeijer, E. T., Schreurs, K. M., & Jukema, J. S. (2025). Digital health interventions for spinal surgery patients: A systematic scoping review. *Digital Health, 11*, 20552076251328549. DOI: 10.1177/20552076251328549 PMID: 40297368

van Deursen, A., & van Dijk, J. (2019). The first-level digital divide. *New Media & Society, 21*(2), 354–375. DOI: 10.1177/1461444818797082 PMID: 30886536

van Dijck, J. (2014). Datafication, dataism and dataveillance: Big data between scientific paradigm and ideology. *Surveillance & Society, 12*(2), 197–208. DOI: 10.24908/ss.v12i2.4776

Van Dijck, J., & Poell, T. (2016). Understanding online health platforms. *Big Data & Society*. Advance online publication. DOI: 10.1177/2053951716654173

Van Dijck, J., Poell, T., & De Waal, M. (2018). *The platform society: Public values in a connective world*. Oxford University Press. DOI: 10.1093/oso/9780190889760.001.0001

Van Dijk, J. (2020). The Digital Divide. Cambridge: Polity Press. *Communication, 2020*.

van Dijk, J. (2005). The deepening divide. *Sage (Atlanta, Ga.)*.

Van Dijk, J. (2005). The deepening divide: Inequality in the information society. *Sage (Atlanta, Ga.)*. Advance online publication. DOI: 10.4135/9781452229812

Van Dijk, J. (2012). *The network society* (3rd ed.). Sage.

Van Dijk, J. (2020). *The digital divide*. Polity Press.

Van Dijk, J. (2020). *The Digital Divide*. Polity Press.

Van Dijk, J. A. (2006). Digital divide research, achievements and shortcomings. *Poetics, 34*(4-5), 221–235. DOI: 10.1016/j.poetic.2006.05.004

Van Dijk, J. A. G. M. (2005). *The deepening divide: Inequality in the information society*. SAGE Publications.

van Toorn, G., Henman, P., & Soldatić, K. (2024). Introduction to the digital welfare state: Contestations, considerations and entanglements. *Journal of Sociology (Melbourne, Vic.), 60*(3), 507–522. DOI: 10.1177/14407833241260890

Vantin, S. (2018). *L'eguaglianza di genere tra mutamenti sociali e nuove tecnologie: Percorsi di diritto antidiscriminatorio*. Pacini Editore.

Vecchi, B. (2020). *Il capitalismo delle piattaforme*. Manifestolibri.

Velkova, J., & Kaun, A. (2021). Algorithmic resistance: Media practices and the politics of repair. *Information Communication and Society*, *24*(4), 523–540. DOI: 10.1080/1369118X.2019.1657162

Veneziano, M. (2020). José van Dijck, Thomas Poell, Martijn de Waal, Platform society. Valori pubblici e società connessa. *Quaderni di Sociologia*, (84-LXIV), 168-170.

Venkatesh, V., Morris, M. G., Davis, G. B., & Davis, F. D. (2003). User Acceptance of Information Technology: Toward a Unified View. *Management Information Systems Quarterly*, *27*(3), 425–478. DOI: 10.2307/30036540

Vermilyea, M., Hall, J. M. M., Diakiw, S. M., Johnston, A., Nguyen, T., Perugini, D., Miller, A., Picou, A., Murphy, A. P., & Perugini, M. (2020). Development of an artificial intelligence-based assessment model for prediction of embryo viability using static images captured by optical light microscopy during IVF. *Human Reproduction (Oxford, England)*, *35*(4), 770–784. DOI: 10.1093/humrep/deaa013 PMID: 32240301

Vicsek, L. (2021). Artificial intelligence and the future of work–lessons from the sociology of expectations. *The International Journal of Sociology and Social Policy*, *41*(7-8), 842–861. DOI: 10.1108/IJSSP-05-2020-0174

Virkki, T. (2007). Emotional capital in caring work. In Charmine E.J. Härtel, Neal M. Ashkanasy, & Wilfred J. Zerbe (editors), *Research on Emotionin Organizations. Volume 3: Functionality, intentionality and morality*. Emerald Group Publishing Limited. Pp. 265-285. https://doi.org/DOI: 10.1016/S1746-9791(2007)3

Vogel, B., Avecedo, M., Appelman, Y., & Noel, B. M.. (2021). The Lancet women and cardiovascular disease Commission: Reducing the global burden by 2030. *Lancet*, *397*(10292), 2385–2438. DOI: 10.1016/S0140-6736(21)00684-X PMID: 34010613

Von Kersbergen, K., & Vis, B. (2014). *Comparative welfare state politics*. Cambridge University Press.

Vuorikari, R., Kluzer, S., & Punie, Y. (2022). DigComp 2.2: The Digital Competence Framework for Citizens – With new examples of knowledge, skills and attitudes. [EN. Publications Office of the European Union.]. *EUR*, *31006*, •••.

Wajcman, J. (2006). Technocapitalism meets technofeminism: women and technology in a wireless world. *Labour & Industry: a journal of the social and economic relations of work*, *16*(3), 7-20.

Wajcman, J., & Young, E. (2023). Feminism confronts AI. *Feminist AI: Critical perspectives on algorithms, data, and intelligent machines, 47*.

Wajcman, J. (2015). *Pressed for time: The acceleration of life in digital capitalism*. University of Chicago Press.

Wajcman, J. (2017). Automation: Is it really different this time? *The British Journal of Sociology*, *68*(1), 119–127. DOI: 10.1111/1468-4446.12239 PMID: 28321856

Wallach, H. (2014, December). Big data, machine learning, and the social sciences: Fairness, accountability, and transparency. In *NIPS workshop on fairness, accountability, and transparency in machine learning*.

Wang, M. T., & Degol, J. L. (2017). Gender gap in science, technology, engineering, and mathematics (STEM): Current knowledge, implications for practice, policy, and future directions. *Educational Psychology Review*, *29*(1), 119–140. DOI: 10.1007/s10648-015-9355-x PMID: 28458499

Wang, S., Li, M., & Ng, S. B. (2022). Research on infant health diagnosis and intelligence development based on machine learning and health information statistics. *Frontiers in Public Health*, *10*, 846598. DOI: 10.3389/fpubh.2022.846598 PMID: 35719653

Warnes, A. M. (1993). Being Old, Old People and the Burdens of Burden. *Ageing and Society*, *13*(3), 297–338. DOI: 10.1017/S0144686X00001069

Webb, C. A., & Fisher, H. (2025). Tracking psychopathology dimensions through passive smartphone sensing—Promises, pitfalls, and pathways to clinical integration. *JAMA Network Open*, *8*(7), e2519054. DOI: 10.1001/jamanetworkopen.2025.19054 PMID: 40608343

Weber, G. M., Mandl, K. D., & Kohane, I. S. (2014). Finding the missing link for big biomedical data. *Journal of the American Medical Association*, *311*(24), 2479–2480. DOI: 10.1001/jama.2014.4228 PMID: 24854141

Weizenbaum, J. (1976). *Computer power and human reason: From judgment to calculation*. W. H. Freeman.

Wenger, E. (1998). *Communities of Practice, Learning, Meaning and Identity*. Cambridge University Press. DOI: 10.1017/CBO9780511803932

Westmarland, N., & Kelly, L. (2013). Why extending measurements of "success" in domestic violence perpetrator programmes matters for social work. *British Journal of Social Work*, *43*(6), 1092–1110. DOI: 10.1093/bjsw/bcs049

Wharton, A. S. (2009). The sociology of emotional labor. *Annual Review of Sociology*, *35*(1), 147–165. DOI: 10.1146/annurev-soc-070308-115944

Whelan, A. (2020). "Ask for more time": Big data chronopolitics in the Australian welfare bureaucracy. *Critical Sociology, 46*(6), 867–880. DOI: 10.1177/0896920519866004

White, R. W., & Horvitz, E. (2009). Cyberchondria: Studies of the escalation of medical concerns in web search. *ACM Transactions on Information Systems, 27*(4), 1–37. DOI: 10.1145/1629096.1629101

WHO. (2019). *RESPECT women: Preventing violence against women* (WHO/RHR/18.19). https://iris.who.int/bitstream/handle/10665/312261/WHO-RHR-18.19-eng.pdf?sequence=1

WHO. (2025). *Violence against women prevalence estimates, 2023: global, regional and national prevalence estimates for intimate partner violence against women and non-partner sexual violence against women.* World Health Organization. https://iris.who.int/handle/10665/383559

Winner, L. (2017). Do artifacts have politics? In *Computer ethics* (pp. 177–192). Routledge. DOI: 10.4324/9781315259697-21

Women, U. N. (2015). *A Framework to Underpin Action to Prevent Violence Against Women.* https://www.unwomen.org/sites/default/files/Headquarters/Attachments/Sections/Library/Publications/2015/Prevention_Framework_unwomen_nov2015.pdf

Women, U. N. (2020). *Overview: How to Use the RESPECT Framework Implementation Guide.* https://www.unwomen.org/sites/default/files/Headquarters/Attachments/Sections/Library/Publications/2020/RESPECT-implementation-guide-Overview-en.pdf

Women, U. N. (2025). *Advancing gender equality through partnerships for gender-responsive artificial intelligence.* https://www.unwomen.org/sites/default/files/2025-01/partnering-for-gender-responsive-ai-003.pdf

Women, U. N. (2025, 13 November). *Digital abuse, trolling, stalking, and other forms of technology-facilitated violence against women and girls.* https://www.unwomen.org/en/articles/faqs/digital-abuse-trolling-stalking-and-other-forms-of-technology-facilitated-violence-against-women

Women, U. N. (2025, 18 November). *Online safety 101: What every woman and girl should know.* https://www.unwomen.org/en/articles/explainer/online-safety-101-what-every-woman-and-girl-should-know

Woodlock, D. (2016). The Abuse of Technology in Domestic Violence and Stalking. *Violence Against Women, 23*(5), 584–602. DOI: 10.1177/1077801216646277 PMID: 27178564

World Bank. (2025). *State of the Art of Social Registries in Latin America and the Caribbean.* World Bank.

World Health Organization Regional Office for Europe. (2025). *Artificial intelligence is reshaping health systems: State of readiness across the WHO European Region.* https://www.who.int/europe/publications/i/item/WHO-EURO-2025-12707-52481-81028

World Health Organization. (2021). Ethics and governance of artificial intelligence for health. World Health Organization. https://www.who.int/publications/i/item/9789240029200

World Health Organization. (2021). *Global strategy on digital health 2020–2025.*

World Health Organization. (2021). *Global strategy on digital health 2020–2025.* https://iris.who.int/handle/10665/344249

World Health Organization. (2021). *Global strategy on digital health 2020–2025.* World Health Organization. https://www.who.int/publications/i/item/9789240020924

World Health Organization. Regional Office for Europe. (2022). *Equity within digital health technology within the WHO European Region: A scoping review.* World Health Organization. https://www.who.int/europe/publications/i/item/WHO-EURO-2022-6810-46576-67595

Wu, X., & Chen, S. (2026). From "Warm Expert" to "Warm Steward": Digital Backfeeding as Everyday Intergenerational GenAI Learning in Chinese Families. *International Journal of Human-Computer Interaction*, •••, 1–28. DOI: 10.1080/10447318.2026.2668041

Xiao, Z., & Han, X. (2023). Evaluation of the effectiveness of telehealth chronic disease management system: Systematic review and meta-analysis. *Journal of Medical Internet Research, 25*, e44256. DOI: 10.2196/44256 PMID: 37103993

Yates, S. J., Kirby, J., & Lockley, E. (2015). 'Digital-by-Default': Reinforcing Exclusion Through Technology. *Defence of welfare, 2*, 158-161.

Yeung, K. (2018). Algorithmic regulation: A critical interrogation. *Regulation & Governance, 12*(4), 505–523. DOI: 10.1111/rego.12158

Yoo, Y., Boland, J. R.Jr, Lyytinen, K., & Majchrzak, A. (2012). Organizing for Innovation in the Digitized World. *Organization Science*, *23*(5), 1398–1408. DOI: 10.1287/orsc.1120.0771

Young, E., Wajcman, J. e Sprejer, L. (2021), *Where are the women? mapping the gender job gap in AI policy briefing* – full report, The Alan Turing Institute, Londra.

Yun, S., Comín-Colet, J., Calero-Molina, E., Hidalgo, E., José-Bazán, N., Cobo Marcos, M., Soria, T., Llàcer, P., Fernández, C., García-Pinilla, J. M., Cruzado, C., González-Franco, Á., García-Marina, E. M., Morales-Rull, J. L., Solé, C., García-Romero, E., Núñez, J., Civera, J., Fernández, C., & Fernández, C. (2025). Evaluation of mobile health technology combining telemonitoring and teleintervention versus usual care in vulnerable-phase heart failure management (HERMeS): A multicentre, randomised controlled trial. *The Lancet. Digital Health*, *7*(5), 100866. DOI: 10.1016/j.landig.2025.02.006 PMID: 40374486

Zajko, M. (2022). Artificial intelligence, algorithms, and social inequality: Sociological contributions to contemporary debates. [Wiley.]. *Sociology Compass*, *16*(3), e12962. DOI: 10.1111/soc4.12962

Zakharova, I., Jarke, J., & Kaun, A. (2024). Tensions in digital welfare states: Three perspectives on care and control. *Journal of Sociology (Melbourne, Vic.)*, *60*(3), 540–559. DOI: 10.1177/14407833241238312

Zarcadoolas, C., Pleasant, A., & Greer, D. S. (2006). *Advancing health literacy: A framework for understanding and action*. John Wiley & Sons.

Završnik, A. (2021). Algorithmic justice: Algorithms and big data in criminal justice settings. *European Journal of Criminology*, *18*(5), 623–642. DOI: 10.1177/1477370819876762

Zhang, B., Chen, C., Lee, I., Lee, K., & Ong, K.-L. (2025). A survey on security and privacy issues in wearable health monitoring devices. *Computers & Security*, *155*, 104453. DOI: 10.1016/j.cose.2025.104453

Zhang, K., Jiang, Y., Xi, K., & Sun, N. (2025). Application of persuasive system design in mobile health interventions for chronic disease management: A mini review. *Frontiers in Public Health*, *13*, 1718371. DOI: 10.3389/fpubh.2025.1718371 PMID: 41358248

Zhang, M., Zhang, Q., Wang, X., Peng, X., Chen, J., & Yang, H. (2025). Prediction of clinical stages of cervical cancer via machine learning integrated with clinical features and ultrasound-based radiomics. *Scientific Reports*, *15*(1), 18862. DOI: 10.1038/s41598-025-03170-w PMID: 40442164

Zhang, Y., Li, X., Wang, H., & Chen, J. (2025). Advanced applications in chronic disease monitoring using IoT mobile sensing devices. *Frontiers in Public Health, 13*, 1510456. DOI: 10.3389/fpubh.2025.1510456

Zhao, Y., Du, Y., Liu, Y., Deng, C., & Li, X. (2025). Artificial intelligence in chronic disease self-management: Current applications and future directions. *Frontiers in Public Health, 13*, 1689911. DOI: 10.3389/fpubh.2025.1689911 PMID: 41358250

Zhu, Z., & Zhu, M. (2023). The usage of Internet of Things in healthcare: A review of mechanisms, platforms, and opportunities from a new perspective. *Journal of Intelligent & Fuzzy Systems, 45*(1), 1–18. DOI: 10.3233/JIFS-224166

Zuboff, S. (2019). *The age of surveillance capitalism: The fight for a human future at the new frontier of power*. PublicAffairs.

Zuboff, S. (2019, January). Surveillance capitalism and the challenge of collective action. [). Sage CA: Los Angeles, CA: Sage Publications.]. *New Labor Forum, 28*(1), 10–29. DOI: 10.1177/1095796018819461

About the Contributors

Gabriella Punziano, Ph.D. in Sociology and Social Research, is an Associate Professor of General Sociology at the Department of Social Sciences, University of Naples Federico II, Italy, where she teaches methodological courses on mixed and digital methods. Her research interests include: social research methodology; mixed and digital approaches; social policies and welfare regimes; analysis of public, institutional, and political communication phenomena; risk communication analysis on social and digital platforms; socioeconomic effects on the Third Sector; changes in individual behaviors; risk governance; science communication; the role of experts in the Covid-19 era; algorithmic feedbackloop in cultural consumption, digital literacy and awerness. Among her recent publications are: with Velotti, L. and Addeo, F. (2022), Covid 19: Government Policies and Human Social Behavior in Italy, CRC PRESS, Routledge, Taylor & Francis Group, UK; with Delli Paoli, A. (2022), Handbook of Research on Advanced Research Methodologies for a Digital Society, IGI Global, Hershey, Pennsylvania, USA; with De Falco, C.C. and Trezza, D. (2022), "Digital mixed content analysis perspective for the study of digital platform social data: an application on the analysis of the COVID-19 risk perception in the Italian Twittersphere," in Journal of Mixed Methods Research, Sage, 16(2); with Padricelli, G.M., Vettori, A. (2025). Algorithmic feedback loops in soft science disciplines. The Lab's Quarterly, 27(3); alone (2025). Adaptive Epistemology: Embracing Generative AI as a Paradigm Shift in Social Science. Societies, 15, 205.

Domenico Trezza holds a PhD in Social Sciences and Statistics from the University of Naples Federico II. He works in the field of monitoring and evaluating educational policies and methods and techniques for data analysis. He is currently assistant professor of Social Research Methodology in the Department of Social Sciences at Federico II and consultant for Ifel Campania for monitoring the Scuola Viva programme.

Giuseppe De Luca Picione is an associate Professor of General Sociology at the University of Naples Federico II, he is a member of the Executive Board of the Italian University Network for Lifelong Learning and Scientific Director of the MIUR Research Centre on Adult Education in Campania. Rector's delegate to the Italian University Network for Lifelong Learning, he teaches Social Innovation and Lifelong Learning, Social Media Data Analysis, Sociology of Criminal Organisations and Security Policies, AI & Public, Social and Political Communication SociaLab.

***

Caterina Ambrosio is a PhD candidate in Social Sciences and Statistics at the University of Naples Federico II. Her PhD scholarship is funded within the framework of the FOSSR – Fostering Open Science in Social Science Research project, led by the National Research Council of Italy. Her main research interests include social research methodology, digital methods, digital sociology, digital awareness, and open science. Among her publications are: with De Falco and Trezza (2025), "Artificial Social Research? AI's Capabilities and Risks in Predicting Values and Attitudes"; with Chianese (2025), "Mapping Technology Usage in Environmental Education"; and with Di Lorenzo (2025), "Digital Twins: Reconstructing Expert Narratives on Emerging Technology".

Kathirvel Ayyaswamy, acquired, B.E.(CSE), M.E. (CSE) from Crescent Engineering College affiliated to University of Madras and Ph. D (CSE.) from Anna University. He is currently working as Professor, Dept of Computer Science and Engineering, Saveetha Engineering College, Chennai. In-charge for CSE Cyber Forensics Research Group. He is a studious researcher by himself, completed 18 sponsored research projects worth of Rs 103 lakhs and published more than 110 articles in journals and conferences. 6 research scholars have completed Ph. D and 7 under progress under his guidance. He is working as scientific and editorial board member of many journals. He has reviewed dozens of papers in many journals. He has author of 13 books. His research interests are protocol development for wireless ad hoc networks, security in ad hoc network, data communication and networks, mobile computing, wireless networks, WSN and DTN. He is a Life member of the ISTE (India), IACSIT (Singapore), Life Member IAENG (Hong Kong), Member ICST (Europe), IAES, etc. He has given a number of guest lecturers/expert talks and seminars, workshops and symposiums.

Noemi Crescentini (PhD in Social Sciences and Statistics) is a Postdoctoral Fellow and Adjunct Professor at the Department of Social Sciences, University of Naples Federico II. Her research interests concern the connections between society and scientific and technological topics, the science communication and the field of social research methodology.

Ciro Clemente De Falco is an Assistant Professor of General Sociology at the Department of Social Sciences, University of Naples Federico II. His research lies in the field of social research methodology and focuses on the development of innovative approaches to the study of contemporary social phenomena through the integration of quantitative and digital methods. His main research interests include the applications and methodological challenges of artificial intelligence in social research, the analysis of digital and geolocated data, and the development of methodological approaches for investigating socio-spatial phenomena. He is a member of the F.A.S.T. Observatory (Future, Algorithms, Society and Technology) at the University of Naples Federico II and of Spoke 3 of the FAIR (Future Artificial Intelligence Research) Extended Partnership.

Giulia De Florio holds an MSc with honours in Digital Sociology and Web Analysis from the University of Naples Federico II. Her research interests include digital sociology, geospatial data, collaborative mapping, digital inequalities, and the analysis of urban transformations through computational and quantitative methods. Her research has been presented at national and international conferences, and her work focuses on the sociological potential of digital and geospatial data, with particular attention to OpenStreetMap, digital welfare, and urban change.

Piero Demetrio Falorsi is a senior statistical expert and social science researcher with extensive experience in public sector data governance and digital transformation. He previously served as a senior executive at the Italian National Institute of Statistics (ISTAT), where he held managerial responsibilities in the development and governance of official statistics. His research focuses on statistical methodologies, data-driven policy analysis, and the transformation of public systems through the use of digital technologies. He collaborates with academic institutions on studies addressing innovation, skills, and institutional change in complex socio-economic environments.

Ahmed Hussein is a senior official statistics expert at the Qatar National Planning Council. Currently, he is at the forefront of a pivotal project focused on modernising official statistics, aligning with the ambitious Sustainable Development Goals 2030. His role involves spearheading efforts to enhance the effectiveness and efficiency of the statistical system through strategic collaborations with the United Nations system. With a remarkable career marked by impactful contributions, Dr Hussein stands as the primary architect of the National Strategy for the Development of Statistics 2008-2013 (NSDS), a seminal document crafted during his tenure with the Qatar Statistics Authority. His leadership during this period left an indelible mark on the statistical landscape of the country.

Emiliana Mangone, Ph.D., is Full Professor of Sociology of Culture and Communication Processes at the Department of Political and Communication Sciences (University of Salerno, Italy). She is Director of the Narratives and Social Changes-International Research Group (NaSC-IRG, 2020-2026) and was Director of the International Centre for Studies and Research on "Mediterranean Knowledge" (2015-2020). Her main research interests are in the field of cultural and institutional systems, with particular attention to social representations, relational processes, knowledge, and narrative as key elements to the human act, in migration studies, and as well as the study of the thought of Pitirim A. Sorokin. For further information please see the personal page: https://emilianamangone.com/ E-mail: emangone@unisa.it - ORCID iD: https://orcid.org/0000-0002-9958-4346.

Giuseppe Masullo, Ph.D, is Associate Professor of Sociology at the University of Salerno (Italy). He is Director of the International Lab for Innovative Social Research (ILIS), laboratory of interdisciplinary studies and research that promote theoretical, epistemological and methodological advances in the field of social sciences through constant dialogue with scholars who are experts in both national and international. His main research interests are in the field of digital methods applied to the study of disadvantaged and discriminated categories due to their gender, cultural and sexual identity. He recently published: Epistemologia e metodi della sociologia italiana. Origini, storia e prospettive, (PM edizioni, 2024), (with M. Coppola), Masculinities and Caring Professions. The Case Study of Students Enrolled in University Courses in Educational Disciplines. FuoriLuogo, 1-14, 2024

Giulia Melis is a post-doc researcher within the Department of Sociology and Social Research of the University of Milano-Bicocca. Her research activity is focused on older adults' digital practices with a life course and gender approach, and qualitative longitudinal methods.

Monica Murero is Associate Professor of Digital Communication, Artificial Intelligence, and Health at the University of Naples Federico II, Italy. Her research focuses on the societal, communicative, and governance implications of artificial intelligence, digital health, and emerging technologies. A pioneer in the field of e-health for more than three decades, she has contributed to the development of research and international debate on digital health, online health communication, and the social impact of emerging technologies. She is the founder of AI for Life and Society (AI4LIVES), an international interdisciplinary research institute dedicated to advancing human-centered approaches to AI, digital health, healthcare innovation, and societal transformation. Her work bridges communication studies, digital health, science and technology studies, and AI governance, with a particular interest in the socio-technical dimensions of data-driven healthcare and welfare systems.

Mino Novello is a Post-doc researcher within the Social Policy Lab at Politecnico di Milano. Their research is focused on risks of social exclusion for older populations, from a perspective of digitisation policy, welfare crisis and crisis of familialism, with a specific focus on policy discourses. They are currently involved in a research project on socio-demographic changes and care poverty in later life. One of their most recent publications is the article "Ageing and technology in the policy discourse on public services digitalisation: a missed opportunity?" written with Emma Garavaglia for the journal Ageing & Society (2026).

Giuseppe Michele Padricelli, PhD in Social Sciences and Statistics, is currently Research Fellow (RTDa) at the Department of Social Science of the University of Naples and adjunct professor in Methodology of social research at University of Campania L. Vanvitelli. His research interests focus on the challenges and advancements of social research methods in light of digital developments, approached through the study of sociology of health, social movements, and collective action.

Dario Russo is a strategic consultant and researcher working at the intersection of digital transformation, public policy, and welfare systems. He is co-founder of RG3 Digital Consulting and collaborates with academic institutions and international organisations on projects related to AI governance, digital finance, and social inclusion. A former senior executive at the Bank of Italy, he has extensive experience in financial infrastructures, payments, and regulatory frameworks. His research focuses on digital welfare, algorithmic governance, and the socio-economic impacts of data-driven decision-making, with particular attention to low- and middle-income countries. He has contributed to policy reports, academic publications, and capacity-building initiatives in Europe, Africa, and the MENA region. His work combines interdisciplinary research with policy-oriented analysis, aiming to bridge the gap between theory and practice in the governance of digital technologies.

Index

A

B

C

D

E

G

H

I

N

O

www.ingramcontent.com/pod-product-compliance
Lightning Source LLC
LaVergne TN
LVHW062325300926
849161LV00007B/1578